Dialysis Technology

A Manual for Dialysis Technicians

Third Edition

Edited by:

Jim Curtis, CHT

Philip Varughese, BS, CHT

Third Edition

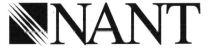
NANT

Foreword

Third Edition

The mission of the National Association of Nephrology Technicians/Technologists (NANT) is to promote education and advance the professional role of the multidisciplinary team in delivering the highest quality of care to the End Stage Renal Disease (ESRD) patient. Dialysis technicians perform basic clinical and technical tasks in the care of the ESRD patient under the direct supervision of a Medical Director, Nephrologist, Chief Technologist or Licensed Personnel. The Nephrology Technologist applies scientific knowledge, dialytic and biomedical theory to practical clinical problems of renal care. As technical professionals, NANT is committed to focus on a comprehensive approach to formalized academic preparation of future technical practitioners.

NANT believes that certification for dialysis technicians and technologists must be uniform for the practitioner to achieve greater professional identity and universal acceptance in the nephrology profession. Education and training standards are essential elements of this process. In order to achieve this goal, NANT produced this third edition of *Dialysis Technology*. It continues to be one of the biggest selling publications to prepare individuals for certification exams in the nephrology community. We are proud to say that this manual has grown from the initial publication of 10 chapters to a total of 23, with three new chapters in this edition. We hope you will take advantage of this valuable resource to assist you in promoting your professionalism in the nephrology community.

The NANT Board of Directors extends its sincere appreciation to RPC, Serim and AMGEN for their financial support of this publication. This monumental project would not be accomplished without the voluntary contributions of the authors and the Board of Directors thankfully acknowledges them. In addition, we extend a special thanks to Philip Varughese, CHT, who was the principal editor for this edition.

Efraim Figueroa, CBNT
2002-2003 NANT President

Preface

Third Edition

"To set forth high quality standards in the dialysis industry; promote the recognition, job security and employment opportunities of nephrology technologists and technicians; educate dialysis practitioners; stimulate research; disseminate new ideas; and address technician and technologist practice issues."

– Goals of NANT

With the release of the third edition of *Dialysis Technology,* we continue to fulfill this vision and provide dialysis technicians with the tools in hand to deliver high quality care to their patients. This edition has been updated with the latest standards of practice and has been revised to include new and updated guidelines. We've also added three new chapters: *Preparation for State Survey, Professional Boundaries, and the History of Dialysis.* These topics were added to educate and increase the technician's awareness on how dialysis started, where it's been, and finally, where it's heading. NANT has been instrumental in enhancing the professionalism of dialysis technologists through educational programs and supporting technician certification exams. It only seemed fitting to include a chapter on how far we have come as an organization to encourage and foster professionalism among technicians nationwide.

This newest edition was a long project, and was made possible because of the tireless efforts of several people. My gratitude and appreciation goes to Jim Curtis, Tangela Monroe, and all the contributing authors, who have devoted countless hours to writing and editing these chapters. It is truly because of their commitment, support, and talents that we are able to provide you with such a comprehensive educational tool. I'd also like to acknowledge the assistance of my daughters, Nancy and Joyce, who were integral in the timely completion of this edition.

I hope this manual provides you with the resources, education, and tools you need to practice dialysis technology with a strong commitment to optimal care for your patients.

Philip Varughese
Co-Editor

Contents

Sponsors

NANT thanks Amgen, Inc., Reprocessing Products Corporation, and Serim Research for their gracious support of the NANT mission to improve the quality of care of the ESRD patient through education and professionalism.

Printing for the third edition was subsidized by:

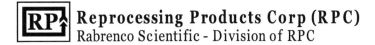 **Reprocessing Products Corp (RPC)**
Rabrenco Scientific - Division of RPC

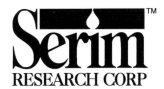

Amgen, Inc graciously subsidized printing and provided funding for the development of the first edition.

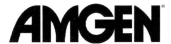

Illustrations

Contributors

Editors

Jim Curtis, CHT
Area Administrator Fresenius
Medical Care NA-
Oregon Kidney Center
Portland, OR

Philip Varughese, CHT
Facility Administrator
Richmond Kidney Center – DaVita
Staten Island, NY

Contributing Authors

Philip Andysiak, BS, MBA, CHT
Renal Consultant
Miami, FL

Matthew J. Arduino, Dr. P.H.
Chief, Dialysis Medical
Devices Section C16
Hospital Infections Program
Centers for Disease Control
and Prevention
Atlanta, GA

Joan Arslanian, MS, MPA, MSN, RN, CS, CHN, PNP
Inservice Instructor
Trude Weishaupt Memorial
Satellite Dialysis
Fresh Meadows, NY

Jerome Beck, BS, CHT
Director of Operations
RENALWEST
Phoenix, AZ

Rick Black, CHT
Chief Technician
Renal Treatment Centers
Littleton, CO

Joanie Brown, CHT
Patient Care Technician
Western Dialysis
Thorton, CO

Ty Cobb, CHT
Technical Supervisor
Ocshner Clinic
Houma, LA

Lina M. Collier, CHT
Dialysis Technician
University of Louisville
Louisville, KY

Danilo Concepcion, CHT
Chief Specialist, Technical Services
St. Joseph Hospital Renal Center
Orange, CA

Karen Crampton, ACSW
Social Work Manager
Greenfield Health Systems
Detroit, MI

Jim Curtis, CHT
Area Administrator Fresenius
Medical Care NA-
Oregon Kidney Center
Portland, OR

Gerald Dievendorf
Regional Medical Care Administrator
New York State Department of Health
Albany, NY

Diane Dolan, CWSV
General Manager
AmeriWater
Dayton, OH

Marsha Evans, CHT
Dialysis Technician, Acute Unit
University of Louisville
Louisville, KY

Lori Fedje, RD, LD
Clinical Manager, Nutrition
Pacific Northwest Renal
Services/RCG
Portland, OR

Clifford Glynn, CHT
Chief Technologist
University of Louisville
Louisville, KY

Bill Hajko, CHT
Senior Training Instructor
Baxter Healthcare Corporation
Pinellas Park, FL

Lorus Hawbecker, RN, CNN
Global Clinical Education Manager
Baxter Healthcare Corporation
Tampa, FL

Kirk M. Lesher, CHT
Bio-Med Technician
Pacific Northwest Renal Services
Portland, OR

Elizabeth J. Lindley, PhD
Clinical Scientist
Renal and Liver Services
St. James's University Hospital
Leeds, UK

Patricia Loughren, RegN, MA(Ed)
Coordinator
Dialysis Technology Program
Georgian College
Barrie, Ontario, Canada

Jenny Orsini, MSN, RN, CNN
Clinical Nurse Specialist
(Transplant)
St. Barnabas Medical Center
Livingston, NJ

Lawrence K. Park, MSPH, CHCM
VP, Corporate Health, Safety,
Environmental Affairs and
Engineering
Fresenius Medical Care
North America
Lexington, MA

Fern Reyes, MPH, RD, LD
Renal Dietician
Pacific Northwest Renal
Services/RCG
Portland, OR

Manual Rivera, CHT
Bio-Med Technician
Pacific Northwest Renal
Services/RCG
Portland, OR

Migdalia Rosario, BS, RN, CPDN
President of M. Rosario DBA
(Nephrology Consultant)
Brooklyn, NY

Byron Roshto, CHT
Director of Operations
Pacific Northwest Renal
Services/RCG
Portland, OR

Patricia Samec, BSN, RN, CNN
Charge Nurse
Oregon Kidney Center
Portland, OR

Ruth Stallard, BSN, RN, CNN
Senior Clinical Research Associate
Renal Division
Baxter Healthcare Corporation
Greensboro, NC

Sharon Stevens, CHT
Chief Technician
Renal Treatment Centers
Denver, CO

John Sweeny, BS, CHT, CBNT
Global Technical Training Manager
Baxter Healthcare Corporation
Pinellas Park, FL

Philip Varughese, CHT
Facility Administrator
Richmond Kidney Center – DaVita
Staten Island, NY

Narayan Venkataraman, MSc, BE
Chief, Department of Biomedical
Engineering
NKF – Singapore

Gail Wick, BSN, RN, CNN
VP Corporate Communications
Fresenius Medical Care
North America
Lexington, MA

Buz Womack, CHT
Technical Manager
CliniShare Dialysis Network
Carmel, CA

Beth Wood, CHT
Area Technical Manager
Renal Treatment Centers
Denver, CO

Chapter 1
Basic Dialysis Theory

Contributing Author:
Lorus Hawbecker, RN, CNN

Chapter Outline

I. Excretory Functions of the Normal Kidney

A. *Maintain Fluid Balance*

B. *Maintain Electrolyte Balance*

C. *Maintain Acid / Base Balance*

D. *Eliminate Toxins*

II. Replacement of Excretory Functions by Dialysis

A. *Maintaining Fluid Balance in Hemodialysis*

B. *Maintaining Electrolyte Balance and Removing Toxins in Hemodialysis*

C. *Maintaining Acid / Base Balance in Hemodialysis*

III. Summary

A. *Replacement of Normal Kidney Function with Hemodialysis*

B. *Normal Kidney Function not Replaced by Hemodialysis*

I. Excretory Functions of the Normal Kidney (Urine Formation)

A. Maintain Fluid Balance
(Water)

1. Non-selective glomerular filtration of blood through capillary walls and membranes of Bowman's capsule into tubular system of the nephron unit.

   a) Hydrostatic pressure differences between blood pressure in capillaries and space in Bowman's capsule force plasma water and solutes dissolved in the water (that are small enough to pass through the membranes) into the nephron's tubular system.

   b) Normal glomerular filtration rate (GFR) = 125 ml / minute (~180 L/ 24 Hours)

2. Selective tubular reabsorption

   a) 99% of water is reabsorbed (approximately 178 L / 24 Hours)

   b) Normal urine output for 24 hours is 1 1/2 to 2 liters.

3. Auto-regulatory mechanisms, controlled by pressure sensing cells (the macula densa and juxtaglomerular cells) in the nephron can increase or decrease blood flow into the nephron depending on the state of hydration thus contributing to maintaining fluid balance.

4. The countercurrent mechanism in the Loop of Henle

   a) Utilizes osmotic forces created by concentration differences in sodium throughout the Loop of Henle to assist in additional water balancing and concentration of the glomerular filtrate.

5. Hormonal regulation

   a) Amount of Aldosterone and Antidiuretic Hormone (ADH) present influence final water balance.

B. Maintain Electrolyte Balance
(Electrolytes are substances which, when dissolved in water, conduct an electrical charge. They perform multiple functions in the body and are needed in very specific amounts.)

1. Non-selective filtration of electrolytes (solute dissolved in the plasma water) occurs in the glomerulus.

Figure 1.1

Excretory Functions of the Normal Kidney

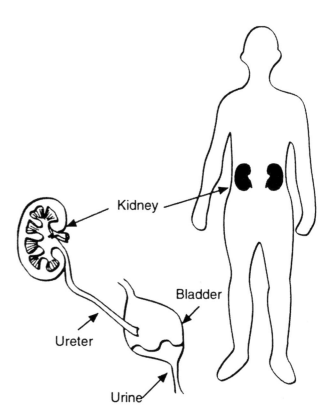

Reprinted with permission from AMGEN *Core Curriculum for Reprocessing of Dialyzers, p. 3, fig. 2.*

---

2. Selective tubular reabsorption

   a.) Most electrolytes which have been filtered, along with other smaller solute substances (such as glucose, amino acids, water soluble vitamins, etc.) needed by the body, are reabsorbed into the blood as they pass through the nephron tubular system to a normal (threshold) level, through both active and passive transport mechanisms.

3. Hormonal regulation

   a) Aldosterone, secreted by the adrenal gland, affects reabsorption and secretion of potassium and sodium.

   b) PTH, secreted by the parathyroid gland, affects reabsorption and secretion of calcium and phosphorus.

C. Maintain Acid /Base Balance
(Hydrogen [H+] and Bicarbonate Balance [HCO₃⁻])

1. Non-selective filtration of bicarbonate occurs in the glomerulus.

2. Reabsorption of bicarbonate occurs throughout the tubular system.

3. Secretion of hydrogen ions occurs through active transport mechanisms.

4. Chemical regulation and interactions in the tubular system promote the conservation of bicarbonate for reabsorption while H+ combines with ammonia and is secreted into the glomerular filtrate.

D. Eliminate Toxins
(Metabolic waste products)

1. Non-selective glomerular filtration of toxins (solutes dissolved in the plasma water) occurs in the glomerulus.

   a) Most filtered toxins remain in the tubular system and are excreted in the urine.

2. A double action of reabsorption and then secretion of urea (a nitrogenous waste) takes place after filtration through the glomerulus. The final result is elimination in the urine of the waste products of protein metabolism and other toxins.

II. Replacement of Excretory Functions by Dialysis

A. Maintaining Fluid Balance in Hemodialysis

1. Ultra-filtration is the mechanism responsible for moving plasma water from the blood into the dialysate through the dialyzer membrane when fluid removal is needed in hemodialysis.

   a) Definition: The movement of solvent (water is the universal solvent) from an area of higher hydrostatic pressure to lower hydrostatic pressure.

   b) Factors affecting ultra-filtration

      (1) Trans-membrane pressure (pressure difference between blood side and dialysate side, most often represented in dialysis by the formula TMP = VP - DP)

Figure 1.2

Filtration and Ultra-Filtration

Filtration:

The passage of a substance through a filter

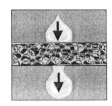

Ultra-Filtration:

The movement of solvent across a semi-permeable membrane from a higher to lower hydrostatic pressure

Reprinted with permission from Althin Academy/Basic Dialysis Theory (1).

(2) Blood side pressure is a positive pressure reflecting the resistance of the blood lines, venous needle, and dialyzer fibers to the flow of blood as it is pushed through the system by the blood pump.

   (a) Blood side pressure is traditionally read at the venous pressure monitor after blood has exited the dialyzer, even though, more accurately, this pressure is an average of the pressure of the blood entering the dialyzer and the pressure of the blood leaving the dialyzer, represented by the formula:
   $$\text{Av. Positive Pressure} = \frac{P\,bi + P\,bo}{2}$$

   (b) Dialysate pressure in conventional dialysis equipment is a negative (vacuum) pressure, generated by pulling dialysate through the dialyzer creating an additional pressure difference across the dialyzer membrane to contribute to fluid removal. Traditionally dialysate pressure is read at the dialysate exit of the dialyzer, although accurately, the dialysate pressure is actually the average of the pressure of dialysate as it enters the dialyzer and the pressure of dialysate as it exits the dialyzer as represented by the formula:

Av. Dialysate Pressure = $\dfrac{P\,di + P\,do}{2}$

(3) Volumetric fluid balancing equipment, (also called UF Control equipment) responds to requests for removal of specific fluid volumes by adjusting the dialysate compartment pressure to maintain just the exact <u>average</u> TMP needed to permit the requested amount of fluid to be pushed / pulled across the membrane. Current accuracy is within 30 to 60 ml per hour. Dialysate compartment pressures in volumetric equipment are often positive, especially with high flux dialyzers, to neutralize higher than needed positive blood side pressure, but <u>net</u> movement of water will be from the blood to dialysate as long as a minimal ultrafiltration rate is set.

(a) The actual pressure affecting fluid removal in volumetric equipment is the average TMP as represented by the formula:

TMP = $\dfrac{P\,bi + P\,bo}{2} - \dfrac{P\,di + P\,do}{2}$

2. Dialyzer coefficient of ultrafiltration (KUF) : amount of fluid per hour that a dialyzer membrane will permit to move through the membrane for every millimeter of mercury pressure (TMP) across the membrane.

a) KUF is expressed as ml (cc) /Hr./ mmHg TMP.

b) KUF performance is published in new dialyzer product literature and is measured and/or approximated during each reuse procedure.

c) Knowledge of the KUF is required to calculate TMP needed on non-volumetric equipment. (Note: the KUF is still the factor controlling the amount of fluid removed by volumetric equipment, but the equipment measures the volume being removed and sets the TMP automatically. The operator does not need the information for calculation.)

3. Fluid removal calculations

a) Today's Weight - Dry Weight = Wt. to be removed + Other Planned Fluid Intake (Prime, Oral Intake, IV's) = Total Weight (Volume) to be removed during dialysis.

Figure 1.3

Osmosis

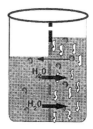

The movement of solvent through a semi-permeable membrane from an area of lesser solute concentration to an area of greater solute concentration.

Reprinted with permission from Althin Academy/Basic Dialysis Theory (1).

b) Enter total to be removed and time of treatment into volumetric machine or if a non-volumetric TMP control machine, continue calculation:

c) Divide total to be removed by # hrs of treatment = Amt. to be removed per hr. This is the ultrafiltration rate (UFR).

d) Divide amount to be removed per hr. by dialyzer KUF = TMP needed.

e) Initiate dialysis and enter TMP needed into TMP controller, or if non-volumetric, non TMP control machine continue calculation:

f) Initiate dialysis, set prescribed blood flow rate, then read the Venous Pressure (VP).

g) From the needed TMP subtract the venous pressure = negative dialysate pressure needed.

h) Set required negative pressure to affect your desired fluid removal over the time of the dialysis.

4. Osmosis, although not a direct mechanism of fluid removal from the blood during hemodialysis, contributes greatly to fluid balance, because it is the mechanism that causes body water to move between the body compartments (intracellular, interstitial, and intravascular). During hemodialysis, the plasma water in the vascular system is the only water that passes through the dialyzer and is subject to removal by the artificial kidney. Maintaining a good refilling rate of the circulatory system

from other body compartments by osmosis, assures there is fluid to be removed while maintaining an acceptable blood pressure and controlling other symptoms.

  a) Definition: The movement of a solvent from an area of lower particulate concentration to an area of higher particulate concentration across a semi-permeable membrane until the dilution (concentration) is equal on both sides of the membrane.

  b) Factors which promote osmosis into the vascular compartment from body cells and tissues:

    (1) Increased hematocrit

    (2) High blood glucose levels

    (3) Keeping serum levels of urea and other toxins high while removing only plasma water. (Sequential Ultrafiltration)

Figure 1.4

Diffusion and Ultrafiltration

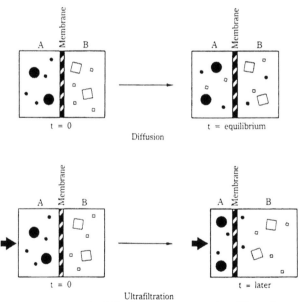

The processes of diffusion (top) and ultrafiltration (bottom). As shown, in both processes, small molecular weight solutes can cross the semi-permeable membrane, whereas larger solutes are held back.

Source: Handbook of Dialysis, *Daugirdas, John T. and Ing, Todd S., Editors. Reprinted with permission of Lippincott-Raven Publishers.*

    (4) Increasing sodium levels in the blood by injecting hypertonic saline.

    (5) Increasing dialysate sodium levels and allowing sodium to diffuse into the blood and raise the serum sodium. (Sodium Modeling / Profiling)

    (6) High albumin levels

    (7) Administration of albumin, mannitol or other volume expanders.

B. Maintaining Electrolyte Balance and Removing Toxins in Hemodialysis

1. Diffusion is the primary mechanism by which solute substances (toxins and electrolytes) move during hemodialysis.

  a) Definition: The movement of solute from an area of greater concentration of solute to an area of lesser concentration of solute until the concentration is equal.

    (1) Diffusion is based on the principal of brownian movement which states that all atoms are in constant random motion at all times.

  b) In hemodialysis, a semi-permeable membrane, which allows the passage of some substances and not others, is placed between two different areas of concentration: the blood and the dialysate.

    (1) Conventional membranes generally allow fairly easy passage of substances up to a molecular weight of 5000.

    (2) High flux membranes, additionally, allow passage of larger substances, currently of molecular weights as high as 40,000 to 50,000.

    (3) The speed at which substances diffuse through a membrane is inversely proportional to their size.

  c) Factors influencing diffusion

    (1) Dialysate composition

      (a) The concentration gradient is the difference in specific solute concentration between blood and dialysate and determines the direction a solute will move.

Figure 1.5

Diffusion

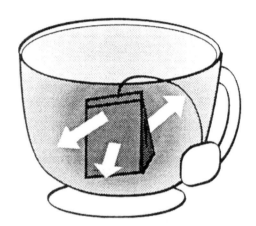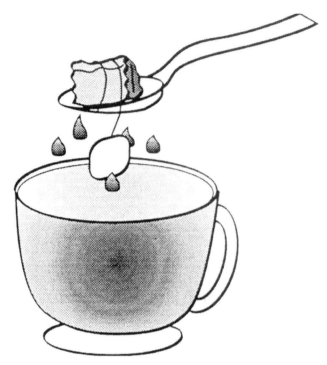

Reprinted with permission from AMGEN Core Curriculum for Reprocessing of Dialyzers, *p. 7, fig. 6.*

(b) Usual composition and range of solute
concentrations found in dialysate:

	Standard	**Range**
Toxins	0	0
Electrolytes:		
Phosphorus	0	0
Sodium	140 mEq/L	160 - 135 mEq/L
Chloride	106 mEq/L	103 - 112 mEq/L
Potassium	2 mEq/L	0 - 3 mEq/L
Calcium	3 - 3.5 mEq/L	2.8 - 4.0 mEq/L
Magnesium	0.5 - 1 mEq/L	0.5 - 1 mEq/L
Bicarbonate	35-38 mEq/L	15 - 42 mEq/L
Dextrose	200 mg/dl	0-200 mg/dl

(c) Increasing Blood Flow Rates and
Dialysate Flow Rates maintains a
greater concentration gradient.

2. Flow geometry

　a) Counter-current flow promotes optimal
diffusion.

　　(1) Blood enters at its highest solute concentration, and dialysate exits at its highest
concentration (but still lower than blood)
at the arterial end of the dialyzer.

　　(a) Blood exits at its lowest solute
concentration as fresh dialysate with
the lowest concentration is entering at
the venous end of the dialyzer.

　b) Dialysate / membrane contact

　　(1) Dialysis can only occur when blood and
dialysate are in direct contact with the
membrane. Reduced contact can result
from:

　　　(a) Blood pump stops and dialysate
bypass alarms.

　　　(b) Unfilled and/or clotted hollow fibers.

　　　(c) Poor dialysate deaeration causing air
in dialysate compartment.

　　　(d) Too wide ID in hollow fibers and too
high a blood channel in plates.

　　　(e) Solute must be within approximately
100 microns of a membrane.

　c) Blood flow rate

　d) Dialysate flow rate

3. Dialyzer characteristics
   a) Membrane pore size and number
   b) Membrane wall thickness
   c) Membrane surface area
   d) Hollow fiber internal diameter

4. Solute drag (convection)
   a) Definition: The movement of solute dissolved in a solvent with the movement of a volume of solvent. In hemodialysis, solute dissolved in the plasma water is removed as water is removed from the blood.
   b) This contribution is considered minimal in conventional dialysis where only small amounts of water move across the membrane. Diffusion is the most effective mechanism for transfer of small molecules across a membrane.
   c) The effect of convection is more important in high flux dialysis, where one of the goals is to remove larger molecules. The movement of larger volumes of water to and through the membrane aids the movement of the larger, heavier molecules. Thus, convection is more effective in moving larger molecular weight substances.

C. Maintaining Acid-Base Balance in Hemodialysis

1. Acetate dialysate
   a) Acetate diffuses into the blood from the dialysate, is carried to the liver, metabolized into bicarbonate, and released into the blood stream.
   b) Advantage(s)
      (1) All electrolytes can be mixed in one liquid concentrate without precipitation.
      (2) Concentrated solution is bacteriostatic.
      (3) All dialysis delivery systems can use the same acetate chemical formulations.
   c) Disadvantage(s)
      (1) It takes 3 to 4 hours for bicarb release and correction of acidosis, so patient actually may become more acidotic during beginning of dialysis due to loss of some bicarbonate ions, increasing dialytic symptoms.
      (2) Acetate has an action of dilating blood vessels, thus contributing to more rapid drops in blood pressure during dialysis for many patients.

   (3) Patients with liver impairment (very young, very old, hepatitis, cirrhosis, etc.) cannot metabolize the acetate into bicarbonate as effectively.
   (4) Some patients have reactions to the acetate.

2. Bicarbonate dialysate
   a) Sodium bicarbonate concentrated solution is added through a separate pathway to the dialysate solution, diffuses into the blood from the dialysate, and acts to neutralize excess hydrogen ions.
   b) Advantages
      (1) Immediate positive effect on acid/base balance by neutralizing hydrogen ions.
      (2) No loss of bicarbonate to the dialysate.
      (3) More stable blood pressures, less symptoms, easier fluid removal.
   c) Disadvantages
      (1) Cannot be stored as concentrate in solution with positive electrolytes such as calcium and magnesium or it will precipitate out, so a third proportioning system pathway is required (3 streams).
      (2) Powdered bicarbonate once mixed has a limited shelf life.
      (3) Bicarbonate solution is NOT bactericidal. All equipment and containers must be well disinfected.
      (4) Precipitation inside dialysis equipment can occur without proper procedures and maintenance. Precipitation can be minimized by:
         (a) Use treated water only in bicarbonate dialysate equipment.
         (b) Use treated water only to mix powdered bicarbonate.
         (c) Mix powdered bicarb well until all powder is dissolved.
         (d) Liquid bicarbonate concentrate must be made with good water.
         (e) Water rinse equipment between acetate and bicarbonate use.
         (f) Water rinse equipment between concentrate use and instilling disinfectant.
         (g) Do not turn equipment off with concentrate in system.

(h) Use acid and vinegar rinses as directed by manufacturer.

(i) Follow recommended cleaning, disinfection, and maintenance procedures.

d) NOTE: Not all dialysis systems use the same chemical formulations and combinations of acid and bicarbonate. Care must be taken that the correct concentrates are used.

III. Summary

A. *Replacement of Normal Kidney Function by Hemodialysis*

1. Fluid Balance

2. Electrolyte Balance

3. Toxin Removal

4. Acid/Base Balance

B. *Normal Kidney Function not Replaced by Hemodialysis and Requiring Medical Management Includes:*

1. Blood pressure regulation by hormonal interaction of the juxtaglomerular cells, renin production, and stimulation of angiotensin.

2. Stimulation of red blood cell production through the production of erythropoietin.

3. Vitamin D metabolism to a metabolite which promotes absorption of calcium from the intestinal tract.

4. Additional removal of phosphorus need through the use of binders.

Suggested Readings

Daugirdas, John T. and Ing, Todd S., Editors: *Handbook of Dialysis,* Second Edition, Little, Brown and Co., 1993.

Gutch, C.F., Stoner, Martha H., and Corea, Anna L.: *Review of Hemodialysis for Nurses and Dialysis Personnel,* Fifth Edition, Mosby, 1993.

Lancaster, Larry E., Editor: *Core Curriculum for Nephrology Nursing,* Third Edition, American Nephrology Nurses Association, 1991.

Man, N.K., Zingraff, J., and Jungers, P.: *Long-term Hemodialysis,* Kluwer Academic Publishers, 1995.

McKinley, Marta R. and Frame, Harriett A., Editors: Section XV, Principles of Hemodialysis, *Certification Review Course Outline,* American Nephrology Nurses Association.

Chapter 2
The Patient

Contributing Authors:
Patricia A Loughren, RegN, MA(Ed)
Gail Wick, BSN, RN, CNN

Chapter Outline

I. Normal Renal Physiology

A. Anatomy of Urinary System

1. Kidneys
   a) Location: Located on posterior abdominal wall just above the waist between the peritoneum and the posterior wall of the abdomen; referred to as retro-peritoneal in location. Right kidney is slightly lower than the left because the liver occupies a large area on the right side superior to the kidney. Three layers cover each kidney. The renal capsule, is a smooth, transparent outer membrane covering the ureter. Over this layer is the adipose capsule (peri-renal fat), a layer of fatty tissue that protects the kidney from trauma and holds it firmly in place. Covering the fatty layer is the renal fascia, a thin layer of dense, irregular connective tissue that anchors kidney to surrounding structures and to abdominal wall.

   b) Appearance: Kidney is reddish and bean shaped, weighs 120 -160 gm in adults, measures 5 - 7 cm wide, 11-13 cm long, about 2.5 cm thick. On medial side of kidney is the hilum, where the renal artery and nerves enter and where the renal vein and ureter exit. The hilum opens into a cavity called renal sinus.

   c) Protection: The kidney is partly protected by the eleventh and twelfth ribs, and posteriorly by large back muscles. Right kidney is protected superiorly by liver and left kidney is protected marginally by the spleen. Each kidney is covered by a thin fibrous capsule composed of connective tissue, blood vessels and lymphatics.

   d) Gross structures:
      (1) Renal cortex: This is a superficial reddish layer about 1 cm wide located just below the protective capsule. About 80 - 85% of nephrons and their blood vessels are located in the cortex. The glomerulus, Bowman's capsule, proximal and distal tubules and collecting tubule of remaining 15 - 20% are located deep in cortex.

      (2) Medulla: This layer is approximately 5 cm wide, and is located in the inner portion of the kidney. It contains the renal pyramids (8 -18 cone-shaped structures located at boundary between cortex and medulla) which project toward the center of the kidney. Tip of each pyramid, the papilla, opens into a minor calyx (a small

Figure 2.1

Internal Structure of Kidney

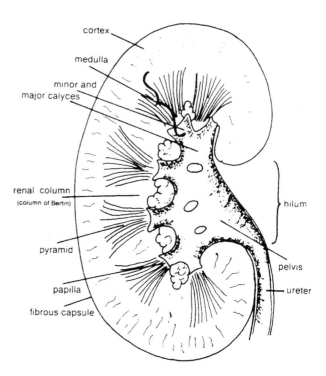

Reprinted with permission of the American Nephrology Nurses' Association, publisher, ANNA Core Curriculum for Nephrology Nursing, *Third Edition 1995.*

duct that collects urine). It contains the renal columns which are the portion of the cortex that extend between the renal pyramids. Together the cortex and renal pyramids constitute the functional portion or parenchyma of the kidney.

(3) Collecting system: Composed of tubules that drain from minor to major calyx into the renal pelvis. The renal pelvis narrows to form the ureter.

(4) Ureter: Small tube leaving the pelvis of each kidney and attaching to the posterior inferior portion of the urinary bladder. Measures about 30 - 33 cm long, 2 - 8 mm in diameter.

(5) Bladder: A hollow muscular bladder that lies in the pelvic cavity just posterior to the pubic bone. Functions to store urine. Its size depends on quantity of urine present. Its typical capacity is 1000 ml of urine.

Figure 2.2

Arrangement of Cortical and Juxtamentry Nephron

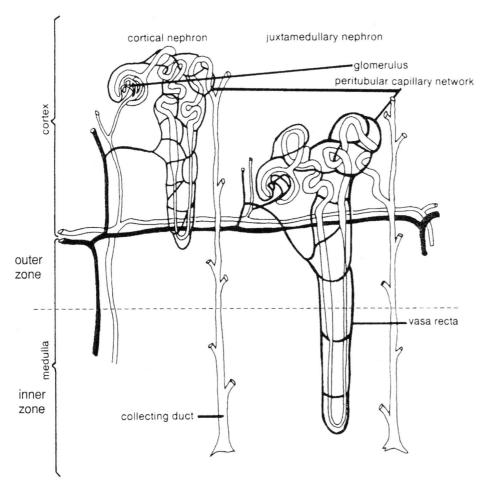

Note the relationship between vascular and tubular components.

Reprinted with permission of the American Nephrology Nurses' Association, publisher, ANNA Core Curriculum for Nephrology Nursing, *Third Edition 1995.*

urinary sphincter, formed of smooth muscle, lies at the junction of the bladder and urethra and is involuntary. External urinary sphincter is formed of skeletal muscle that surrounds urethra, giving voluntary control.

B. Blood Supply

1. Kidneys receive approximately 20 - 25% (about 1200 ml/min) of total cardiac output, referred to as the renal fraction. Body's total blood supply circulates through kidneys approximately 12 times/ hour. Approximately 90% of renal blood supply circulates through the cortex at a rate of about 4.5 ml/min., and 10% circulates through medulla at about 1 ml/min.

2. Blood enters kidneys through left and right renal arteries, which branch off the abdominal aorta. Renal arteries divide into interlobular arteries which pass between renal pyramids. Interlobular arteries give rise to arcuate arteries, which arch between the cortex and medulla. Afferent arterioles arise from branches of interlobular arteries and divide into tufts of about 12 capillaries called glomerular capillaries. These rejoin to form the efferent arterioles which form the peritubular capillaries which surround the proximal and distal convoluted tubules and the loop of Henle. Blood from peritubular capillaries enter interlobular veins. Veins of the kidney run parallel to arteries and have similar names, with the exception that there are no lobar or segmental veins. Renal vein exits through hilum and joins inferior vena cava, for return to liver.

(6) Urethra: A tube that exits from the urinary bladder inferiorly and anteriorly to the outside of the body. Triangle shaped portion of the bladder located between the opening of the ureters and the opening of the urethra is called the trigone. Length of urethra in males is about 20 cm, for females about 4 cm.

(7) Sphincters: When bladder reaches a volume of a few hundred ml, a reflex is activated, (micturition reflex) which causes the smooth muscle of the bladder to contract, causing urination. The internal

Figure 2.3

Summary of Nephron Structure

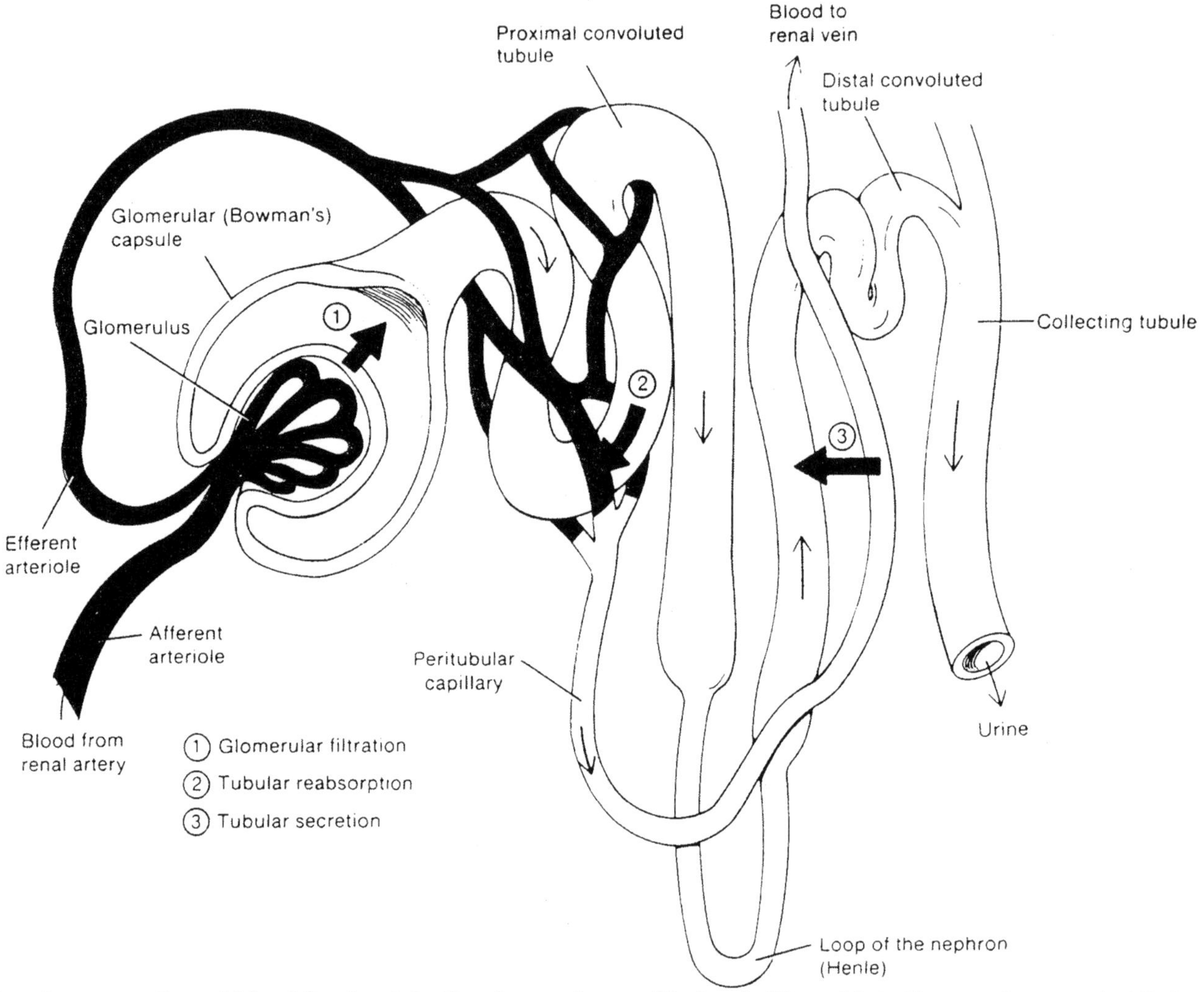

The plasma portion of blood flowing into the glomerular capillaries is filtered into Bowman's capsule (1). As the filtrate flows through the lumen of the tubule some substances are reabsorbed from the filtrate into the peritubular capillaries (2), and other substances are secreted from the peritubular capillaries into the lumen of the tubule (3).

Reprinted with permission of the American Nephrology Nurses' Association, publisher, ANNA Core Curriculum for Nephrology Nursing, *Third Edition 1995.*

C. Nerve Supply

1. Kidneys are innervated by sympathetic branches from celiac plexus, upper lumbar splanchnic and thoracic nerves, and inter mesenteric and superior hypogastric plexus. These join to form the renal nerve plexus.

D. Lymphatic Flow

1. Lymphatic drainage from kidneys and upper ureters flows into aortic and para-aortic lymph nodes, then into thoracic lymph duct, which empties into systemic circulation.

The Patient *Chapter 2*

13

E. Microscopic Structure of the Kidney: The Nephron

1. There are two types of nephrons: 20% (juxta medullary nephrons) lie close to the medulla and have long loops of Henle that penetrate deep into the medulla. The remaining 80% (cortical nephrons) have short loops of Henle and are located almost entirely in the cortex.

2. Nephrons process approximately 180 L of filtrate per day, and normally can reabsorb all the filtrate's essential constituents because they have a considerable reserve for reabsorption capacity. Filtration is a function of the Bowman's capsule, whereas reabsorption and secretion are functions of the tubules and collecting ducts.

3. A nephron is composed of:
   a) Renal corpuscle or Bowman's capsule (where blood plasma is filtered),
   b) Renal tubules - Proximal Convoluted Tubule, Loop of Henle, Distal Convoluted Tubule,
   c) Collecting Ducts (into which the filtered fluid or filtrate passes).

4. Renal Corpuscle/Bowman's capsule: Shaped like a double walled cup, in which the glomerular capillaries fit snugly. The endothelial cells of the glomerular capillaries have large pores, and there are gaps or slits between the podocytes that form the inner wall of Bowman's capsule. These pores and the connective tissue between them form a semi-permeable membrane that allows water and small molecules to pass through easily but prevents plasma proteins and blood cells from being lost.
   a) Approximately 20% of plasma passing through the glomeruli filters into Bowman's capsule. This is equal to a glomerular filtration rate (GFR) of approximately 125 ml/min. Volume of filtrate depends on net filtration pressure, which is the difference between the outward push of hydrostatic pressure and the inward attraction of the colloidal osmotic pressure of the blood in the glomerular capillaries.
   b) Glomerular hydrostatic pressure forces filtrate out of the glomerulus into Bowman's capsule. Glomerular hydrostatic pressure in the capillaries is about 60 mmHg.
   c) Colloidal osmotic pressure of blood is approximately 28 mmHg as it enters the glomerular capillaries. Colloidal osmotic pressure opposes the formation of glomerular filtrate, so conditions that reduce it tend to increase the quantity of fluid filtering into the tubule. Blood albumin concentration, which is kept constant by the liver, is largely responsible for colloidal osmotic pressure. However, this may decline for short periods when fluid intake is high or when albumin is lost during period of starvation or in renal disease.
   d) Capsular hydrostatic pressure is the pressure exerted by fluids in the glomerular capsule (about 15 mmHg).
   e) Net filtration pressure is estimated to be about 17 mmHg, which can be calculated by subtracting capsular hydrostatic pressure and colloidal osmotic pressure from glomerular hydrostatic pressure, as follows:

   60 mmHg - (28 mmHg + 15 mmHg) = 17 mmHg

F. Renal Tubules

1. Proximal convoluted tubule
   a) Reabsorption in this part of the nephron requires active transport and consumes energy. Approximately 66% of water from the filtrate entering Bowman's capsule is reabsorbed. Sodium, chloride, potassium, calcium and magnesium are reabsorbed. Glucose and amino acids are also reabsorbed into the tubules. Hydrogen ions are secreted in exchange for sodium.

2. Loop of Henle
   a) Approximately 25% of glomerular filtrate is reabsorbed by the Loop of Henle (LH) although only the ascending limb actively reabsorbs electrolytes, mostly chloride and sodium. The descending limb has a passive role. Because it is very permeable to water and salts, some of the NaCl reabsorbed from the ascending limb diffuses across the interstitial space, re-enters the descending limb of the LH and recycles through the loop many times, creating a high concentration of Na in the medulla, especially in the tips of the pyramids and their vasa recta. This plays an important role in water conservation during times of dehydration.
   b) As hypertonic filtrate moves along ascending limb, no more water is reabsorbed, as the walls are impermeable to water. Filtrate becomes increasingly dilute as NaCl is reabsorbed.

Dialysis Technology Third Edition © National Association of Nephrology Technicians/Technologists 2003

Hypotonic filtrate enters the distal convoluted tubule (DCT) with an osmotic pressure that is only 1/3 that of the blood and 1/12 that of the medullary tips.

3. Distal convoluted tubule and collecting ducts General mechanisms: Approximately 9% of the glomerular filtrate enters the DCT from the LH, more than 18 L/day. Unlike other portions of the collecting system, the DCT's reabsorption is accomplished by intrinsic and extrinsic mechanisms that adjust excretion to maintain the homeostasis of plasma, electrolytes, and pH.

   a) Intrinsic Control Mechanisms: Intrinsic mechanisms include all the local tissue mechanisms that do not require nervous or hormonal stimulation to make changes. These are related to sodium reabsorption in exchange for hydrogen ions and the action of the juxtaglomerular apparatus in control of the diameter of the afferent arteriole which, in turn, controls the GFR and the quantity of sodium in the DCT.

   b) Extrinsic Control Mechanisms: Extrinsic mechanisms involve the stimulation or inhibition of the active transport mechanisms by the nervous system or by hormones. They are: the renin-angiotensin-aldosterone system and atrial natriuretic hormone.

   c) The renin-angiotensin-aldosterone system acts to increase BP when it falls below normal. The enzyme renin is secreted by cells in the juxtaglomerular apparatus when they are stimulated by a fall in the afferent arteriole BP. Renin initiates a series of complex reactions by splitting angiotensin I from a plasma molecule called angiotensinogen. Angiotensin I is rapidly converted to angiotensin II as it passes through the lungs in general circulation, forming a potent vasoconstrictor. This, in turn stimulates cells of the adrenal cortex to produce and secrete aldosterone. Aldosterone stimulates the Na/K pump and ATP-ase enzymes of the DCT to reabsorb more Na and secrete more K+. The extra reabsorbed Na increases the secretion of ADH from the hypothalamus and the reabsorption of water. This increases plasma blood volume and BP.

   d) Atrial natriuretic hormone acts to reduce BP when it rises above normal levels. It is secreted by cells of the atrial wall when they are stretched by an increase in venous volume on the right side of the heart. ANH reduces the reabsorption of Na by the kidney tubules, and as a result, more Na is excreted, decreasing the osmolality of plasma. This in turn, reduces the secretion of ADH which causes more filtrate to be lost, ultimately returning BP to normal.

G. Function of the Nephron

1. The active physiology of the nephron performs three basic functions: glomerular filtration, tubular secretion, and tubular reabsorption. By performing these functions, nephrons maintain homeostasis of the blood.

2. Glomerular filtration: Substances in blood that are small enough, pass across the wall of the glomerular capillaries into the renal tubule. Water and small molecules readily pass through, but blood cells and most proteins do not. Trace amounts of albumin (a small size blood protein) enter. Formation of filtrate depends on pressure difference between glomerular capillaries and Bowman's capsule, called filtration pressure, which forces fluid through. When pressure increases, the volume of filtrate increases. Filtration pressure is influenced by blood pressure, blood protein concentration and concentration of solutes.

3. Tubular reabsorption: As fluid moves along the renal tubule, many useful materials are reabsorbed into the blood in peritubular capillaries. About 98% of filtrate is normally reabsorbed and is returned to general circulation. Involves both passive transport mechanisms (requiring no energy as it follows concentrate gradient) and active transport mechanisms (requiring energy in the form of ATP to move elements against a concentration gradient). Sodium, potassium, glucose, calcium, bicarbonate, chloride, phosphate, and amino acids are actively reabsorbed. Most reabsorption (65%) occurs in proximal convoluted tubule (PCT), smaller amounts in Loop of Henle and DCT. Descending Loop of Henle further concentrates the filtrate by removing more water (about 15%). Ascending Loop of Henle functions to dilute the filtrate by removing solutes. Sodium and chloride are reabsorbed here. In DCT, further NaCl is removed and water moves out by osmosis, reducing the filtrate by another 19%. Only about 1% of the original filtrate is excreted as urine.

4. Tubular secretion: As fluid passes along tubule, it also gains some additional materials (potassium, hydrogen, ammonia, uric acid, and other wastes) from the adjacent cells and capillaries. This can be active or passive. Ammonia diffuses passively because of its high concentration. Hydrogen, potassium, and creatinine are actively transported into the filtrate for secretion.

H. Regulation of Acid-Base Balance

1. Concentration of hydrogen ions in body fluids as a measure of pH, usually maintained between 7.35 and 7.45. Mechanisms that regulate pH are critical for survival. pH is controlled by: a) buffers, b) respiratory system, i.e., exhalation of carbon dioxide, and c) kidney excretion.

2. Buffers
   a) Buffers are chemicals that resist change in pH of a solution when either acids or bases are added. Buffers function to prevent rapid, drastic changes in the pH of body fluid by changing strong acids and bases to weak acids and bases. Buffers work within fractions of a second.
   b) Three principal buffers are: protein buffers, bicarbonate buffers, and the phosphate buffers.
      (1) Protein buffers: Most abundant buffer in cells and plasma. At least three-quarters of all buffering power resides within cells, as intracellular proteins. Proteins are composed of amino acids that have one amino group, which can act as a base by picking up an H ion (when pH falls), and one carboxyl group, which can act as acid by releasing an H ion (when pH rises). Both of these groups are able to function as buffers because of the following reactions:

      For organic acid (carboxyl) groups:

      $- COO$ + H = $- COOH$
      Carboxyl group (ionized)   H+ ion   Cardoxyl group

      For amino groups:

      $- NH_2$ + H = $-NH_3$
      Amine group   H+ ion   Ammonium group

      Consequently, the same protein molecules can function reversibly as either acids or bases depending on the pH of the environment. Hgb is an excellent example of a protein that functions as an intracellular buffer. CO_2 released from tissues forms carbonic acid, which

dissociates, liberating H+ and H_2CO_3 in the blood. At the same time, Hgb is unloading O_2, which leaves it carrying a negative charge. This allows excess H+ to bind to Hgb, minimizing changes in pH.

(2) Bicarbonate buffers: This is the most important extra cellular fluid buffer. Basis of the reaction is:

$CO_2 + H_2O \longleftrightarrow H_2CO_3 \longleftrightarrow H= + HCO_3$

An enzyme, carbonic anhydrase, increases the rate of reaction about 5,000 times. Reaction moves in either direction depending on concentration of molecules on either side. CO_2 concentration is regulated by respiration. HCO_3 is regulated by the kidneys. If more H+ is added to the system, it is buffered by the HCO_3 and forms H_2CO_3 (a weak acid), ensuring that the pH changes only minimally. The H_2CO_3 breaks down into H_2O and CO_2 and the CO_2 is exhaled, returning pH closer to normal.

(3) Phosphate buffers: Operation of the phosphate buffers is nearly identical to bicarbonate buffers. Components are the sodium salts of dihydrogen phosphate (H_2PO_4) and monohydrogen phosphate (HPO_4-). H_2PO_4- acts as a weak acid. N_2HPO_4 acts as a weak base.

Hydrogen ions released by strong acids are tied up in weak acids:

HCl + N_2HPO_4 =
Strong acid   Weak base

$Na_2H_2PO_4$ + $NaCl$
Weak acid   Salt

Strong bases are converted to weak bases:

$HaOH$ + Na_2HPO_4 =
Strong base   Weak acid

$NaHPO_4$ + H_2O
Weak base   Water

Because the phosphate buffer system is present in low concentration in the ECF (1/6 that of the bicarbonate buffers system), it is relatively unimportant for buffering blood plasma. However, it is very effective in buffering urine and intracellular fluid where phosphate concentrations are usually higher.

3. Respiratory system regulation
   a) Respiratory system eliminates carbon dioxide from blood while replenishing its stores of oxygen. Carbon dioxide generated by cellular

respiration enters RBCs and is converted to bicarbonate ions for transport in plasma Reversible equilibrium exists between dissolved CO_2/water and between carbonic acid/hydrogen/bicarbonate ions.

$$CO_2 + H_2O = H_2CO_3 = H+ + HCO_3$$

b) An increase in any of these chemicals will push the reaction in the opposite direction. In healthy individuals, CO_2 is expelled from lungs at the same rate it is formed in tissues. Respiratory system regulation of acid-base balance provides a physiological or functional buffer. Although it acts more slowly than the chemical buffers, it has 1-2 times the buffering power of all the chemical buffers combined. Changes in alveolar ventilation can produce dramatic changes in blood pH. Either doubling or halving alveolar ventilation can raise/lower blood pH by about 0.2 pH units. Because normal arterial pH is 7.4, a change of 0.2 pH units would yield blood pH of 7.6 or 7.2- both outside the normal limits. Alveolar ventilation can be increased about 15 fold or reduced to 0; this respiratory control of blood pH has a tremendous reserve capacity.

4. Kidney Excretion

a) Nephrons of the kidneys regulate urine pH directly by secreting hydrogen ions into the urine. The kidney is a powerful regulator of pH, but responds more slowly than does the respiratory system. As pH of body fluids decreases below normal, (acidosis), the rate of H+ ion secretion increases, and bicarbonate ion is reabsorbed, increasing pH to normal levels. On the other hand, as body fluid pH increases above normal (alkalosis), the rate of H+ ion secretion by the kidneys declines and bicarbonate ions are secreted, thus decreasing pH towards normal levels.

I. *Hormone Secretion by the Kidney and Other Functions*

1. The kidneys are responsible for production of erythropoietin factor, an enzyme that activates erythropoietin, a glyco-protein formed in the liver and other tissues. Erythropoietin promotes the production and maturation of red blood cells in the bone marrow. Erythropoietin is produced in response to decreased blood oxygen tension and decreased renal perfusion which may be caused by anemia, hypoxia, or renal ischemia.

Red blood cells are responsible for the oxygen carrying capacity of the blood. Fatigue and poor exercise tolerance are early symptoms of anemia.

2. Renal prostaglandins are synthesized in the renal cortex and medulla. They are produced in response to both renal ischemia and vasoconstriction. These prostaglandins contribute to balanced blood pressure by controlling vascular resistance and GFR.

3. The kidneys also play a role in the metabolism of vitamin D. Vitamin D3 is formed in the skin and metabolized in the liver and kidneys into an active form. The system is activated in response to hypocalcemia or hypophosphatemia. It acts in conjunction with the parathyroid hormone to increase intestinal absorption of calcium and phosphate, to mobilize calcium from bones, and to increase renal tubular reabsorption of calcium and phosphate. Production of D3 is suppressed by elevated calcium and phosphorus levels in the blood and also develops in chronic renal failure. In this case, it is the most significant factor contributing to renal osteodystrophy.

4. Lastly, the kidneys serve to excrete bacterial toxins and water soluble drugs, and although most drugs and toxins are biometabolized and inactivated by the liver, some inactivation also takes place in the kidneys.

II.Overview of Renal Failure

A. *Acute Renal Failure*

1. Acute renal failure (ARF) is characterized by a sudden, severe impairment in renal function, causing an acute uraemic episode, usually associated with oliguria (<500 ml/day) and azotemia (retention of nitrogen containing substances in the body). It may result from both metabolic or pathologic damage to the kidneys. Acute renal failure is usually associated with a defined period of acute illness, followed by a period of recovery, and although the mortality rate is still high, the prognosis for patients with ARF is improving.

2. Major causes of ARF include acute tubular necrosis, acute glomerulonephritis, acute urinary tract obstruction, occlusion of the renal artery or vein, acute pyelonephritis, bilateral cortical necrosis, and nephrotoxic agents, including drugs. A wide variety of drugs may be nephrotoxic, including: antibiotics (aminoglycosides), anesthetics, (methoxyflurane), antineoplastics (metho-

trexate), and non-steriodal anti-inflammatory drugs (ibuprofen). Radiographic contrast medium, organic solvents, heavy metals, and endogenous toxins have also been implicated.

3. Causes of ARF can be further subdivided based on location: pre-renal, renal, and post-renal. Pre-renal problems arise from inadequate perfusion of an otherwise normal kidney. This can be caused by congestive heart failure and hypovolemia (caused by hemorrhage or burns), and altered vascular resistance (caused by sepsis, antihypertensive medications, anaphylactic reactions and neurogenic shock). Renal causes for ARF stem from primary damage to the kidneys, leading to loss of nephron functioning. This can be caused by thrombosis/stenosis, acute tubular necrosis, glomerulonephritis, pyelonephritis, and diabetic sclerosis. Post-renal causes involve obstruction of the urinary tract distal to the kidneys, which results in interference with the flow of urine. Renal calculi, benign prostatic hypertrophy, and malignant tumors of the prostate are common contributing causes.

4. Regardless of its cause, ARF follows a common clinical course with the following stages being seen: initiating, oliguric, diuretic, and recovery stage.

5. The initiating stage begins when the kidney is injured and lasts from hours to days. The first signs and symptoms of renal impairment become evident. The oliguric stage lasts from 5 to 15 days, but can persist longer. In this stage renal healing begins, cells regenerate along the damaged basement membrane causing scar tissue development, and the nephron becomes clogged with inflammatory products. This leads to decreased glomerular filtration, decreased tubular transport of toxins, decreased renal clearance and urine formation. The most frequent causes of death in this stage are due to cardiac arrest from hyperkalemia, severe GI bleeding, and overwhelming infection. The diuretic stage usually lasts 1-2 weeks, sometimes longer. In this phase, there is a return of renal function with large losses of accumulated fluids because renal tubular patency has been restored. The high concentration of urea and sodium act as osmotic diuretics and the kidney's ability to concentrate urine is not yet optimum. With continued healing, most functions are regained, depending on the severity of the initial insult to

the kidney. The signs of azotemia lessen towards the end of this stage. In the recovery stage, which can last several months to a year, the healing process is completed with a few non-reversible changes taking place. A scar tissue layer replaces the damaged basement membrane, though the functional loss is not always measurable or significant. As well, the nephrons return to full patency, and tubular cells regenerate to allow essentially normal renal function. Body fluid and electrolyte balance return to essentially normal.

6. The goal of treatment of ARF is to prevent further progression, to determine and correct the cause of the insult, to manage the patient's fluid volume problems and electrolyte acid-base imbalances. Dialysis is used to remove nitrogenous wastes and fluid, to control pH, and to regulate electrolyte balance. Blood transfusions may be considered if the patient becomes clinically anemic. Nutritional support is important to prevent loss of lean muscle mass. In most situations, there is considerable weight loss during the time of acute illness due to anorexia.

7. The prognosis for ARF depends on the cause and extent of damage. The mortality rate continues to be about 50%, and this will worsen with the occurrence of sepsis, respiratory problems, and other multi-system failure. Obviously advancing age and other preexisting medical conditions also affect the prognosis unfavorably.

B. Chronic Renal Failure

1. Chronic renal failure is a slow, progressive deterior-ation in the functioning of the kidneys, developing over a period of years. The kidneys lose their ability to maintain the normal volume and composition of body fluids in the presence of normal dietary intake. Despite the wide variety of causes, the clinical symptoms are remarkably similar.

2. Causes of CRF include congenital disorders (kidney malformation or absence), cystic disorders (polycystic kidney disease), tubular disorders (renal tubular acidosis), neoplasms (benign and malignant cancers), infectious disease (pyelonephritis, renal tuberculosis), chronic glomerulonephritis, obstructive disorders (chronic renal calculi), and chronic systemic disease (diabetes mellitus, amyloidosis, scleroderma, systemic lupus erythematosus, hypertensive nephropathy or Goodpasture syndrome).

3. The condition, regardless of its many causes, usually follows the following three-stage progression.

   a) Stage I shows signs of decreased renal reserve, with 40 - 75% of normal function. At this point the patient is usually asymptomatic, has essentially normal BUN and creatinine. Excretory and secretory functions are satisfactory and homeostasis is maintained. Symptoms are usually not evident until about 80% of nephrons are affected.

   b) In stage II, residual renal function of about 20 - 40% of normal. Signs include a decrease in glomerular filtration rate, poor solute clearance, lessened ability to concentrate urine, and lowered hormone secretions. Other symptoms include rising BUN and creatinine, mild azotemia, polyuria, and clinical anemia.

   c) In stage Ill, commonly called End Stage Renal Failure (ESRF), residual kidney function is less than 15% of normal. The excretory, secretory and other regulatory functions of the kidney are severely impaired, with evidence of severely elevated BUN and creatinine, anemia, fluid overload, electrolyte imbalances (sodium, potassium, phosphate, and calcium) and uremic syndrome. The patient may also demonstrate hypertension, pulmonary edema, altered nutrient metabolism, and renal osteodystrophy. The mental status, peripheral nerve conduction, and platelet aggregation of the patient may be significantly impaired.

4. Generally speaking, though symptoms may differ depending on the wide variety of causes, the signs and symptoms of ESRD (Uremic Syndrome) are quite similar across most disease processes. These include, but are not limited to:

   a) Fluid and electrolyte problems: hypertension, engorged neck veins, liver enlargement, dependent edema, electrolyte imbalance.

   b) Acid-base imbalances: increased rate and depth of respiration, altered mental status, alterations of plasma bicarbonate <22 mEq/L with pH below 7.4.

   c) Neurological problems: "restless legs," burning sensation on soles of feel, apathy, confusion, stupor, flapping tremor of hands (asterixis).

   d) Gastrointestinal problems: anorexia, nausea, vomiting, diarrhea or constipation, uremic breath odor, melena (blood in stools).

   e) Cardiovascular problems: hypertension, arrhythmias, CHF, pericardial friction rub, atherosclerosis

   f) Respiratory problems: uremic fetor, dyspnea and crackles over the lung fields, pulmonary edema

   g) Skeletal problems: soft tissue calcifications, joint swelling, pain, osteodystrophy.

   h) Integumentary problems: edema in extremities with poor skin turgor elsewhere, pruritus, brittle nails and hair, easy bruising, altered pigmentation, bleeding gums/nose

   g) Anemia: symptoms include pallor, fatigue, poor exercise tolerance - may be related to decreased erythropoietin production, inadequate dietary intake, ongoing losses with blood sampling and dialysis.

   h) Endocrine malfunction, e.g., loss of growth hormone (in children with ESRD), changes in production of hormones and regulation of reproductive functioning and libido (LH and FSH and testosterone in men and estrogen and progesterone in women).

5. Conservative management of CRF is initiated when there is a measurable decrease in kidney functioning and continued until more aggressive management is indicated. Dietary changes might include low protein, high carbohydrate, moderate fat diet, low sodium and potassium intake, vitamin supplementation, and fluid intake to balance output according to residual function.

6. When conservative management no longer controls progressive symptoms, hemodialysis or peritoneal dialysis prescriptions are initiated depending on the needs of the patient and preference of the attending physician. Dialysis is a chronic treatment and therefore is not considered a cure for the disease. Transplantation is considered the only long-term solution to the problem of ESRD, and in itself, has selected associated problems.

III. Causes of Renal Failure

A. Infections

1. Infections of the urinary tract area are a significant cause of renal morbidity. Generally, they do not progress to ESRD unless there is a major structural problem such as obstruction.

2. Pyelonephritis (PLN) is an infection of the kidney and renal pelvis and is usually caused by bacteria (gram-negative bacilli and enterococci) ascending from the lower urinary tract when contamination of the urinary meatus may occur with fecal bacteria. Abscesses can occur as a result of PLN or systemic transport of bacteria from other infections. Common predisposing factors to developing pyelonephritis include: kidney stones, chronic urinary reflux, pregnancy, neurogenic bladder, surgical instrumentation, and female sexual trauma. Most of these conditions cause an acute infection. Lifestyle factors such as inadequate fluid intake and inattention to the need to void also contribute. Chronic infection results in tissue inflammation, fibrosis and scarring, leading to poor function. Patient complaints commonly include fever, chills, dull, constant flank pain, hematuria, pyuria, dysuria, and frequency of urination. General management includes: treatment of infection with antibiotics, fluid intake of 3500-4000 ml/day, analgesics and antipyretics to control fever and pain, rest, and follow-up in 7 to 10 days to determine the adequacy of treatment. The patient should also receive health teaching to prevent re-infection.

3. Renal and peri-renal abscesses can occur as a complication of infection elsewhere in the body, especially sub-acute bacterial endocarditis. Commonly, abscesses form at the lower pole of the kidney where drainage collects. Rupture of the abscess within the kidney or through the capsule can spread the infection and cause damage to other structures/organs. Common complaints for the patient with renal abscess include chills, fever, flank tenderness with mass sometimes palpable, nausea and vomiting, anorexia, and abdominal pain with guarding. Common treatment for renal abscess is similar to PLN, except that surgical incision and drainage may be required if the abscess is localized and painful. Care of the surgical site requires aseptic technique and care in the handling of contaminated dressings to prevent cross contamination. Since the patient may also experience nausea and vomiting, anti-emetics may be prescribed. Follow-up is required to ensure healing is complete.

4. Renal tuberculosis, though not common, is currently on the increase as a result of immigration from areas where the TB is endemic. Further, it is associated with risk factors such as homelessness, poverty and co-existing HIV infection. The TB bacillus is carried from the lung and seeded in the kidney where it forms cysts which can rupture. Damage to the kidney, as shown on dye studies, gives the kidney a "moth eaten" appearance. Common complaints for the patient with renal tuberculosis include fever, diaphoresis, weight loss, urgency, frequency, flank pain, generalized fatigue, and lethargy. Tuberculin skin test is positive. Common treatments include administration of anti-TB drugs, isolation precautions while sputum and urine cultures are positive, and general measures to reduce fever and pain and to maintain adequate hydration/nutrition. Additionally, lab test follow-up should be done to determine that acid-fast bacilli have disappeared from the urine. Renal TB can be prevented with aggressive treatment of pulmonary TB.

B. Autoimmune Disorders

1. Glomerulonephritis: This disease also accounts for the greatest number of patients who enter chronic dialysis and transplant programs. (Price and Wilson, 1992.) Origin may be acute or chronic. The acute form is most often seen as post streptococcal glomerulonephritis.

2. Acute post streptococcal glomerulonephritis: Onset of APSGN usually occurs 1 - 2 weeks after a beta - hemolytic streptococcal throat/ skin infection. Antigen-antibody complexes deposit on the glomerular basement membrane, initiating an inflammatory response. Damage to the basement membrane allows RBCs and proteins to escape into the filtrate. Most common age is school age children and young adults. Males outnumber females 2:1. The most common patient complaints include headache, low back pain, malaise, nausea, vomiting, fever, and chills. Urine volume is decreased and urine is dark brown or rust in color, commonly called "brick colored". Hypertension and edema are found in the most significant cases. Common treatments include control of edema and treatment of hypertension (through diuretics and antihypertensives) and presenting infection (with antibiotics). Limit fluids to 500 ml/day + urine produced for previous 24 hour period. Limiting sodium, potassium, and protein intake while still taking in 2500-3000 calories per day can become a challenge for the anorexic patient. Phosphate binding agents are sometimes administered if phosphate levels are high. Bed rest is indicated during the febrile period.

3. Interstitial nephritis: Nephritis is the second most common cause of acute glomerulonephritis. It can be a complication of drug toxicity, irradiation, or systemic lupus erythematosus, which in themselves cause very significant illnesses. The most common patient complaints with interstitial nephritis include polyuria, nocturia, allergic skin rash, headache, low back pain, weight gain or loss, fever, and chills. Interstitial nephritis results in tissue scarring and loss of function. Common treatments include treating underlying infection and discontinuing any drugs associated with nephotoxicity. Other treatments are symptomatic as listed above.

C. Renovascular Disorders

1. Renovascular disease encompasses several significant pathologies that can lead to ESRD. These are: diabetic nephropathy, nephosclerosis, and renal artery/vein occlusion. The kidneys are highly vascular organs that process about 1200 ml of blood per minute. When occlusive processes lead to alterations in flow to or from the kidney, the damage to the filtration system is usually irreversible.

2. Diabetic nephropathy (DN) is a consequence of diabetes mellitus. The glomeruli are affected by sclerosis of the afferent and efferent arterioles and thickening of the basement membrane through deposition of hyaline fibrous material. The glomerular filtration rate decreases and azotemia occurs. The symptoms of DN may not develop for years after the onset of diabetes. Control of blood pressure and serum glucose levels appear to be significant contributing factors. Patient symptoms include: Changes in BP hyper or hypotension, nausea, anorexia, thirst, oliguria, dehydration, increased specific gravity of urine, and weight loss. Common treatments include optimum control of the underlying condition - diabetes. Weight control and dietary counseling, in keeping with both the diabetic and renal diet, may make compliance a challenge. Nutritional modifications are made to maintain adequate nutritional status while reducing the workload on diseased kidneys. Fluid intake should balance output, and needs to be carefully regulated to equal insensible water losses (400 - 600 ml) plus output/24 hours. Antihypertensives and diuretics can be used to control blood pressure, and antibiotics may be helpful in the treatment of co-existing infections. Insulin or oral hypoglycemics are necessary to control blood glucose levels.

3. Nephrosclerosis is the damage caused by prolonged hypertension on the renal arterial and arterioles. Several factors contribute to the condition: the age at which hypertension develops, the severity and the presence of other risk factors, e.g., race, family history, cardiovascular disease, obesity, smoking and sedentary lifestyle. The pathology of the condition includes spasm, thickening, hypertrophy and hyaline degeneration of the renal arterial supply. The nephrons slow/stop production of substances that lower BP. Common patient complaints include hypertension, tachycardia, palpitations, extra heart sounds, headache, fatigue, blurred vision, retinal changes. Nocturia, hematuria and proteinuria are also found. Common treatments include combined drug therapies (with antihypertensives and diuretics) to control BP. Monitoring the patient's BP, daily weight, intake and output, monitoring lab values and cardiac response are key to successful treatment.

4. Renal artery/vein occlusion or thrombosis can contribute to sudden complete blockage of blood flow to/from the kidney. When thrombosis, sclerosis, or occlusion occurs in a renal artery, oxygen rich blood supply to the kidney is compromised and the tissues quickly become anoxic. An embolism can occur with mitral valve stenosis, subacute bacterial endocarditis, or as a secondary to myocardial infarction. Stenosis is usually caused by atherosclerosis, and the consequent decreased pressure stimulates the juxtaglomerular apparatus to secrete renin which can lead to a complex series of events that will cause angiotensin and aldosterone to be secreted, favoring sodium and water retention and increasing BP. Occlusion of a renal vein causes an outflow problem, with subsequent swelling or hydronephrosis of the kidney. Common patient complaints include: hypertension, flank pain, oliguria, gross hematuria, proteinuria, and foamy, deep yellow colored urine. Common treatment includes control of the underlying cardiac disease and hypertension through anti-hypertensives, prevention of further embolic disorders through anti-coagulation, and analgesics to control pain. Surgical intervention, e.g., embolectomy or nephrectomy are considered when other less invasive treatments are unsuccessful. Careful monitoring of the other healthy kidney is essential.

D. Metabolic Disorders

1. Metabolic disorders contribute to the growing number of conditions that can impact on kidney function. These include renal calculi and acute renal tubular acidosis.

2. Renal calculi affect a significant percentage of the population, most commonly men, and there are regional/geographic differences. While some stones do pass spontaneously, most are extremely painful and can cause obstruction and infection. The peak incidence is in the 30s to 50s for most patients. Factors contributing to the incidence of renal calculi include: long term ingestion of calcium carbonate containing antacids, vitamin D, megadoses of vitamin C and ingestion of drugs -acetazolamide, probenecid, and triamterene. Dietary patterns and limited fluid intake can also foster stone formation. Intake of highly mineralized water may also be a cause. Hyperparathyroidism can lead to hypercalcemia and hypercalciuria, a major cause of stones. Common patient complaints include fever, severe colicky flank pain radiating to the groin, nausea, vomiting, dysuria, and urgency. Common treatment begins with relief of pain (analgesics), removal of the calculi (passively or through surgical means), maintenance of fluid balance (through IV fluids), and treatment of any causative factors; e.g., obstruction, infection, or metabolic conditions. Surgical intervention may take the form of pyelolithotomy, nephrolithotomy, ureterolithotomy, cystoscopic basket extraction, or lithotripsy. As a prevention to further stone development, dietary modification with low calcium, low oxalate, or low purine - depending on the analysis of the offending stone. High fluid intake, 3500 - 4000 ml/day is recommended using demineralized water.

3. Acute renal tubular acidosis occurs when the kidneys are unable to excrete acid urine because of a tubular defect. Renal tubular acidosis (RTA) may affect the full age spectrum, from infants to adults, and is commonly associated with cystinosis and hyperparathyroidism. Either the proximal or distal convoluted tubules can be involved.

   a) With proximal RTA, there is a defect in reabsorption of HCO_3, producing hyperchloremic metabolic acidosis with hyponatremia and hypokalemia. ECF volume depletion occurs due to significant water loss.

   b) With distal RTA, a decrease in secretion of H+ ions is seen, with similar K + loss and polyuria. Common patient complaints for patients with RTA include weakness, lethargy, anorexia, bone pain, hyperchloremic metabolic acidosis, hypokalemia, hypercalciuria. Common treatments focus on control of metabolic acidosis with moderate doses of bicarbonate and electrolyte replacement. Acidosis must be corrected slowly to avoid lowering potassium levels further. Diuretics may be helpful in some patients to decrease calcium excretion. Potassium supplementation is usually required. Symptomatic treatment is utilized for other symptoms.

E. Renal Carcinomas

1. Renal cell carcinoma accounts for about 90% of kidney cancers. As with all cancers, renal cell carcinoma is on a dramatic increase, possibly due to earlier diagnosis, and also related to ongoing concerns about environmental contaminants.

2. In the US in 1993, an estimated 27,000 new cases of adenocarcinoma of the kidney were diagnosed and approximately 11,000 deaths occurred in the same year related to this condition. (Tanagho and McAninch, 1995.) Renal cell carcinomas are therefore a significant cause of morbidity and mortality among men and women in the fifth and sixth decade of life. The life expectancy of a patient with metastases is poor, e.g., only 5-20% are alive one year after diagnosis. The condition is most often one - sided, with left and right kidneys being equally affected. The tumor can arise anywhere in the kidney, causing compression of surrounding tissues and affecting urine production. Metastases are found most commonly in the lungs, lymph nodes, liver and bones. The adjacent pelvic organs, e.g., bladder, ovaries, etc. are commonly affected. Common patient complaints include chronic aching pain in the flank region, unexplained weight loss, palpable mass in the flank area, hematuria, and anemia. Common treatment focuses on control of tumor development. No radiation or chemotherapy has been found to conclusively prevent tumor growth. Nephrectomy, which involves removal of the affected kidney, surrounding fat, fascia, lymph nodes, and adrenal gland is the usual treatment. The prognosis is poor if there is involvement beyond the capsule. Post operative management includes pain control,

maintenance of fluid and electrolyte balance, prevention of complications of abdominal surgery, e.g., pneumonia and thrombotic disorders, prevention of wound infection by use of aseptic technique, early mobilization, and emotional support to the patient and family.

F. Obstructive and Congenital Disorders

1. Obstruction contributes significantly to stasis of urinary flow, which leads to hydro nephrosis, a type of atrophy that may lead to renal insufficiency and, in later stages, renal failure. Additionally, obstruction and stasis can lead to urinary tract infection, which worsens the clinical picture. In hydro nephrosis, the renal pelvis and ureter dilate and hypertrophy. Back pressure of urine causes compression leading to ischemia, in most cases without pain as a significant symptom. Common patient complaints include dull, inconsistent backache, fever and pyuria with infection, and hematuria. Common treatment consists of antibiotics to treat infection, and surgical intervention to relieve obstruction and preserve renal function. Nephrectomy may be indicated if the damage is extensive. Post operative care is similar to that listed above.

2. Congenital disorders include a wide variety of structural deformities occurring in prenatal development. These include polycystic kidney disease, hypoplasia and, dysplasia.

   a) Polycystic Kidney Disease is a genetically transmitted disorder, with an incidence of 1 - 1,000, which has two forms: the autosomal recessive type in infants and autosomal dominant type in adults. Children affected have a significantly reduced life span and poor prognosis. The only reasonably successful treatments are intermittent dialysis or renal transplantation. Genetic counseling is suggested for parents of affected children.

   b) The adult onset form accounts for 5 - 10% of adult dialysis patients, with symptoms showing between age 30 - 50 and as late as the 70s. In both forms of this condition, normal kidney tissue is replaced by clusters of fluid filled cysts. These cysts enlarge and become persistently infected, compressing surrounding structures. Poor perfusion may prevent antibiotics from reaching pockets of infection and abscesses and septicemia

may occur. Symptoms include: hematuria, abdominal fullness with palpable mass, polyuria and dull flank pain. Hypertension and renal failure follow the onset of symptoms within 5 - 15 years. Nephrectomy is suggested with persistent infection, or rupture of the cysts with bleeding.

3. Hypoplasia is a condition in which fewer than the normal number of nephrons is present. Dysplasia is a condition where areas of the kidney have remained underdeveloped from birth. Often these two coexist and are then termed hypodysplasia. If both kidneys are severely malformed, death usually will occur in the neonatal period. Common patient complaints are consistent with renal failure and uremic syndrome. Common treatment includes surgical removal of the affected kidney. Careful assessment of the other kidney is indicated. If CRF ensues, dialysis is undertaken. Transplantation is considered when the patient is stable and able to withstand surgery. Post operative care is similar to that of nephrectomy. Additional care is taken since the patient following transplantation is also immunosuppressed and is therefore susceptible to infections.

IV. Vascular Access

Vascular accesses are the life lines of hemodialysis patients, providing access to the patient's circulation. Blood is channeled from them via the bloodlines through the extra-corporeal circuit of the dialysis machine. Vascular accesses serve as the foundation for hemodialysis. These accesses also provide the greatest day to day challenge to providers of hemodialysis services. It is estimated that over 70% of patients on dialysis for over two years have had at least one hospitalization for access related complications. Conservative estimates are that access related hospitalizations account for over $150 million in annual costs. Additionally, malfunctioning accesses are a major potential cause of inadequate delivery of the dialysis prescription. It is impossible to over emphasize the importance of the role of the direct caregiver in caring for, assessing, and preventing complications in the patient's access.

A. Internal Accesses

Arteriovenous fistula (AVF) is the preferred access for chronic hemodialysis due to reduced complication rates, but it is not always possible to create them because of inadequate vascular anatomy. Small, atherosclerotic or calcified arteries result in low flow into the venous limb of the fistula, preventing maturation into an access that is adequate to provide sufficient flow for hemodialysis.

Figure 2.4

Different Types of Accesses

A-V *Fistula*

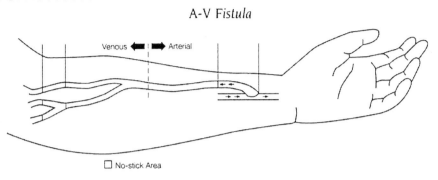

Loop Graft — Non-Reinforced

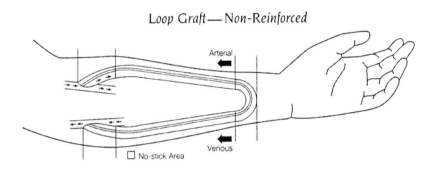

Loop Graft — Reinforced

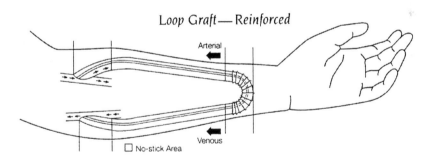

Reprinted from the IMPRA Stick with Us *workshop guide, p. 11*

An native fistula that matures (is still functioning after 6 weeks) well has the best chance for long-term survival of any internal access.

Arteriovenous grafts are also very suitable accesses for hemodialysis patients, and at present is the most common. They are the best choice if a patient must be dialyzed soon after placement of the access. Overall, the incidence of complications from grafts is twice that of AVFs: rates of thrombosis and infection are 6 times and 10 times higher, respectively.

1. AV Fistula:
   a) Anastomosis between artery and vein
   b) Advantages of AV Fistula:
      (1) Lower incidence of clotting
      (2) Lower incidence of infection
      (3) Minimal daily care
      (4) 70% patency after three years
      (5) Avoids potential for allergic response to synthetic materials

c) The greatest disadvantage is the 6 to 12 week maturation period required before use

d) Types of anastomosis

   (1) Side (A) to side (V)

   (2) End (A) to end (V)

   (3) Side (V) to end (A)

e) Common vessels used

   (1) Radial artery to cephalic vein

   (2) Brachial artery to cephalic vein

f) Maturation time: 6 - 12 weeks

g) Complications

   (1) Poor flow

     (a) Inadequate anatomy

     (b) Multiple needle punctures - fibrosis

   (2) Thrombosis

     (a) Early (4-6 weeks), usually technical in nature

     (b) Late:

       i) Usually associated with venous stenosis. Central venous stenosis may be present. Accounts for 80% of thrombotic episodes.

       ii) Low flow (hypotension, hypercoagulability, dehydration, access compression)

       iii) Hemodialysis related (platelet activation, hemoconcentration)

     (c) Signs and symptoms: decreased thrill, diminished bruit, increased venous pressure or decreased arterial pressure, recirculation, decreased adequacy of hemodialysis treatment

     (d) Treatment: declot, thrombolytic agents, surgical revision, percutaneous transluminal angioplasty, new access

   (3) Pseudoaneurysms

     (a) Extravasation of blood after needle removed is primary cause

     (b) Signs and symptoms: dilitation, pounding, sensitive

     (c) Infection, compression of fistula, erosion of skin, and hemorrhage may occur

     (d) Treatment: avoid puncture area, repair skin when it thins

   (4) Infection

     (a) Rare, usually staphylococcal when present

     (b) Causes: break in aseptic technique, seeding from another site, poor hygiene

     (c) Signs and symptoms: those of local inflammation

     (d) Complications: thrombosis, erosion of skin, septic emboli

     (e) Treatment: antibiotics, surgical revision, new access

   (5) Steal syndrome

     (a) Caused by ischemia of distal portion of limb that is deprived of oxygenated blood when blood takes the path of least resistance through the access

     (b) Most commonly seen in diabetic patients and other patients with small vessel disease

     (c) Signs and symptoms: affected limb is colder and pale; cyanotic nail bed; pain in the distal limb, worse with dialysis

   (6) Aneurysms

     (a) "One-site-itis," repeated use of same site is primary cause.

     (b) Signs and symptoms: dilatation of vessel, pounding, sensitive

     (c) Complications: recirculation, thrombi, rupture

     (d) Treatment: surgical revision

2. AV Grafts

  a) A graft is interposed between an artery and a vein. Synthetic, biological, or semibiological material may be used.

  b) Advantages

   (1) Can be used in two weeks, sooner if necessary

   (2) Larger cannulation site

   (3) Useful when natural vessels aren't suitable

   (4) Size and blood flow are not dependent on maturation

  c) Maturation: 2 weeks or longer is preferred, but can be used immediately if absolutely necessary

  d) Placement is variable, the most common initial site is the non-dominant forearm from the radial artery; end of graft to the side of artery or vein.

   (1) Arm is preferred

   (2) Avoid thigh if possible

   (3) Loop preferred

Figure 2.5

Needle Placement

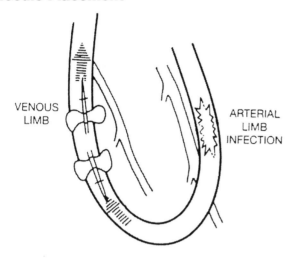

Needle placement if only one portion of the graft can be used for cannulation.

Reprinted from Vascular Access for Hemodialysis, *p. 133, fig. 11-5.*

e) Complications:

   (1) Thrombosis is primary complication

      (a) Cause: commonly anatomic lesions in the vascular system. Majority associated with stenosis, most often in the venous system.

   (2) Infection is second most common complication.

      (a) Incidence rate decreases if you can wait 2 weeks before use.

      (b) May be localized or systemic

      (c) Is more serious than with native fistula - disintegration of synthetic material and subsequent hemorrhage may result. May have to remove.

      (d) Signs and symptoms: redness, drainage, tenderness, swelling, febrile episode, sudden development of false aneurysm

      (e) Treatment: antibiotics for at least 6 weeks, resection of infected prosthesis

   (3) Steal syndrome – see fistulas

   (4) Pseudoaneurysms – see fistula

   (5) Stenosis and thrombosis

      (a) Most common reason is poor flow at anastomotic site

      (b) Early detection is critical

Figure 2.6

Confirm Direction of Blood Flow

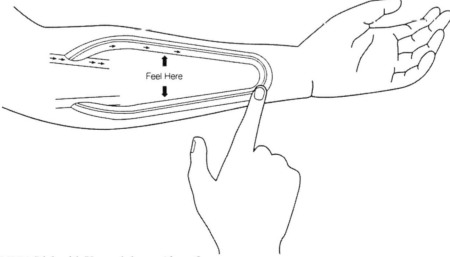

Reprinted from the IMPRA Stick with Us *workshop guide, p. 9.*

3. Detection of stenosis and thrombosis (AVF and grafts)

   a) Venous pressure > 150 mm/hg at 200-225 ml/min blood flows

   b) Intragraft pressures > 50 mm/hg with blood pump off

   c) Recirculation > 15%

   d) Physical findings – discontinuous, systolic harsh high-pitched bruit vs continuous, soft, low-pitched bruit of normally functioning access

   e) Color doppler ultrasound

   f) Angiography

4. Venipuncture considerations

   a) Always assess the access for signs of infection before needle insertion.

   b) Palpate the access to determine the direction of bloodflow, strength of flow, integrity of wall and straightness of potential sites.

   c) Never insert needle into an infiltrated, bruised, of infected site.

   d) Rotate insertion sites to maintain integrity of access; rotation should allow for at least two to three weeks of healing.

   e) Select sites so that needle tips are at least two inches apart.

   f) Attempt to leave enough room above the venous needle site for another insertion in case the first one infiltrates.

   g) Prepare sites appropriately:

      (1) Wash the access limb with microbial soap, preferably one containing lotion to minimize skin irritation.

      (2) Follow with 10% povidone iodine solution, 2% chlorhexidine, or 70% alcohol, applied to cannulation site in a circular motion while increasing the radius of the circle. Allow to dry.

      (3) Do not palpate the sites after the povidone iodine has been applied.

   h) Apply a non-occlusive tourniquet to both AV fistulas and grafts to maintain maximum distention of vessel.

   i) The venous needle must always be pointed in the direction of the flow.

   j) The arterial needle may be pointed up or down, depending on which direction gives the best blood flow and ease of insertion.

   k) Pull the skin taut in the opposite direction of the needle insertion. This compresses peripheral nerve ending to decrease pain.

   l) Common angle of insertion:

      (1) 20-35 degrees for AVF

      (2) 45 degrees for grafts

         (a) NOTE: a 45 degree angle is important for grafts because a smaller angle may separate the reinforcing layer of graft, thus weakening it.

Figure 2.7

Select Cannulation Site

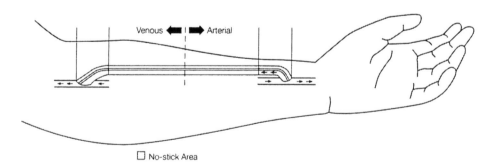

Straight Graft

Venous ⬅ | ➡ Arterial

☐ No-stick Area

Reprinted from the IMPRA Stick with Us *workshop guide, p. 10.*

---

m) Never force a needle, it should slide easily in. A more distinctive "pop" may be felt with grafts.

n) Always release the tourniquet to ensure that a good flow exist before infusing fluids.

o) Needles should not be routinely rotated or "flipped."

   (1) Slicing of the bottom of the vessel may occur.

   (2) The axis of the needle will be flat against the top of the vessel, potentially traumatizing it.

   (3) The hole in the skin and vessel my be stretched, making hemostasis more difficult.

p) Once placed, do not flatten the angle of the needle when applying tape. A 2X2 may be placed under the wings of the needle to maintain position. Avoid constricting or obstructing flow through the access when taping.

5. Hemostasis

   a) Mild to moderate pressure should be applied to the site after the needle is removed, rather than applying pressure as the needle is being pulled out. The entire shaft of the needle must be out of the skin first.

   b) Use of two fingers to hold pressure is recommended, one finger on the skin site, and one finger where the needle entered the vessel. Because the needle is inserted at an angle, the vessel insertion site is not directly under the skin insertion site.

   c) While holding pressure, always palpate above the site to assure that blood flows through the vessel.

   d) Three basic rules of compression with prolonged bleeding:

   (1) Direct compression with two fingers

   (2) Elevate arm to improve outflow

   (3) Do not check site for 7 to 10 minutes to allow for fibrin formation. Remove pressure slowly to prevent dislodging clot.

6. Infiltration during dialysis

   a) If a hematoma or infiltration occurs while dialysis is being initiated, firm pressure should be held over the site until bleeding stops. If the hematoma is large, apply a tight dressing and an ice pack over the site for 15 minutes before trying the site again.

Figure 2.8

Subclavian Catheter

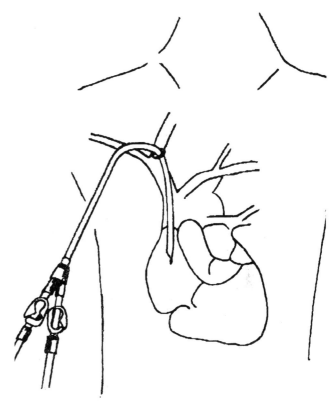

Drawing showing temporary vascular access using subclavian vein catheter.

Reprinted with permission of the American Nephrology Nurses' Association, publisher, ANNA Core Curriculum for Nephrology Nursing, *Third Edition 1995.*

b) If a needle infiltrates while the patient is on dialysis, turn the blood pump off and insert another needle. The original needle must be left in place until the treatment is over unless hematoma enlarges. Apply ice to the area of infiltration.

c) The patient should be instructed to use an ice pack on the hematoma on the day it occurs to minimize further bleeding into the tissue. Warm compresses can be used the following day to increase circulation and reduce swelling.

B. External Accesses

Temporary angioaccess is frequently necessary in the following situations: loss of internal access resulting in replacement; no internal access can be created;

and for acute dialysis or plasmapheresis. While external accesses offer circulation to the vascular compartment, use of them is frustrating to personnel trying to achieve high blood flow rates and prevent the numerous complications that accompany their use.

Dual lumen central venous hemodialysis catheters are the temporary accesses of choice. Three common locations for the cannula are the subclavian, femoral, and internal jugular veins.

1. Comparison of the three locations:
   a) Subclavian
      (1) Can be left in place several weeks
      (2) Extended function
      (3) Allows ambulation
      (4) Complications can be major and life threatening
      (5) Use is cautioned with respiratory conditions
      (6) Incidence of catheter associated bacteremia is high
      (7) Risk of thrombosis and stricture of SC vein or superior vena cava is high
   b) Femoral vein
      (1) Usually removed within 24-48 hours
      (2) Short term function
      (3) No ambulation
      (4) Complications usually minor
      (5) Incidence of catheter associated bacteremia is low if new catheter is used for each treatment
   c) Internal jugular vein
      (1) Can be left in place several weeks, longer if soft cuff catheter is used
      (2) Extended function
      (3) Limited ambulation
      (4) Complications usually minor
      (5) Incidence of catheter associated bacteremia is high
      (6) Stricture rate is low, thrombotic rate is similar to SC

2. Complications
   a) Insertion related
      (1) Arrhythmias
      (2) Arterialpuncture
      (3) Pneumothorax, risk is greater on the left side
      (4) Hemothorax
      (5) Perforation, greatest risk with SC
      (6) Air embolism
   b) Later complications
      (1) Infection (major complication)
         (a) Sources: migration from skin down catheter, contamination of connections or infused fluids, seeding
         (b) Staphylococcus aureus or epidermis the most common organisms
         (c) Prevention:
            i) Chlorhexidine disinfection pre-placement
            ii) Silver impregnated collagen cuffs
            iii) Antiseptic bonded catheters
            iv) Antibiotic ointment at exit sites
            v) Use of dry gauze dressings
            vi) Limited duration
         (d) Treatment
            i) Antibiotics
            ii) Removal of catheter
      (2) Thrombosis
         (a) Types
            i) Intracatheter (decreased function)
            ii) Fibrin (potential source of infection)
            iii) Mural (infection, occlusion)
         (b) Management
            i) Intracatheter
         (c) Intralumenial thrombolytics
            i) Urokinase
            ii) Streptokinase
         (d) Avoid forced irrigation
            ii) Fibrin sleeve
         (e) Catheter replacement if function impaired
         (f) Consider catheter venogram to document thrombosis
         (g) Low dose thrombolytics
         (h) Catheter stripping
            i) Mural
         (i) Catheter removal
         (j) Anticoagulation
         (k) Direct infusion of thrombolytics
         (l) Surgical thrombectomy
      (3) Central venous stenosis
         (a) Develops in 20-50% of patients with SC catheters. When this occurs, fistula creation is precluded. It is associated with prolonged cannulation and with stiff, non-silicone catheters.

(b) Usual manifestation: swelling of the arm

(c) Treatment: anticoagulation may help edema; angioplasty; placement of venous stent

(4) Perforation

(a) Cause: vascular erosion with prolonged cannulation or rigid catheters. Repetitive catheter movement may also be a factor.

V. Patient Rights

The American Hospital Association has created "A Patient's Bill of Rights" with the expectation that care providers will observe and protect the rights of the patient. It is also felt that observance of these rights will contribute to better patient care and greater patient satisfaction with treatment.

1. The patient has the right to considerate and respectful care.

2. The patient has the right to obtain from his physician complete, current information concerning his diagnosis, treatment, and prognosis in terms the patient can be reasonably expected to understand. When it is not medically advisable to give such information to the patient, the information should be made available to an appropriate person on his behalf. He has the right to know, by name, the physician responsible for coordinating his care.

3. The patient has the right to receive from his physician information necessary to give informed consent prior to the start of any procedure and/or treatment. Except in emergencies, such information for informed consent should include but not necessarily be limited to, the specific procedure and/or treatment, the medically significant risks involved, and the probable duration of incapacitation. Where medically significant alternatives for care or treatment exist, or when the patient requests information concerning medical alternatives, that patient has the right to such information. The patient also has the right to know the name of the person responsible for the procedures and/or treatment.

4. The patient has the right to refuse treatment to the extent permitted by law and to be informed of the medical consequences of his action.

5. The patient has the right to every consideration of his privacy concerning his own medical cane program. Case discussion, consultation, examination and treatment are confidential and should be conducted discreetly. Those not directly involved in his care must have the permission of the patient to be present.

6. The patient has the right to expect that all communications and records pertaining to his care should be treated as confidential.

7. The patient has the right to expect that, within its capacity, a hospital must make reasonable response to the request of a patient for services. The hospital must provide evaluation, service, and/or referral as indicated by the urgency of the case. When medically permissible, a patient may be transferred to another facility only after he has received complete information and explanation concerning the needs for and alternatives to such a transfer. The institution to which the patient is to be transferred must have accepted the patient for transfer.

8. The patient has the right to obtain information as to any relationship of his hospital to other health care and educational institutions insofar as his care is concerned. The patient has the right to obtain information as to the existence of any professional relationships among individuals, by name, who are treating him.

9. The patient has the right to be advised if the hospital proposes to engage in or perform human experimentation affecting his care or treatment. The patient has the right to refuse to participate in such research projects.

10. The patient has the right to expect reasonable continuity of care. He has the right to know in advance what appointment times and physicians are available and where. The patient has the right to expect that the hospital will provide a mechanism whereby he is informed by his physician, or a delegate of the physician, of the patient's continuing health care requirements following discharge.

11. The patient has the right to examine and receive an explanation of his bill, regardless of source of payment.

12. The patient has the right to know what hospital rules and regulations apply to his conduct as a patient.

Further, no catalogue of rights can guarantee for the patient the kind of treatment he has a right to expect. A hospital has many functions to perform, including the prevention and treatment of disease, the education of both health professionals and patients, and the conduct of clinical research. All these activities must be conducted with an overriding concern for the patient, and above all, the recognition of his dignity as a human being. Success in achieving this recognition ensures success in the defense of the rights of the patient

From the Patient's "Bill of Rights," American Hospital Association, 1972.

The Consumer Bill of Rights and Responsibilities, November 1997, has been presented in a report prepared by the Advisory Commission on Consumer Protection and Quality in the Health Care Industry. It is available from the US Government Printing Office. This document attempts to capture significant points of legislation in the Patient's Bill of Rights, from a consumer perspective.

VI. Professional Ethics

Ethics is a systematic reflection on the morally accepted principles of right and wrong in the conduct of a profession. Professional ethics act as a guide for behavior and decision making in the health care field.

There are several theories related to ethics.

Deontological theories relate to our "duties" as professionals, followed by rights and responsibilities. The basis of this theory is that some actions are immoral, no matter how positive and beneficial the consequences may be and some actions are moral, no matter how negative the consequences may be. Basically, one cannot judge the morality of an action on the basis of its consequences alone. Rather, the "means" counts in justifying the "ends".

Teleological theories place more focus on the consequences of actions in a more practical manner. The basis of this theory is that the moral thing to do in any situation is to bring about the best balance of benefits to the individual or group. In this case, the actions are goal driven and the "ends" count in justifying the "means".

There are five ethical duties that guide our behavior as health care professionals.

1. Non-maleficence: the duty to "do no harm". In this case, we are also obligated to inform the patient of direct/indirect harm, to remove the patient from harm.

2. Beneficent: the duty to "do good". In this case, we are obligated to provide care in a manner that benefits the patient.

3. Fidelity: the duty to be "faithful" to the patient. In today's terms, this means meeting the patient's reasonable expectations for safe and competent care, showing respect for the patient, following policies of the agency in providing care, honoring the patient's right to consent, and to privacy/confidentiality. It also means following through on the work agreement, where the professional has a duty to perform job competencies to the best of his/her ability and to remain current in the field so that safe practice can be ensured.

4. Autonomy: the duty to support the patient's right to self-determination and to follow through on the patient's informed, competent wishes. In the event that we cannot support the patient's wishes, (if it goes against our religious principles), then we are obligated to withdraw and to find another professional who can do so. This has significant implications for end-of-life issues and withdrawal from treatment.

5. Veracity: the duty to tell the truth. This means that professionals are obligated to be honest in reporting, charting or discussing information related to the patient or with the patient. In health care, there are arguments for and against disclosure in specific situations, depending on where the greatest good would be served.

6. Justice: the duty to ensure fairness in situations. This means preventing discrimination, providing equitable arrangements when priorities are set, and ensuring that decisions are impartial and with the best interests of the patient in mind.

In recognizing that an ethical dilemma exists, we must examine which duty best serves the interests of the patient, and therefore over-rides others. For example, there can be a dilemma for the care provider when a diagnosis is shared with family, and they indicate adamantly that they do not wish this information to be given to the patient and that to do so would significantly compromise the patient's health and well being. The duty to fidelity and autonomy may not be primary in this case. Rather, the duty to "do no harm" might be seen as the most significant concern, especially in light of underlying harm to the patient. Decision making in ethical situations should not occur in isolation, but rather with input from the multi-disciplinary team, ethics committee and pastoral care at the hospital/agency. Documentation in these situations should be detailed, so that it is clear how the decision was derived.

Suggested Readings

AMGEN, Inc. (1992), *Core Curriculum for Dialysis Technicians,* Wisconsin: Medical Media Publishing, Inc.

Brouwer, D. (1664, November), *Cannulation Camp: Basic Needle Cannulation Training for Dialysis Staff, Dialysis and Transplantation* Magazine.

Brundage, D., (1992), *Renal Disorders,* St. Louis: Mosby -Year Book.

Burrows-Hudson, S., editor. (1993), *Standards of Clinical Practice for Nephrology Nursing,* ANNA, Pitman, NJ.

Daugirdas, JT and Ing, TS, editors, (1994), *Handbook of Dialysis,* Boston: Little, Brown and Co.

Edge, R., and Groves, 3., (1994), *The Ethics of Health Care: A Guide for Clinical Practice,* Albany, NY: Delmar Publishing.

Hamilton, E., Whitney, E., and Sizer, F., (1991), *Nutrition: Concepts & Controversies,* St. Paul: West Publishing Co.

Hawkins, CT (1995, April), *Nurses' Roles in Influencing Positive Vascular Access Outcomes,* ANNA Journal.

Lancaster, L., (1995), *ANNA Core Curriculum for Nephrology Nursing,* Third Edition, Pitman, New Jersey: Anthony J. Jannetti, Inc.

Nissenson, A., Rind, R., and Gentile, D., (1995), *Clinical Dialysis,* Third Edition, Norwalk, Connecticut: Appleton & Lange.

Nissenson, et al, editors (1993), *Dialysis Therapy,* St. Louis: Mosby Year - Book, Inc.

Poleman, C., and Peckenpaugh, N., (1994), *Nutrition: Essentials and Diet Therapy,* Sixth Edition.

Price, S., and Wilson, L., (1992), *Pathophysiology: Clinical Concepts of Disease Processes,* Fourth Edition, St. Louis: Mosby - Year Book, Inc.

Purtilo, R., (1993), *Ethical Dimensions in the Health Professions,* Second Edition, Philadelphia: W.B. Saunders Co.

Sands, J. and Miranda, C. (1996, February), *Optimizing Hemodialysis Access: A Teaching Tool, Nephrology News and Issues* Magazine.

Schwab, 53, guest editor. (1994, July), *Advances in Renal Replacement Therapy,* National Kidney Foundation, WB. Saunders Company.

Seeley, R., Stephens, T., and Tate, P., (1996), *Essentials of Anatomy & Physiology,* Second Edition, St. Louis: Mosby-Year Book, Inc.

Wilson, B., Shannon, M., and Stang, C., (1997), *Nurses Drug Guide,* Stamford, Connecticut: Appleton & Lange.

Chapter 3
Dialyzers

Contributing Authors:

Lina M. Collier, CHT　　*Clifford F. Glynn, Sr., CHT*

Jim Curtis, CHT　　*Lorus Hawbecker, RN, CNN*

Marsha Evans, CHT

Chapter Outline

I. Dialyzer Design

There are three basic dialyzer configurations. Each design has the four necessary parts: a casing, a membrane, a blood compartment, and a dialysate compartment.

A. Coil Dialyzers

1. Coil dialyzers were the first type of hemodialyzer to be mass produced. Cellulose tubing concentrically wound with a mesh support screen around a central core. The blood channel was very long to obtain the needed surface area, and resistance was high. Ultrafiltration was unpredictable, and blood leaks were frequent.

2. Coil dialyzers are no longer available.

B. Parallel Plate Dialyzer

1. The original plate dialyzer was the Skeggs Hemodialyzer. It was followed by the Kiil and its modifications. The dialyzers were large and heavy. Cleaning assembly, leak-testing, and sterilization were performed by hand before each use. Gambro in the mid-1960s developed a lightweight, multi-layer, disposable dialyzer. A variety of small, compact parallel plate dialyzers followed.

2. Advantages of parallel plate dialyzers are:
   a) Heparin requirements usually are low. There is minimal clotting in the blood compartment.
   b) Ultrafiltration is reasonable, predictable, and controllable.
   c) They are very inexpensive.

3. Disadvantages of the plate dialyzer are:
   a) The uneven blood flow around the inlet parts, outlet parts, and in the corners of the blood compartment could produce local thrombi.
   b) They are resistant to rinsing and are potential sources of bacterial growth and endotoxin formation.
   c) Plate dialyzers are very compliant, the volume of blood they hold increases as the TMP increases.
   d) Plate dialyzers do not reuse well, and efficacy of reprocessed plates cannot be determined by total cell volumes due to their compliancy.

C. Hollow-Fiber Artificial Kidney (HFAK)

1. Hollow-Fiber Kidneys are the most common type of dialyzer in use. They are marketed in a variety of sizes and membranes. They are constructed

Figure 3.1

Examples of Dialyzers

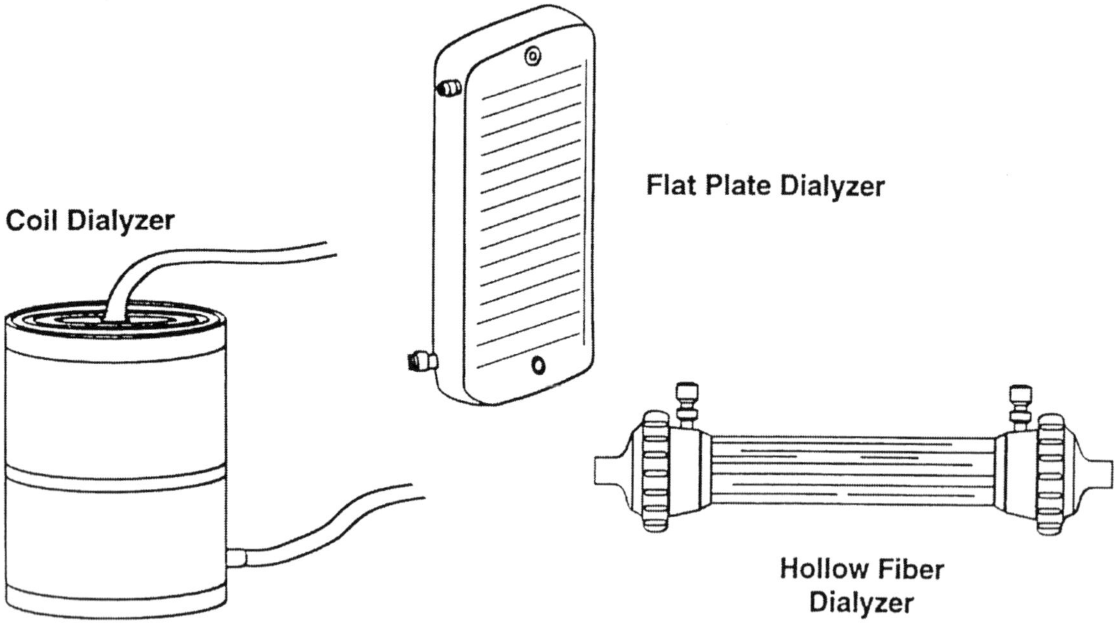

Source: NANT Core Curriculum for Reprocessing of Dialyzers, *p. 4, fig. 3.*

Figure 3.2

Parallel Plate Hemodialyzer

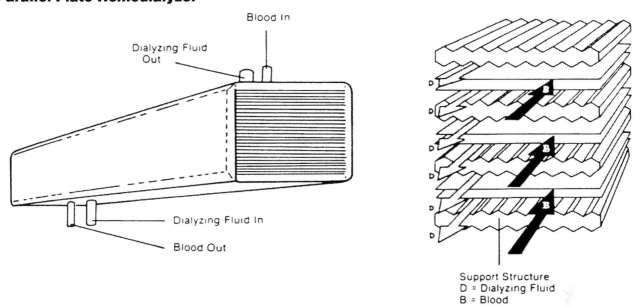

Blood In

Dialyzing Fluid
Out

Dialyzing Fluid In

Blood Out

Support Structure
D = Dialyzing Fluid
B = Blood

Reprinted with permission of the American Nephrology Nurses' Association, publisher, ANNA Core Curriculum for Nephrology
Nursing, *Third Edition 1995.*

Figure 3.3

Hollow-fiber Dialyzer

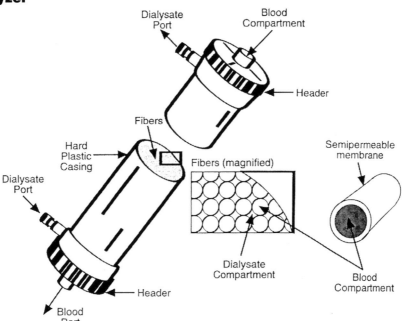

Dialysate
Port

Blood
Compartment

Header

Fibers

Hard
Plastic
Casing

Semipermeable
membrane

Dialysate
Port

Fibers (magnified)

Dialysate
Compartment

Blood
Compartment

Header

Blood
Port

Source: NANT Core Curriculum for Reprocessing of Dialyzers, *p. 5, fig. 4.*

of rigid hollow tubes that are made of semi-permeable materials.

2. The number of fibers in each dialyzer ranges from 10,000 to 20,000 or more, depending upon length, kind of membrane, and surface area of the dialyzer.

3. Advantages to using the HFAK are:

    a) Resistance to blood flow is low because of the large number of blood passages.

    b) They are non-compliant; that is, they hold the same volume of blood at high pressures as they do at low pressures.

c) Ultrafiltration can be controlled very precisely.

d) HFAKs are well adapted to reuse and the efficacy of reprocessed HFAKs can be predicted by total cell volumes.

4. Disadvantages of the HFAK are:

    a) Meticulous deaeration of the fiber bundle is necessary during the priming procedure. Otherwise fibers may airlock and not admit blood.

    b) There can be uneven distribution of blood at the inflow header space. Relative stagnation occurs in some areas with reduced perfusion of some fibers.

Figure 3.4

Blood and Dialysate Flow

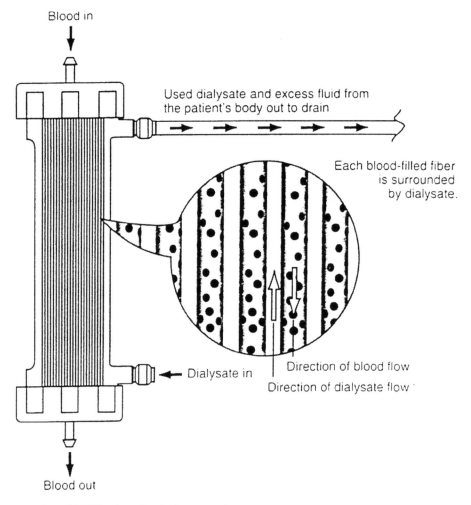

Reprinted with permission from AMGEN *Core Curriculum, p. 9, fig. 3.*

---

c) Dialysate channeling can occur in the dialysate compartment, reducing effective surface area.

d) Most patients require more heparin.

e) Residual toxic products of sterilants or disinfectants (ethylene oxide, Renalin, formaldehyde) in the absorptive potting material of the headers can cause adverse patient reactions.

II. Membranes for Hemodialysis

A. Hemodialysis Membrane Material

1. Membranes for hemodialysis are manufactured from polymer material.

   a) A polymer is a chemical term. It can be defined as a compound formed by the combination of simple repeating molecules

2. Description of polymer materials used in hemodialysis membranes

   a) Cellulose

   (1) The cellulose polymer is natural plant fiber derived from cotton and/or wood.

   (2) Chemical composition is a complex carbohydrate with glucose in the backbone of the molecule.

   (3) Cellulose was the most common material used in early dialyzer.

   (4) Examples: Cuprophan,® Cupammonium Rayon, Regenerated Cellulose

   (5) Generally accepted advantages:

   (a) Consistent small molecule transport characteristics

   (b) Low ultrafiltration coefficients do not require fluid control equipment

   (c) Generally inexpensive

   (d) Usually reuse well

   (6) Generally accepted disadvantages:

   (a) Reduced biocompatibility compared to other membrane types

   (b) No significant removal of larger molecules (above 5,000 MW)

   b) Substituted Cellulose (sometimes called Semi-Synthetic or Modified Cellulose)

   (1) Polymer is a cellulose base that has been chemically altered.

   (2) Chemical composition of the cellulose is modified such that the hydroxyl groups on the glucose backbone (thought to

be responsible for some of the severe membrane reactions seen with pure cellulose) are replaced (substituted) with other functional groups, most often acetate.

   (3) Examples: Cellulose Acetate, Cellulose Diacetate, Cellulose Triacetate, Polysynthane,® Hemophan® (replacement uses an amino group).

   (4) Generally accepted advantages:

   (a) Improved biocompatibility.

   (b) Performance characteristics can be easily varied during manufacturing so semi-synthetic membranes are available with a wide range of solute and water permeability. (Conventional / High Efficiency / High Flux)

   (c) High flux semi-synthetics offer better capability to limit backfiltration than many synthetic high flux membranes due to somewhat lower KUF's.

   (5) Generally accepted disadvantages:

   (a) More expensive than cellulosic

   (b) Reusability varies.

   (c) High Flux semi-synthetics require ultra-filtration control equipment

   c) Synthetic

   (1) Polymer consists of compounds synthesized from petrochemicals and processed into membranes.

   (2) Chemical composition is made up of thermoplastic compounds, similar to those commonly used in creating many different plastics and fabrics.

   (3) Examples: Polysulfone(PS), polymethylmethacrylate (PMMA), polyacrylonitrile (PAN, AN69), polyamide, and EVAL.

   (4) Generally accepted advantages:

   (a) Improved biocompatibility

   (b) Performance characteristics can be varied to provide good removal of larger molecular weight substances (high flux), and some synthetics are also now available with conventional (low flux) and high efficiency permeability.

   (c) Excellent reusability

(5) Generally accepted disadvantages:
  (a) Most expensive.
  (b) High flux synthetics require ultra-filtration control equipment.
  (c) High flux synthetics may have undesirable protein loss.
  (d) High flux synthetics have greatest risk of back-filtration.

B. Membrane Manufacturing Processes

1. Liquification

Hemodialysis membrane processing begins by creating a thick viscous material from the polymer, either by dissolving it with chemicals, or melting it with heat. This thick slurry or polymer dope can then be drawn out into hollow fibers (much like a spider spins a web) or pressed into thin sheets. The greater blood / membrane exposure in the hollow fiber design provides the most efficient solute transfer. Thus more than 95% of today's hemodialysis membranes are hollow fibers. Only a few companies continue to produce plate (flat sheet) membrane dialyzers.

2. Extrusion

Refers to the spinning or drawing out of the fiber. To maintain the open core of the fiber, most processes pump either a chemical substance or a gas down the center as the fiber is spun.

3. Coagulation

The walls of the fiber must be solidified so the fiber holds its shape. This is done in solution spun membranes with either a water or chemical bath of the fibers. Melt spun fibers solidify by air cooling.

4. Extraction

This is the stage during which the actual membrane porosity is created. The potential pore structure is determined by the preceding processing steps. Picture the membrane wall as being composed of a mixture, much as you get when you mix oil and vinegar together, only it is now solidified. The extraction step removes one or more elements of the original mixture, thus creating spaces or openings throughout the membrane wall. These are the pores. The size, shape, number, and characteristics of the pores vary, depending on the polymer used and variations in the manufacturing processes.

Figure 3.5

The Fiber Spinning Process

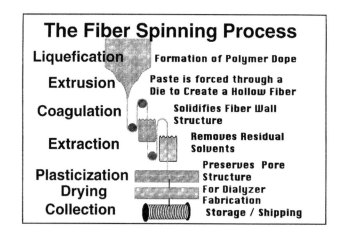

Reprinted with permission of Althin Academy

5. Plasticization

The pore structure of many membranes is fixed by filling the membrane wall with glycerin and then drying. The glycerin remains in the fiber wall until the dialyzer is primed and can sometimes be visualized in the first saline entering the venous drip chamber from a dry (non-reuse) dialyzer.

C. Membrane Characteristics

1. Porosity
  a) Pore size
    (1) Cellulosic and Substituted Cellulosic membranes are said to have a homogenous "gel matrix" type porosity. The polymer strands are twisted (much like twisted strands of spaghetti), and the pores are tortuous tunnels, through which molecules must weave in order to diffuse through the membrane. How tightly or loosely the strands are twisted determine the pore size. Cellulosic membranes are always very tight providing the small molecule removal of conventional low flux or high efficiency dialyzers. High efficiency dialyzers simply have more small pores to increase the removal of small size molecules such as urea. The pore size of substituted cellulosic

Figure 3.6

Molecular Weight Chart

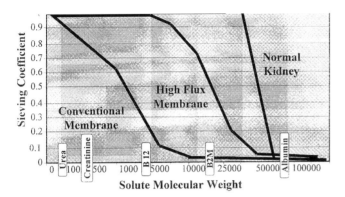

Reprinted with permission of Althin Academy

membranes may be varied during manufacturing to produce porosity for conventional, high efficiency or high flux (removal of molecules greater than 5000 molecular weight).

    (1) Synthetic membranes tend to have a more frank "straight through" type pore, and molecules move by either diffusion or are carried through as water crosses the membrane (convection). The original synthetics were large pore membranes allowing passage of the higher molecular weight substances. Today synthetics can be manufactured with smaller pores as well, creating conventional and high efficiency membranes with diffusive properties.

  d) Pore structure

    (1) A symmetric structure means the membrane has the same size pore openings on both the blood side and the dialysate side of the membrane. Semi-synthetic and cellulosic membranes tend to be homogenous and symmetric.

    (2) Asymmetric membranes are those with pores which expand from small inner lumen pore openings in a smooth thin skin layer, through a widening spongy, micro-porous sub-layer to a larger opening on the dialysate side.

  e) Number of pores per square meter (m^2) surface area.

    (1) One upon a time, performance was simply defined by the amount of square meter surface area of membrane because all membranes had comparable permeability. Today the number and size of pores in any amount of membrane depends on the polymer type and the fabrication process, and the clinician must examine the performance specifications of the membrane once it is incorporated into a dialyzer to determine if it will meet the patient's individual needs.

2. Membrane Wall Thickness

  a) Membrane thickness varies from one type of membrane to another. Usually synthetics and semi-synthetics are thicker than the cellulosic type. Generally thinning a membrane, especially the gel matrix type, improves diffusion because the distance molecules must travel through the tortuous tunnels is decreased.

  b) Some membranes become thicker during clinical use either due to swelling of the fiber wall or to adherence of protein material to the inside of the wall.

    (1) Increasing wall thickness can decrease the expected diffusive performance of the membrane, and is thought to be responsible for the drops in performance that have been noted from published in-vitro (laboratory testing) clearances to in-vivo (actual clinical performance) measurements.

    (2) Protein adsorption can contribute to improved biocompatibility of the less biocompatible membranes during reuse, and to the removal of some of the larger low molecular weight proteins such as complement and Beta 2 Microglobulin. Generally synthetic membranes are the most adsorptive, polyacrylonitrile having the greatest adsorptive capability.

3. Membrane Hydraulic Permeability

  a) How easily water moves through a membrane is a function of the size of the pores, the number of pores, and the tortuosity of the path through the membrane wall.

b) Cellulose and substituted cellulosic membranes, characterized by smaller size pores with a tortuous, homogenous structure, generally have low fluid removal capability. The synthetic asymmetric membranes with their more open pore structure have the highest hydraulic permeability. This explains why it is possible for two different membranes to have comparable pore size openings, but different fluid removal characteristics.

D. Membrane Permeability Descriptions

1. **Clearance** (K) is a VOLUME measurement and must always be stated in relation to a specific blood flow rate.

   a) It is a term that describes the volume of blood that will be totally cleared of a specific substance in a specified period of time in relation to the volume of blood that has passed through the system.

   b) Dialyzer membrane clearances are always stated as the milliliter (ml.) volume that will be cleared in relation to the Blood Flow (Qb) Rate per minute (ml/min).

c) For example: "A Urea Clearance of 182 at 200 Qb" means: At a blood flow rate of 200 ml. per minute, the membrane in this dialyzer should totally clear all the urea from 182 of those 200 ml of blood.

d) Clearances can be stated and measured either in-vitro or in-vivo.

e) Clearance is the most commonly used description of a membranes permeability to small solute substances such as urea and creatinine.

f) Clearance Formula: (with ultrafiltration at 0)

$$\frac{\text{Concentration of the blood in} - \text{Concentration of the blood out}}{\text{Concentration of the blood in}} \times \text{Blood Flow Rate}$$

2. **Sieving Coefficient** (S.C.) is a conceptual mathematical expression of the way membrane pore structure interferes with the transfer of a specific solute into the dialysate.

   a) It describes the percent of a given solute you would expect to be able to pass from the blood into the dialysate based only on convective flow through the membrane.

Figure 3.7

Membrane Pore Structure

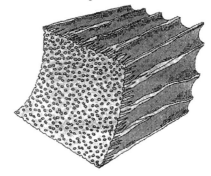

Symmetric

Typical of Cellulosic and
Substituted Cellulosic Membranes

Pore openings are the same size on blood and dialysate sides of the membrane wall.

Asymmetric

Common Structure of Synthetic Membranes

Pore openings through the membrane wall widen as they go from blood side to dialysate side.

Reprinted with permission of Althin Academy

b) It is expressed as a decimal from 0.1 to 1.0. The higher the number, the more of the solute you would expect to pass.

c) For example:

(1) The S.C. of every dialysis membrane for urea is 1.0, indicating that given the size of the molecule compared to the pore size of the membrane, you would expect 100 % to be able to pass through the membrane.

(2) On the other hand, conventional low flux membranes have very low (less than 0.2) S.C.'s for larger molecules such as Beta 2 Microglobulin, while high flux membranes have Sieving Coefficients up to 0.8; indicating that the pore size of the membrane could permit up to 80% to pass through.

d) S.C. is used most often to describe membrane permeability to larger molecules such as Beta 2 Microglobulin and albumin.

e) S.C. Formula:

$$S.C. = \frac{\text{Solute Ultrafiltrate Concentration}}{\text{Solute Blood Concentration}}$$

f) Clinical Sieving Coefficients vary with dialysis conditions and blood (hematocrit) chemistries.

3. **KOA** is a numerical description of the solute transport efficiency of a dialyzer membrane. It is referred to as the "mass transfer coefficient."

a) It takes into account the amount (m^2) of membrane and all three resistances a

substance must overcome to be dialyzed.

(1) Solute must get through the blood to the membrane. This resistance changes mainly depending on the blood flow rate and the internal diameter of the fiber.

(2) Solute must move through the pores of the membrane. The membrane resistance for a solute in any given dialyzer will be a constant.

(3) Solute must be carried away by the dialysate. This resistance is influenced by changing the dialysate flow rate.

b) KOA is expressed as a whole number: the higher the number, the lower the resistance to solute passage and the greater the permeability of the membrane for that solute. In hemodialysis membranes, the KOA for urea can range from 200 to as much as 900 at high blood and dialysate flow rates.

c) KOA information is entered into computerized urea kinetics programs and used to calculate expected clearances as blood and dialysate flows are increased.

d) KOA Formula: The KOA formula is a very involved calculation requiring specific membrane information and a calculator with an exponential function.

4. **KUF** is the coefficient of ultrafiltration and describes the permeability of a membrane to fluid (plasma water) passage.

a) It is expressed as the volume in milliliters that a membrane will permit to pass per hour for every millimeter of mercury hydrostatic pressure applied across the membrane (Trans-Membrane Pressure).

b) KUF is expressed as ml/hr/mmHg TMP.

c) KUF Ranges

(1) Conventional membranes: 3 to 10 ml/hr/mmHg TMP

(2) High efficiency membranes: 7 to 12 ml/hr/mmHg TMP

(3) High flux membranes: 12 to 90 ml/hr/mmHg TMP

Figure 3.8

KOA

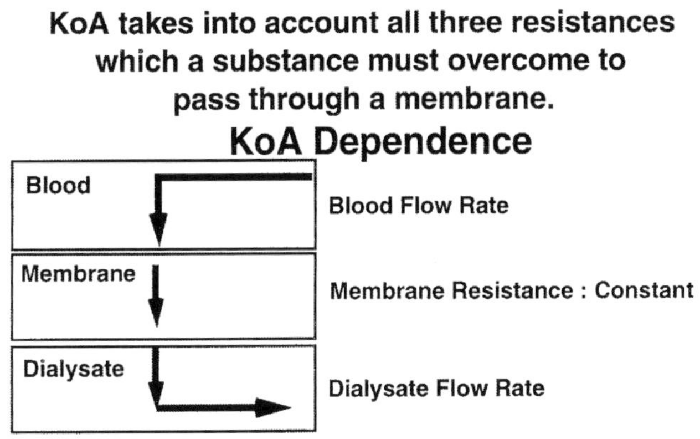

KoA takes into account all three resistances which a substance must overcome to pass through a membrane.

KoA Dependence

Reprinted with permission of Althin Academy

Figure 3.9

Review of Membrane Characteristics Affecting Diffusion

Membrane Characteristics Affecting Solute Transport

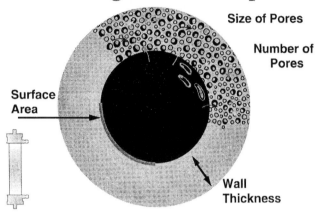

Size of Pores

Number of Pores

Surface Area

Wall Thickness

Reprinted from Althin Academy/Basic Dialysis Theory (1).

Figure 3.10

Convection (Solute Drag)

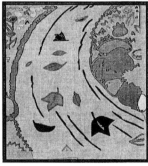

The Movement of Solute by Means of Water Currents

As water moves across the semi-permeable membrane, it pulls solute with it.

Reprinted from Althin Academy/Basic Dialysis Theory (1).

III. Dialyzer Characteristics

To understand dialyzers and to be able to compare one dialyzer to the next, it is important to understand basic dialyzer characteristics.

A. Solute Removal

Dialyzers vary in their ability to remove solutes from the blood of dialysis patients. There are three primary means of removing solutes:

1. Diffusion: Conductive solute transfer, or diffusion, is the movement of solutes across a semi-permeable membrane from an area of greater concentration to an area of lesser concentration, until both sides of the membrane have equal concentrations (equilibrium). The majority of solutes are moved during dialysis by diffusion.

   a) Most effective method of removing small molecular weight solutes

   b) Clearance specifications of a dialyzer are given as ml/min at a given blood flow (Qb) and dialysate flow (Qd) rate. If a dialyzer has a stated urea clearance of 250 ml/min at a 300 Qb, it means that conceptually, 250 mls will be completely cleared of urea, while the remaining 50 mls will have the same urea level as before.

   c) Diffusive clearance capabilities are dependent on blood flow rate, membrane surface area, and dialysate flow rate.

2. Convection: Convective solute transfer occurs along with fluid movement. As fluid containing solutes crosses a semi-permeable membrane, it drags solutes along with it. This process is also called *solute drag*.

   a) Most effective for removing large molecular weight solutes.

   b) Convective specifications for certain solutes will be given as a sieving coefficient. If a dialyzer has a sieving coefficient of 0.5 for a solute, that means that 50% of the solute in a solution that is ultrafiltered through the membrane will pass through to the dialysate side. The remaining 50% might remain in the blood or be absorbed to the membrane.

   c) Convective clearance capabilities are dependent on the molecular weight cutoff, the surface area, and the ultrafiltration rate.

3. Adsorption: This is simply the adhesion of material to the wall of the dialyzer membrane. All dialyzers adsorb materials to some extent,

Figure 3.11

The Relationship Between Blood Flow (Qb) in ml/min. and Clearance in ml/min. in a Typical Dialyzer

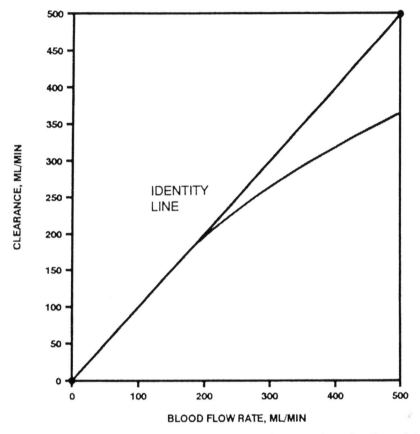

Clearance increases with blood flow; at some point it diverges from the identity line with Qb as a function of membrane permeablitiy (Ko) and area (A).

Reprinted with permission of the American Nephrology Nurses' Association, publisher, ANNA Core Curriculum for Nephrology Nursing, *Third Edition 1995*

usually small proteins. The hydrophobic synthetic membranes are more adsorptive than cellulosic membranes.

a) Adsorption is advantageous to the extent that the adsorbed protein creates a "secondary membrane" which isolates the membrane from the blood. This improves biocompatibility, and happens much more rapidly with most synthetics than it does with cellulosics.

b) Adsorption is disadvantageous in that adsorbed material can interfere with diffusion and convection in some circumstances. Reuse of highly adsorptive

membranes can lead to lower diffusion because fouling within the membrane wall itself is not detected by TCV testing.

c) Adsorptive characteristics of dialyzers are not given in product literature.

d) Adsorptive capabilities are dependent on the membrane material, surface area, and the amount of material already adsorbed to the membrane.

B. Ultrafiltration Rates

1. Another important function of dialysis is ultrafiltration of water across the membrane. Water moves across the membrane in response to hydraulic pressure, in either the blood or

dialysate compartment. This pressure can be varied by the dialysis machine to control the rate and amount of water removed.

2. Each dialyzer has a manufacturer's specified ultrafiltration coefficient (KUF). Dialysis staff members can calculate the actual ultrafiltration rate (UFR) of a dialyzer with this formula:

a) UFR = KUF x TMP

Where: UFR is the ultrafiltration rate
KUF is the dialyzer's ultrafiltration coefficient.
TMP is the average transmembrane pressure.

C. Biocompatibility

All the materials used in the manufacture of dialysis membranes are associated with some degree of blood-material interaction.

1. Free hydroxyl radicals on the membrane surface may instigate the complement activation that occurs during dialysis with cellulose membranes. A leachable cellulose material, called limulus-amebocyte-lysate-reactive-material (LALRM), may also be involved in activation of the complement.

Figure 3.12

Ultrafiltration vs. TMP, cellulosic and high-flux membranes. UF starts at about 25 mm HG because of plasma oncotic pressure.

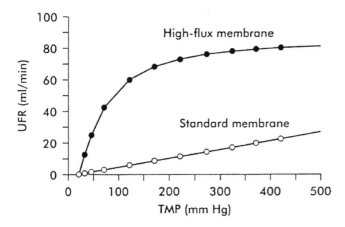

Redrawn from Jacobson HR, Striker GE, Klahr S: Principles and Practice of Nephrology, *Philadelphia, 1991, B.C. Decker. In Gutch CF, Stoner MH, and Corea AL:* Review of Hemodialysis for Nurses and Dialysis Personnel, *ed 5, St. Louis, 1993, Mosby-Year Book, Inc.*

2. Release of histamine, thromboxane, and monokines such as interleukin-1 and tumor necrosis factor, as well as direct changes in leukocyte activity and numbers, probably result from complement activation.

3. The clinical manifestations vary from unnoticed, to minimal intradialytic symptoms, to major anaphylactic reaction.

4. First-use syndrome, a reaction to a new dialyzer, may come from ethylene oxide retained in the dialyzer header.

5. The ability of a membrane to adsorb proteins to the fiber wall is a primary mechanism in membrane biocompatibility. These adsorbed proteins, called a secondary membrane, effectively isolates the blood from the membrane such that the blood no longer is exposed to the "foreign substance." This is the reason that reprocessed dialyzers are more biocompatible than are new ones. Synthetic membranes are more adsorptive than cellulose membranes due to their hydrophobic nature

IV. Categories of Dialyzers

All categories of dialyzers may be made from cellulosic or synthetic membranes.

A. Conventional Dialyzers

1. Generally made of cellulosic materials

2. Moderate diffusion, with surface areas of 0.5 to 1.3 square meters

3. Low ultrafiltration rates, with KUFs ranging from 2.4 to 6.5

4. Low molecular weight cutoff (~3,000 daltons)

5. Minimal adsorption

6. High complementation activation

B. High Efficiency Dialyzers

1. Generally made of cellulosic materials

2. Higher diffusion, with surface areas of 1.4 to 2.2 square meters

3. Moderate ultrafiltration rates, with KUFs ranging from 5 to 12

4. Low molecular weight cutoff (~3,000 daltons)

5. Minimal adsorption

6. High complementation activation

7. In many respects, high efficiency dialyzers are the same as conventional, but with more fibers, therefore more surface area.

C. High Flux Dialyzers

1. Generally made of synthetic materials

2. High diffusion with surface areas of 1.1 to 2.2 square meters

3. High ultrafiltration rates with KUFs up to 90.

4. High molecular weight cutoff (~15,000 daltons)

5. Moderate to very high adsorption

6. Low complement activation

7. High яux dialysis differs greatly from conventional and high efficiency dialysis. These dialyzers use a membrane permeable to a broad range of molecular weight solutes, up to and including beta 2 Microglobulin (11,800 daltons). Beta 2 Microglobulin, or B_2M is a large molecular weight solute which plays an important role in Dialysis Associated Amyloidosis, a potentially crippling build up of protein in bones and body tissue. The major difference between high яux and high efficiency dialysis is the permeability of the membrane to larger solutes such as B_2M.

V. Dialyzer Flow Characteristics

The flow of blood and dialysis fluid in their individual compartments can be guided in two configurations.

A. Concurrent flow, blood and dialysate travel in the same direction.

1. Concurrent flow is less efficient, but it will give more gentle dialysis suited to pediatric dialysis or for first dialysis of a potentially unstable adult.

B. Countercurrent flow, blood яows in one direction, dialysate flows in the opposite direction.

1. Advantages of countercurrent flow is that as blood progresses through the dialyzer it is exposed to a constant flow of fresh dialysate, which better maintains the concentration gradient for more efficient dialysis.

Suggested Readings

Amgen, Inc. (1992), *Core Curriculum for Dialysis Technicians.* Wisconsin: Medical Media Publishing, Inc.

Curtis, J., (1992), *Dialyzer Membranes: Clinical Applications. NANT News,* Summer and Fall Issues.

Daugirdas, JT and Ing, TS, editors, (1994), *Handbook of Dialysis.* Boston: Little, Brown and Co.

Gutch, C.F., Stoner, M.H., Corea, A.L. (1993), *Review of Hemodialysis for Nurses and Dialysis Personnel,* Fifth Edition, Mosby.

Man, N.K., Zingraff, J., Jungers, P. (1995), *Long-Term Hemodialysis.* Kluwer Academic Publishers.

Chapter 4
The Dialysis Procedure

Contributing Authors:

Jerome Beck, CHT

Beth Wood, CHT

Sharon Stevens, CHT

Rick Black, CHT

Joan Brown, CHT

Chapter Outline

I. Initiation of Dialysis

A. Predialysis Safety Checks

B. Initiation of Dialysis

C. Drawing Blood Work

D. Calculating TMP

E. Setting Machine Parameters

F. Charting

II. Monitoring during the Treatment

A. Blood Related Complications

B. Patient Related Complications

C. Dialysate Related Complications

D. Pressures in the Extracorporeal Circuit

E. Treatment Factors and Their Impact on Dialyzer Clearance

F. Heparinization and Clotting Times

G. Charting

III. Discontinuation of Dialysis

A. Termination of Treatment

B. Removing Needles

C. Maintaining Catheter Patency

D. Post Assessment of the Patient

E. Documentation

F. Dismantling the Delivery System

G. The Delivery System Hydraulic Flow Path

IV. Machine Troubleshooting

A. Alarm Actions

B. Power Source Problems

C. Water Supply Problems

D. Machine Monitors

I. Initiation of Dialysis

A. Predialysis Safety Checks

1. Ensure proper functioning of water system through performing on-site chemical testing and gauge readings.

2. Ensure absence of chemical used to disinfect dialysis machine.

3. Correct concentrate(s) present
   a) Adequate amount for entire dialysis treatment

4. Correct patient dialyzer is present.

5. Ensure proper functioning of dialysis machine through checking alarm and/or pressure holding tests.

6. Ancillary testing of conductivity and/or pH of the dialysate

7. Check integrity of extracorporeal circuit.

8. If reuse is practiced ensure presence then absence of sterilant in dialyzer.
   a) Formaldehyde less than 5 ppm
   b) Renalin less than 3 ppm

B. Initiation of Dialysis

1. Aseptic Technique

Figure 4.1

Access Preparation: Aseptic Technique

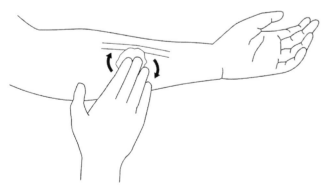

Scrub in a circulation motion.

Reprinted from the IMPRA Stick with Us *workshop guide, p. 12.*

---

a) Absence of contamination

b) Universal precautions must be followed.
   (1) Gloves
   (2) Mask
   (3) Protective eye wear
   (4) Gown
   (5) Hand washing

2. Types of Accesses
   a) Surgically created by connecting an artery to a vein thereby increasing blood flow sufficiently to enable the initiation of the dialysis procedure
      (1) AVF: arteriovenous fistula, connection of one's own artery to vein
      (2) Graft: synthetic material connected between patient's artery and vein
   b) Surgically implanted accesses
      (1) Temporary dual lumen catheter, for temporary access to patient's circulatory system. Femoral, jugular, or subclavian vein used for this purpose.
      (2) Permanent dual lumen catheter, implanted when other avenues of access are not possible; higher risk of infection and clotting.

3. Preparing the Access
   a) Evaluate access
   b) Check for signs of infection
      (1) Redness
      (2) Tenderness
      (3) Hot to the touch
      (4) Purulent drainage
   c) Check for patency
      (1) Grafts & AVF: bruit, thrill
      (2) Catheters: blood easily aspirates from each limb (done once catheter is aseptically cleaned); sutures intact
   d) Check for correct direction of flow; or which limb is arterial/venous (catheter)
      (1) Occlude graft in the middle, and feel for pulse. Arterial is the side on which the pulse is felt.

4. Graft & AVF Cannulation
   a) Use aseptic technique and universal precautions

Figure 4.2

Direction of Blood Flow

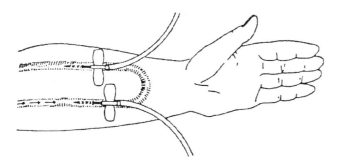

Direction of blood flow determines needle placement.

Reprinted from Vascular Access for Hemodialysis, *p. 133, fig. 11-3.*

b) Select needle sites; rotate sites, avoid surgical scars, aneurysms, hematomas, inflamed and infected areas, also stay at least one inch away from anastomosis.

c) Clean selected sites with disinfectant starting in the center of site, using a circular motion outward.

d) Anesthetize sites if necessary.

e) Insert fistula needle with bevel up at a forty-five degree angle until a flashback of blood is observed, level needle out and thread into access to the hub of the needle, tape needle securely.

 (1) Avoid rotation of needle once it is inserted.

f) Administer any required heparin bolus to the venous needle 3-5 minutes before initiation of dialysis treatment.

5. Catheters

a) Clean limbs of catheter with disinfectant using aseptic technique and universal precautions, allowing time for disinfectant to work.

b) Aspirate anticoagulant from limbs of catheter, check for patency.

C. Drawing Blood Work

1. Use aseptic technique and universal precautions.

2. Draw lab work prior to the administration of anticoagulant.

Figure 4.3

Calculation of TMP Worksheet

1. **Calculation of weight loss**
   Pre-dialysis weight☐ _____ lb or _____ kg
   – Desired post-dialysis weight☐ _____ lb or _____ kg

   = Required weight loss☐ _____ lb or _____ kg

2. **Calculation of total fluid removal**
   Required weight loss _____ kgx1000 = _____ ml
   + Saline prime given to patient
   + Estimated oral intake☐☐ _____ ml
   + Saline rinseback given to patient☐ _____ ml
   + Other (IVs, blood, drugs, etc)☐☐ _____ ml

   = Total required fluid removal☐☐ _____ ml

3. **Calculation of ultrafiltration rate**
   Total fluid removal☐☐ _____ ml
   √ Hours of dialysis☐☐ _____ hr

   = Required ultrafiltration rate☐☐ _____ ml/hr

4. **Calculation of transmembrane pressure**
   Untrafiltration rate☐☐ _____ ml/hr
   √ Dialyzer ultrafiltration factor☐☐ _____ ml/hr/mmHg

   = Required transmembrane pressure☐ _____ mmHg

3. Draw lab work from arterial port or arterial fistula needle.

4. Lab tubes remain upright, proper labeling of tubes and proper handling of specimens must be observed.

D. Calculate TMP (Transmembrane Pressure)

1. Necessary if equipment is not fluid control type

2. TMP is calculated for proper fluid removal.

3. Basic formula:

a) Total volume to be removed divided by number of hours of treatment equals volume of fluid to be removed hourly

b) Hourly volume of fluid divided by the coefficient of the dialyzer being used equals TMP needed for fluid removal

Figure 4.4

Computerized Dialysis Treatment Log

GSH ACUTE
HEMODIALYSIS RUN SUMMARY

Treatment Date: 01/29/97	Center: GSH Acute	Patient name:
Station: ____	Modality: Incenter HD	Med Record No.: 57-30-50
Schedule: T1 R1 S1	Bld Group:	Birthdate: 12/18/1920
Diabetic Status: Yes	Page: 1	Nephrologist: STAFF, Doctor

Access Status   **PRE-ASSESSMENT**   Other Notes

Type: AV Goretex | Access: normal |

Site: Left Upper arm | Admitted: wheelchair |

Access site: staples intact | Cardiac: rate irregular | Signature: _____

Access: peripheral access not used | Complaints: bone pain | RIVERA, Manuel

                         | Dialysis initiated without difficul |

                         | Lungs: crackles bilateral |

                         | Respirations: labored |

Date: 01/29/97   **HEMODIALYSIS WORKSHEET**   Dry Weight: 77.50 kg

         Ordered Goal Achieved   Today's Wt: 83.50

Runtime in mins: 180   180   Bath: K+   Na   Ca   Glc   Buff

T.Fluid removed: 5.80 5.80   3.0   140. 2.50 200

Blood flow: 400   400   Other bath:

Dialysate flow: 500   500

                         Machine type: Fresenius   Prime: Saline

Needles: 15g Twin   Heparin Load: 2000   Tie off: 0 min

Dialyzer: CT190   Maint: 0 to PT

Dialysate: Bicarbonate   Na modeling: Step 145 mEq/L

Lidocaine: BP Support: L: 100/ 40 H: 200/100

Other notes: wc weight=19.5 kg; pressure held by clamps;

Physician: Dr. John, SMITH   Staff: RIVERA, Manuel

Test/Procedure	ICD-9	Status	Staff	Medication	Dose	Units	Given?	Staff
Hemo: Chem, CBC, Post Bun		Done	MRR	Epogen*	10000.000	unit	Yes	MRR
Admin - Bloods		Done	MRR	Calcijex*	0.500	mg	Yes	MRR
				Albumin 5%	250.000	cc	Yes	MRR

DIALYSIS FLOW SHEET

>Date	Time	*Attr	BP Sitting	BP Standing	Pulse	Temp	>Wgt	!Wt chg	Hct	Glc	ArtP	VenP	Qb	TMP	UFR	COND	*Air	Comment
01/29/97	14:24	POST	120 / 55	/	55	98.0	77.7	-5.8										tx dcd withou
01/29/97	14:17	INT	138	72	64						160	180	400	100	1.40		Y	
01/29/97	14:14	INT	124	85	64						160	180	400	120	1.40		Y	5%albumin 250
01/29/97	14:11	INT	116	53	64						160	180	400	140	1.70		Y	
01/29/97		INT	118	56	64						160	180	400	140	104.0		Y	
01/29/97	14:08	INT	144	60	88						160	180	400	120	107.0		Y	
01/29/97	14:04	PRE	136	63	64	97.3	83.5	3.5	31.4	184								

Status   **POST ASSESSMENT**

                                           Other Notes

In/Out: Out patient | Discharged: vital signs stable |

Discharge: D/C Wheelchair |

Service Code: Incenter HD | Signature: _____

Machine S/N: 1651 FRESENIUS | RIVERA, Manuel

             1651 |

Source: Legacy Health System, Portland Oregon (diPROTON).

Figure 4.5

Manual Dialysis Treatment Log

DAILY DIALYSIS LOG

Legacy Good Samaritan Hospital & Medical Center

PATIENT ID PLATE

	WEIGHT		VITAL SIGNS BLOOD PRESSURE

DATE _____
DIALYZER _____
BATH _____
NA _____
HOURS _____
BFR _____
HEPARIN _____
ACCESS   L   R
CATH   GRAFT   FIST
NEEDLES   A ___ V ___

WEIGHT
PRE _____ POST _____
EDW _____ GOAL _____

LABS

VITAL SIGNS
BLOOD PRESSURE
PRE   POST

APICAL PULSE _____ _____
TEMP _____ _____

ASSESSMENT	PRE	POST	UNCHANGED ☐
ARRIVED			☐
LUNGS			☐
HEART			☐
EDEMA			☐
ACCESS			☐

UF CALCULATION

DESIRED WT LOSS _____ cc   +   FLUIDS _____   =   GOAL _____   +   HOURS _____   =   UFR _____

PRE CBG = _____

TIME	B.P.	BFR	PRESSURE		HEP	ACTS	TMP OR NEG	UF REM /	N/S ADMIN	COMMENTS, MEDICATIONS AND SIGNATURES
			ART	VEN		ART / VEN		UFR		

TIME _____
LITERS PROCESSED _____

MACHINE #	RENALIN NEG	BLEACH NEG	PRESS TEST	ALARM TEST	CONDUC	SIGNATURE	CALCIJEX

EPO _____

REUSE LABEL

105290 (800-055) 1/95

Source: Legacy Health System, Portland Oregon.

Figure 4.6

Blood and Dialysate Circuits

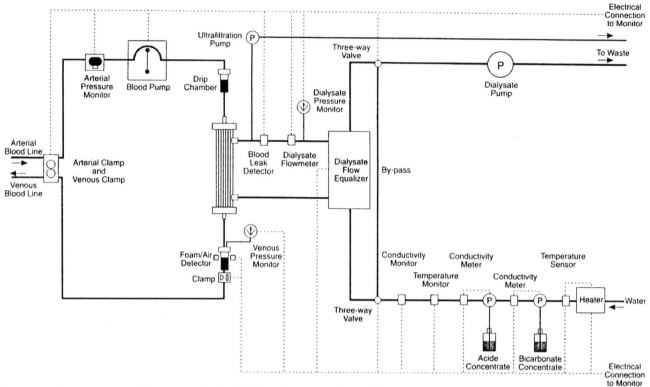

Reprinted with permission of Kluwer Academic Publishers Long-term Hemodialysis, p. 34, fig. 4-2.

E. Setting Machine Parameters

1. Ensure alarm limits are set.

2. Ensure proper fluid removal parameters are set.

3. Ensure proper blood flow rate is set.

4. Ensure proper anticoagulant rate is set.

5. Ensure proper dialysate temperature is set.

6. Ensure proper dialysate flow rate is set.

F. Charting

1. Documentation of treatment

    a) Physician-prescribed treatment parameters

    b) Pre- and post-patient assessment

       (1) Patient weight gain/loss

       (2) Access assessment

       (3) Vital signs

       (4) Assessment of fluid status

       (5) Overall patient status

    c) Medications given

    d) Vital signs during treatment

    e) Treatment parameters

       (1) Arterial/venous pressures

       (2) Blood and dialysate flow rates

       (3) TMP/Ultrafiltration rate

       (4) Patient or machine complications

       (5) Signatures of patient care staff

       (6) Complete and legible

II. Monitoring during the Treatment

A. Blood Related Complications

Those complications which result from the flow of blood through the extracorporeal circuit.

1. Air in blood
   a) Causes:
      (1) Inadequate blood flow (in relation to blood pump setting) through arterial needle
      (2) Kink in the arterial blood tubing pre-blood pump
      (3) Poor connections in the extracorporeal circuit circuit pre-blood pump
      (4) Latex injection port pre-blood pump not self-sealing.
      (5) Low levels in the drip chambers
      (6) Not priming the heparin administration line prior to initiating infusion
      (7) Not removing all air during dialyzer priming (dialyzers disinfected with peracetic acid solutions are prone to this when exposed to high storage temperatures or rinsing dialysate side first when preparing for dialysis)
      (8) Empty IV containers pre-blood pump left opened to the extracorporeal circuit.
      (9) Inadequate deaeration of the dialysate (particularly if using high negative dialysate pressures for fluid removal)
      (10) Cold normal saline exposed to dialysate can form a type of condensation resulting in air bubble formation.
   b) Signs and symptoms:
      (1) Air-in-blood alarm
      (2) Air bubbles or foaming in the blood
      (3) Pre-blood pump blood tubing may collapse and/or jump when related to inadequate blood flow through the arterial needle.
   c) Prevention:
      (1) Identify access problems which may influence blood flow.
      (2) Ensure effective cannulation and adequate anticoagulation to maintain good flow through the arterial needle throughout the treatment.
      (3) Ensure proper connection of all fittings and that lines remain unkinked.
      (4) Ensure correct dialyzer priming procedures including heparin administration line.
      (5) Ensure correct drip chamber levels are maintained at all times.
      (6) Ensure IV containers are not empty and that they remain clamped when not in use.
      (7) Use IV solutions at room temperature only.
      (8) Use a tempering valve in the water treatment systems when incoming water temperatures to the facility are very low.
      (9) Ensure correct function of the dialysate delivery system's deaeration system.
   d) Treatment:
      (1) Correct cause of air entering the extracorporeal circuit.
      (2) Small amounts of air may be removed by the drip chambers and then readjusting their levels as necessary.

2. Air embolism
   a) Causes:
      (1) Disarmed or defective air-in-blood detector with air in the extracorporeal circuit
   b) Signs and symptoms:
      (1) Air in the extracorporeal circuit
      (2) Chest pain, dyspnea, coughing, and cyanosis
      (3) Visual disturbances including double vision and blindness
      (4) Neurologic complications including confusion, restlessness, fear, hemiparesis, seizures, and coma
      (5) Death
   c) Prevention:
      (1) Always use the air-in-blood detector when the patient is connected to the extracorporeal circuit.
      (2) Carefully visualize the venous blood line if disarming the alarm.
   d) Treatment:
      (1) Stop blood flow immediately.
      (2) Place patient in the Trendelenburg position on his/her left side.
      (3) Assess vital signs.
      (4) Administer oxygen.
      (5) Notify the physician.
      (6) Activate the EMS.

3. Blood loss (exsanguination)

a) Causes:

(1) Blood line separation or needles dislodging from circulatory access

(2) Dialyzer membrane leak

(3) Dialyzer casing becomes cracked or the header cap is improperly fitted

(4) Fistula aneurysm or anastomosis ruptures

b) Signs and symptoms:

(1) Visual observation of blood, e.g., on patient clothing or skin, chair, floor, etc.

(2) Blood leak detector alarm and possible red-tinged dialysate post dialyzer (if a dialyzer membrane leaks)

(3) Arterial and/or venous pressure alarms may occur.

(4) Hypotension, vomiting, and/or convulsions

(5) Death

c) Prevention:

(1) Ensure all bloodline and needle connections are secure; only luer-lock connections should be used (tape connections which are not luer-lock).

(2) Tape needles to minimize movement and/or the potential for dislodgment.

(3) Ensure that the entire extracorporeal circuit including the access is visible.

(4) Perform a visual inspection of the dialyzer pre-dialysis and ensure the header caps are properly connected and that there are no signs of damage.

(5) Ensure the blood leak detector is properly maintained and calibrated.

d) Treatment:

(1) Stop blood pump immediately and clamp blood lines.

(2) Apply pressure to access if a needle has dislodged.

(3) Tighten and secure loose fittings if no separation has occurred.

(4) If a dialyzer membrane leak has occurred, return blood based on severity of the leak.

(5) Assess severity of blood loss and treat patient accordingly including administration of oxygen and administration of a volume expander for hypotension.

4. Access recirculation

a) Causes:

(1) Needles are too close together – less than 2 inches apart

(2) Inadequate access flow for the desired blood flow rate

(3) Access outflow stenosis and less often inflow stenosis

(4) Access thrombosis

(5) Tourniquet placed above the venous needle

(6) Bloodlines placed backwards, e.g., the arterial line placed on the venous needle

(7) Fistula aneurysm

b) Signs and symptoms:

(1) Increased pre and/or post dialysis chemistries

(2) Progressive darkening of the blood during dialysis

(3) Lightening of the arterial blood during saline infusions through the venous line

(4) Change in quality of bruit

(5) Possible increase in venous pressures and/or reduction in arterial pressures

(6) Possible difficulty in establishing prescribed blood flow rates

(7) Reduced clotting times and need for increased anticoagulation

c) Prevention:

(1) Ensure proper cannulation and bloodline connection.

(2) Prompt reporting and follow-up of patient assessment findings and intradialytic observations

5. Clotting in the extracorporeal circuit

a) Causes:

(1) Incorrect and/or inadequate anticoagulation therapy

(2) Low blood flow rates

(3) Hemoconcentration resulting from access recirculation or ultrafiltration continuing when the blood pump is off

(4) Increased hematocrit

(5) Air in the extracorporeal circuit

(6) Change in the patient's status or medications

(7) Clotting disorder

b) Signs and symptoms:

(1) Fibrin or clot formation in the extracorporeal circuit

(2) Blood becomes darker in color

(3) If clotting is occurring in the dialyzer, an increase in the post blood pump arterial pressure and a decrease in the venous pressure; if clotting is occurring in the venous drip chamber, an increase in the venous pressure

(4) Progressively lower hematocrit/hemoglobin

(5) Air in the extracorporeal circuit

(6) Poor rinse-back at the end of dialysis

(7) Dialyzer volume loss (if performing volume measurements for dialyzer reuse)

c) Prevention:

(1) Correctly administer adequate anticoagulation based on patient parameters and clinical observation.

(2) Perform ongoing assessment for signs of clotting throughout the treatment and adjust anticoagulation as needed.

(3) Adjust anticoagulation according to changes in patient status or treatment parameters.

(4) Maintain prescribed blood flow rates.

(5) Prevent and/or promptly correct causes of blood related alarms to minimize the time the blood pump is off.

(6) Correct causes of access recirculation.

(7) Correct causes of air in the extracorporeal circuit.

6. Poor blood flow

a) Causes:

(1) Poor venipuncture technique resulting in the bevel being pushed up against the vessel wall or incorrect placement of the catheter resulting in the side holes being pushed up against the vessel

(2) Infiltration

(3) Improper needle gauge for blood flow required

(4) Vessel spasms

(5) Vessel thrombus or stenosis

(6) Clotted needle or catheter

(7) Catheter has moved since placement

(8) Sutures are constricting catheter

(9) Needle/catheter or blood tubing is kinked or clamped

(10) Blood pump calibration or roller occlusion is incorrect

b) Signs and symptoms:

(1) Collapsed arterial blood line

(2) Air or foam present beginning in the arterial blood line

(3) Jumping arterial blood line

(4) High pre-blood pump negative pressure

(5) High venous pressure if the problem is on the venous end

(6) Poor lab values resulting from blood pump calibration and/or occlusion

c) Prevention:

(1) Correct venipuncture technique or catheter placement.

(2) Correct anticoagulation technique.

(3) Correct selection of needle gauge.

(4) Ensure all appropriate clamps are opened and no kinks are present in tubing.

(5) Ensure proper maintenance of the blood pump according to manufacturer recommendations.

d) Treatment:

(1) Reposition needles or catheter.

(2) If the needle is clotted or infiltrated, insert a new needle.

(3) Correct kinks or open clamps.

(4) Refer patient for correction of access/vessel problems.

(5) If encountering problems with a catheter, lower patient's head to increase central vein pressure, have the patient take a deep breath and cough forcefully, change the patient's position, reverse blood line connections on the catheter, and/or manually apply pressure over the catheter.

(6) Use fibrinolytic agents to declot catheter.

(7) Refer patient for removal of catheter.

7. Needle infiltration

a) Causes:

(1) Improper venipuncture technique

(2) The needle moves after insertion generally from poor or no securing.

(3) The patient moves the access extremity.

b) Signs and symptoms:
  (1) Burning and/or tenderness at the access site
  (2) Swelling, hardness, and bruising of the access
  (3) Increased pre-blood pump pressure if the arterial needle is infiltrated, increased venous pressure if the venous needle is infiltrated

c) Prevention:
  (1) Correct venipuncture technique.
  (2) Securing the needles to prevent movement or displacement.

d) Treatment:
  (1) Remove needle if necessary and insert a new needle above original site.
  (2) A cold pack can be applied to reduce swelling, afterwards, 24 hours warmth should be applied to the site.

B. Patient Related Complications

Complications the patient may experience during the hemodialysis procedure.

1. Hypotension
  a) Etiology:
    (1) Excessive ultrafiltration or sodium removal
    (2) Antihypertensive medications
    (3) Eating meals during treatment
    (4) Low sodium dialysate
    (5) Unstable cardiovascular status
    (6) Dehydration
    (7) Anemia
    (8) Hypoalbuminemia
    (9) Incorrect weight loss goal or ultrafiltration rate
  b) Signs and symptoms:
    (1) Gradual or sudden drop in blood pressure which may be associated with dizziness; nausea and vomiting; pallor; perspiration or cold, clammy skin
    (2) An early warning sign may be complaints of feeling warm and fanning him/herself.
    (3) Yawning
    (4) Feeling faint
    (5) Dizziness upon standing
    (6) Tachycardia
    (7) Loss of consciousness

c) Prevention:
  (1) Reliable ultrafiltration control systems
  (2) Patient education regarding early recognition of signs and symptoms
  (3) Maintain adequate hematocrit.
  (4) Treat cardiovascular problems.
  (5) Accurate estimates of dry body weight including assessment of fluid volume prior to each treatment
  (6) Accurate measurement pre-dialysis weight
  (7) Encourage fluid restrictions interdialytically generally <1kg/day.
  (8) Withhold antihypertensives immediately prior to and during treatment.
  (9) Dialysate sodium levels at or above plasma levels
  (10) Withhold food during dialysis to hypotensive-prone patients.

d) Treatment:
  (1) Place patient into Trendelenburg position.
  (2) Stop or reduce ultrafiltration.
  (3) Administer 100-200 cc normal saline or a volume expander, e.g., hypertonic saline, mannitol, albumin.

2. Hypertension
  a) Etiology:
    (1) Disequilibrium syndrome
    (2) Fluid overload
    (3) Noncompliance with antihypertensive medications
    (4) Erythropoietin therapy
    (5) Renin response
  b) Signs and symptoms:
    (1) Dizziness
    (2) Headache
    (3) Nausea and vomiting
    (4) Edema
    (5) Patients may be asymptomatic.
  c) Prevention:
    (1) See Dialysis Disequilibrium Syndrome.
    (2) Control fluid overload by limiting fluid and sodium intake interdialytically.
    (3) Adhere to antihypertensive medication requirements.
    (4) Establish and maintain an accurate dry body weight.

d) Treatment:

    (1) Aggressive ultrafiltration in the presence of fluid overload

    (2) Therapy should be directed to the pathogenesis and acute target organ effects including antihypertensive medication therapy.

    (3) Phlebotomy if the hematocrit is >38%

3. Muscle cramps

    a) Etiology:

        (1) Hypotension

        (2) Excessive fluid removal or hypo-osmolality usually late in the treatment.

        (3) Low dialysate sodium compared to serum sodium

        (4) May be associated with hypokalemia

    b) Signs and symptoms:

        (1) Cramping predominately in the lower extremities

        (2) Hypotension

    c) Prevention:

        (1) Proper dietary management

        (2) Prevent hypotensive episodes (see hypotension).

        (3) Correct dialysate sodium levels.

        (4) Carnitine supplementation

        (5) Administer oral quinine.

        (6) Stretching exercises targeted at the affected muscle groups may be useful.

    d) Treatment:

        (1) Bolus of hypertonic saline or glucose

        (2) Infusion of normal saline may be helpful.

4. Nausea/vomiting

    a) Etiology:

        (1) Hypotension (most common)

        (2) Dialysis Disequilibrium Syndrome

        (3) Pyrogen reaction

        (4) Influenza or intestinal virus

    b) Signs and symptoms:

        (1) Nausea

        (2) Vomiting

        (3) Headache

        (4) Hypotension

c) Prevention:

    (1) Avoidance of hypotension (see Hypotension)

    (2) Avoidance of disequilibrium (see Dialysis Disequilibrium Syndrome).

    (3) Avoidance of pyrogenic reactions (see Fever and/or chills)

d) Treatment:

    (1) Treat any associated hypotension.

    (2) Administer an antiemetic as ordered.

5. Headache

    a) Etiology

        (1) Dialysis Disequilibrium Syndrome

        (2) Acetate containing dialysate.

        (3) Caffeine withdrawal as the blood caffeine concentration is acutely reduced during dialysis

        (4) Hypertension

        (5) Fluid shifts

        (6) Change in sodium levels

        (7) Anxiety/nervous tension

    b) Signs and symptoms:

        (1) Pain in the head or face

    c) Prevention:

        (1) See Dialysis Disequilibrium Syndrome.

        (2) Use bicarbonate containing dialysate.

        (3) See Hypertension.

    d) Treatment:

        (1) Administer acetaminophen during dialysis.

6. Angina

    a) Etiology:

        (1) Hypotension

        (2) Anemia

        (3) Arteriosclerotic cardiovascular disease

        (4) Coronary artery spasm

        (5) Severe vascular volume depletion in susceptible patients

        (6) Anxiety

    b) Signs and symptoms:

        (1) Chest pain

    c) Prevention:

        (1) See Hypotension.

        (2) Maintain hematocrit.

        (3) Administer nitroglycerin or related drugs.

d) Treatment:

    (1) Discontinue dialysis if necessary.

    (2) Administer oxygen and drugs as ordered.

    (3) Decrease ultrafiltration.

    (4) Assess and treat volume depletion.

7. Pruritus

  a) Etiology:

    (1) Uremia

    (2) Decreased sweat and sebaceous gland activity leading to dry skin

    (3) Elevated calcium-phosphorus product and hyperparathyroidism leading to deposition of calcium phosphate crystals

    (4) Histamine release due to an allergic response to such things as heparin, blood tubing plasticizers, and ethylene oxide

    (5) Iron deficiency

    (6) Increased calcium levels of water used to prepare dialysate or dialysate concentrate

  b) Signs and symptoms:

    (1) Severe generalized itching on and off dialysis, if due to an allergic reaction, itching will be only during dialysis

    (2) Reddened skin

    (3) Crusting

  c) Prevention:

    (1) Keep skin clean and moisturized.

    (2) Adequate dialysis therapy

    (3) Control hyperphosphatemia.

    (4) Control hyperparathyroidism.

    (5) Correction of iron deficiency

    (6) Switch from ethylene oxide sterilized dialyzers.

  d) Treatment:

    (1) See prevention.

    (2) Antihistamines

    (3) Phototherapy

8. Fever and/or chills

  a) Etiology:

    (1) Infection (commonly of the access)

    (2) Introduction of pyrogenic material or endotoxins via the dialysate or poorly reprocessed dialyzer

    (3) Poor aseptic cannulation technique

    (4) Contaminated new dialyzer

  b) Signs and symptoms:

    (1) The patient feels cold after initiating dialysis which may include involuntary shaking. Chills will lead to temperature elevation.

    (2) Fever – patients with access site-related septicemia are often febrile prior to dialysis and, in the absence of treatment, fever persists during and after dialysis; patients experiencing a pyrogenic reaction are afebrile prior to dialysis but become febrile during dialysis with the fever resolving spontaneously with cessation of dialysis.

    (3) Patients experiencing an iatrogenic intro-duction of pyrogenic material or endotoxin will display signs and symptoms generally within the first hour of dialysis.

    (4) Hypotension

    (5) Redness, swelling, and drainage from the access if related to an access infection

  c) Prevention:

    (1) Proper water treatment and system disinfection procedures

    (2) Proper dialyzer reuse procedures

    (3) Proper bicarbonate preparation, storage, and handling procedures as well as bicarbonate container cleaning and disinfection procedures. Other concentrate containers should be cleaned and disinfected as well.

    (4) Aseptic technique utilized in the preparation of the dialyzer and blood lines. Preparation should not occur more than two hours prior to the planned treatment.

    (5) Proper cleaning and disinfection procedures for dialysis equipment inclusive of external surfaces and the fluid path

    (6) Aseptic technique used to initiate dialysis

    (7) Protection of the patient from known infectious agents

  d) Treatment:

    (1) Assess for sources of signs and symptoms.

    (2) Obtain blood cultures.

    (3) Obtain dialyzer inlet and outlet dialysate cultures as well as a water culture of the water entering the delivery system.

(4) Administer acetaminophen as ordered.

(5) Administer antibiotics as ordered.

9. Dialysis Disequilibrium Syndrome

   a) Etiology:

      (1) Rapid removal of BUN in comparison to urea nitrogen removal in brain tissue and cerebral spinal fluid (CSF) causing water movement into the brain and CSF

   b) Signs and symptoms:

      (1) Headache

      (2) Nausea and vomiting

      (3) Hypertension

      (4) Restlessness

      (5) Increased pulse pressure

      (6) Convulsions

      (7) Coma

      (8) Death

   c) Prevention:

      (1) Short, frequent dialyses with lower urea removal rates

      (2) Higher sodium dialysate

      (3) Use of mannitol as a volume expander

   d) Treatment:

      (1) Same as prevention

      (2) Termination of the dialysis procedure when signs and symptoms are identified

10. First-use syndrome

   a) Etiology:

      (1) Complement activation by new cellulosic membrane with reduced occurrence in reused dialyzers

      (2) Ethyene oxide in dialyzer

   b) Signs and symptoms

      (1) Chest pain which may or may not be accompanied by back pain

      (2) Hypotension

      (3) Pruritis

      (4) Vague discomfort

      (5) Shortness of breath

      (6) Nausea and vomiting

   c) Prevention:

      (1) Use of synthetic membranes

      (2) Dialyzer reuse procedures which do not remove the protein coat on the membrane, e.g., sodium hypochlorite

      (3) Rinse new, "dry" dialyzers according to manufacturer recommendations

      (4) Use gamma sterilized dialysis

   d) Treatment:

      (1) Supportive management of signs and symptoms

      (2) Oxygen should be given.

      (3) Myocardial ischemia should be considered, and if angina pectoris is suspected, it should be treated. Symptoms generally abate after the first hour of dialysis and treatment can usually be continued.

11. Anaphylaxis

   a) Etiology:

      (1) Bradykinin system activation by AN69 membranes with patients taking ACE inhibitors

      (2) Ethylene oxide sensitivity

      (3) Iron dextran administration

      (4) Sodium azide (used to package some water treatment ultrafilters)

      (5) Heparin.

   b) Signs and symptoms:

      (1) Initial onset may be immediate or delayed up to 30 minutes.

      (2) Acute bronchoconstriction

      (3) Anxiety and a feeling of warmth at the access site or throughout the body

      (4) Followed by agitation, tightness in the chest, and nausea

      (5) Followed by shortness of breath, coughing, wheezing, urticaria, pruritis, facial edema, flushing, or respiratory stridor

      (6) Vasodilation and hypotension or hypertension

      (7) Gastrointestinal disturbances such as abdominal cramping or diarrhea may also occur

      (8) Cardiac arrest and death may supervene

   c) Prevention:

      (1) Rinse new, "dry" dialyzers according to manufacturer recommendations

      (2) Use of a different dialyzer membrane

      (3) Use an initial test dose with iron dextran

      (4) Thorough rinsing of ultrafilters prior to being placed into service

d) Treatment:

(1) Supportive management of signs and symptoms

(2) If the patient is suffering a severe reaction, immediately terminate dialysis and do not return the blood.

(3) Depending upon the severity of the reaction, treatment with oxygen and IV antihistamines, steroids, and epinephrine can be given.

(4) Immediate cardiorespiratory support may be required.

12. Dysrhythmia

a) Etiology:

(1) Rapid electrolyte and pH changes brought about by dialysis, especially potassium

(2) Hypotension

(3) Underlying heart disease

(4) Dialyzing off antiarrhythmic medications during dialysis

(5) Low potassium level or rapid drop in potassium in conjunction with digitalis therapy

(6) Hypoxemia

b) Signs and symptoms:

(1) Slow or rapid irregular pulse

(2) Skipped or extra beats

(3) Patient complains of palpitations

c) Prevention:

(1) Use a higher dialysate potassium concentration if the patient is on digitalis therapy while restricting dietary potassium to avoid predialysis hyperkalemia

(2) Administer antiarrhythmic medications as ordered.

(3) Control of hypotension

(4) In patients with myocardial ischemia, antianginal prophylaxis may be necessary in addition to alterations in dialysate potassium and calcium levels.

(5) Appropriate monitoring of heart rate and rhythm

d) Treatment:

(1) Antiarrhythmic medications as required

(2) Discontinue dialysis for severe, symptomatic dysrhythmias

(3) Monitor ECG

13. Dialysis-associated pericarditis, pericardial effusion, and/or cardiac tamponade

a) Etiology:

(1) Intercurrent bacterial or viral infection

(2) Hypercatabolism, volume overload, hyperparathyroidism, hyperuremia, and malnutrition have all been proposed.

(3) Inadequate dialysis can usually be partially incriminated.

(4) If pericarditis occurs in a stable patient, the etiologic agent may be cytomegalovirus or other viral infection.

b) Signs and symptoms:

(1) Chest pain with or without dyspnea, cough, or constitutional symptoms often worsened in recumbency and relieved by sitting upright or leaning forward

(2) Pericardial friction rub

(3) Paradoxical pulse

(4) Jugular venous distention

(5) Hypotension

(6) An abnormal ST wave segment noted on ECG.

(7) Fever

(8) Muffled heart sounds

(9) Absent apical impulse

(10) Pulse alternations, where there is a regular alternation of weak and strong beats

c) Prevention:

(1) Osculate for a friction rub and for a paradoxical pulse when the patient has chest pain or unexplained hypotension.

(2) In patients with known pericarditis, dialyze without heparin or with regional or tight heparin protocols

(3) Maintain intravascular volume to avoid hypotension in patients with known pericarditis

d) Treatment:

(1) Minimal or no heparin during dialysis

(2) Intensive dialysis usually by increasing the frequency of treatment

(3) Surgical drainage by either subxiphoid pericardiostomy, procedure of choice, or pericardiocentesis may be required

14. Seizures
   a) Etiology:
      (1) Dialysis Disequilibrium Syndrome
      (2) Electrolyte imbalances
      (3) Hypotension
      (4) Dialysate composition errors
   b) Signs and symptoms:
      (1) Change in level of consciousness
      (2) Jerking movements of the arms and leg.
   c) Prevention:
      (1) Avoid large, rapid drop in BUN during dialysis.
      (2) Monitor blood pressure and support during treatment.
      (3) Administer anticonvulsant medication.
   d) Treatment:
      (1) See Dialysis Disequilibrium Syndrome.
      (2) Frequent blood pressure monitoring.

15. Internal access infection
   a) Etiology:
      (1) Infection is more serious in an AV graft than fistula due to the potential disintegration of synthetic materials and subsequent hemorrhage of the AV graft.
      (2) Break in aseptic technique
      (3) Poor hygiene and care of access
      (4) Bacterial seeding from another infected site within the body
   b) Signs and symptoms:
      (1) Redness, swelling, tenderness, pain, and drainage from any area of the access
      (2) Fever with or without any other signs if the infection is in the interior of the graft
      (3) Fever and/or chills as hemodialysis treatment progresses
   c) Prevention:
      (1) Proper aseptic technique during cannulation
      (2) Patient education regarding care and hygiene of the access
   d) Treatment:
      (1) Do not cannulate any inflamed areas.
      (2) Culture any drainage.
      (3) Draw blood cultures if the patient becomes symptomatic.
      (4) Immediate antibiotic therapy
      (5) Surgical revision

16. Central venous catheter infection
   a) Etiology:
      (1) Poor connection technique between the catheter and external connections
      (2) Colonization of the catheter fibrin sheath during bacteremia from a distant focus, e.g., infected diverticuli
      (3) Colonization of the catheter exit site or the tunnel
   b) Signs and symptoms:
      (1) Redness, swelling, tenderness, and drainage
      (2) Fever
      (3) Exit site warmth
   c) Prevention:
      (1) Aseptic handling of the catheter
      (2) Application of an occlusive local dressing every treatment
      (3) Application of povidone-iodine ointment at each dressing change
      (4) Soak the exit site with povidone-iodine solution intradialytically.
      (5) Teach patient how to keep site clean and dry
   d) Treatment:
      (1) Based on culture data
      (2) Antibiotics
      (3) In most cases removal of the catheter is necessary if the patient becomes septic or no positive response to antibiotics is observed within 2-3 days

17. Internal access thrombus
   a) Etiology:
      (1) Poor arterial blood flow
      (2) Stenosis
      (3) Hypotension
      (4) Prolonged pressure on the access either externally, e.g. sleeping on access arm, constrictive clothing, excess compression to achieve hemostasis post dialysis, or internally, e.g., from hemorrhage into graft tunnel or pseudoaneurysm
      (5) Repeated infiltration compresses the vessel
      (6) Repeated venipuncture of the same sites particularly in grafts
      (7) Infection
      (8) Development of a pseudodiaphragm

b) Signs and symptoms:

(1) Absence of bruit and thrill

(2) Difficult venipuncture

(3) Able to aspirate only very dark blood

(4) Patient may complain of pain at the arterial anastomosis prior to complete thrombosis.

(5) In a fistula, poor to no dilation of the venous branches of the fistula when a tourniquet is applied to the upper arm

(6) Increased venous pressure during dialysis

(7) Increased access recirculation

c) Prevention:

(1) Ongoing assessment of access

(2) Correct venipuncture technique designed to preserve access

(3) Management of hypotension intra and interdialytically

(4) Patient education regarding access care

(5) Use proper pressure to achieve hemostasis.

d) Treatment:

(1) Report flow problems to a vascular surgeon.

18. Central venous catheter thrombus and or vessel stenosis

a) Etiology:

(1) Inadequate heparinization of the catheter interdialytically

(2) Blood remaining in the catheter post dialysis

(3) Epithelial injury of the vein wall

(4) Catheter composition and stiffness appear to correlate with thrombogenicity

b) Signs and symptoms:

(1) Difficult or unable to aspirate blood from either side of the catheter

(2) Difficulty in maintaining blood flow

(3) Edema of the ipsilateral arm

c) Prevention:

(1) Thoroughly flush catheter with normal saline post treatment to remove blood.

(2) Instill heparin into both lumens of catheter after flushing with saline.

d) Treatment:

(1) Use of fibrinolytic agents, e.g., urokinase

(2) Refer patient to the physician.

19. Aneurysm

a) Etiology:

(1) Occur most often at the anastomosis in the AV fistula

(2) Infiltration

(3) Repeated cannulation at the same site of the access

(4) Shearing of the walls of the vessel during cannulation

b) Signs and symptoms:

(1) Dilation of the vessel wall

(2) Bounding pulse in the area of dilation

(3) Area may be more or less sensitive to pain than remaining fistula.

c) Prevention:

(1) Proper cannulation technique

(2) Rotation of cannulation sites

(3) Avoid probing with cutting edge of needle.

d) Treatment:

(1) Avoid area during cannulation.

(2) Surgical revision

20. Pseudoaneurysm

a) Etiology:

(1) Occurs with AV grafts where blood pools with no communication with blood in the active vessel

(2) Unsealed puncture site and poor hemostasis

(3) Repeated cannulation of same sites

b) Signs and symptoms:

(1) Unusual dilation of graft anywhere along its course

(2) Difficulty cannulating that specific area

c) Prevention:

(1) Rotation of cannulation site

(2) Ensure pressure applied to insertion site is also compressing site where the needle entered the graft.

(3) Ensure cannulation sites have completely stopped bleeding before discharging patient.

d) Treatment:

(1) Avoid area during cannulation.

(2) Assess area every treatment for changes on inspection and palpation and signs and symptoms of infection.

(3) Surgical revision

21. Steal syndrome

a) Etiology:

(1) Normal arterial blood supply to the distal extremity is shunted through the access depriving the distal extremity of needed oxygenation.

(2) Occurs most often in patients with compromised distal circulation prior to access placement

b) Signs and symptoms:

(1) Weak or absent pulse in affected limb compared to the other

(2) Cold, pale, and/or cyanotic distal extremity

(3) Pain in the distal extremity made worse by initiation of hemodialysis

(4) Atrophy of muscles in distal extremity

(5) Necrosis of distal extremity if not corrected

c) Prevention:

(1) Placing a small lumen prosthetic graft and/or graft that is tapered at the arterial anastomosis

(2) Banding of the graft at the arterial anastomosis

d) Treatment:

(1) Place affected extremity in dependent position to afford distal circulation some assistance from gravity.

(2) Keep distal extremity warm.

(3) Assess distal extremity for: pulses distal to access, color, temperature, motor function, sensory function, and areas of skin breakdown.

(4) Meticulous attention to skin care of distal extremity

(5) Instruct patient in all of the above.

(6) Surgical revision.

22. Cardiac arrest

a) Etiology:

(1) Electrolyte imbalance, especially hyperkalemia.

(2) Dysrhythmias.

(3) Myocardial infarction

(4) Cardiac tamponade

(5) Large air embolism

(6) Hemolysis

(7) Exsanguination

(8) Hyperthermia

b) Signs and symptoms:

(1) Absence of apical or carotid pulse

(2) Lack of respiration

(3) Nonresponsiveness

(4) Asystole or ventricular fibrillation on ECG

c) Prevention:

(1) Prevent conditions which could precipitate any of the conditions listed in etiology.

(2) Careful assessment predialysis and during dialysis

(3) ECG monitoring of patients considered at risk during dialysis

d) Treatment:

(1) Assess for signs of cardiac arrest and call for assistance.

(2) Initiate cardiopulmonary resuscitation.

(3) Discontinue dialysis and return blood to patient if appropriate. (If cardiac arrest occurs immediately at the beginning of treatment and the cause is unknown, do not return the blood to the patient. Dialyzer membrane incompatibility or infusion of dialyzer disinfectant may have occurred.).

(4) Access lines should remain in place to provide a route for administration of saline and medications.

(5) Dialysate and patient blood samples should be sent to the lab.

(6) Retain the dialyzer and blood lines for later analysis.

(7) The dialysis machine should be replaced and its safety features evaluated for possible malfunction.

23. Dialysis encephalopathy

a) Etiology:

(1) Accumulation of aluminum in the body from water used to prepare dialysate or from administration of large quantities of aluminum-containing binders

b) Signs and symptoms:

   (1) Speech disturbances including apraxia, dysarthia, and aphasia

   (2) Myoclonic jerks

   (3) Seizures

   (4) Poor gait

   (5) EEG changes

   (6) Intellectual deterioration

   (7) Anemia

   (8) Osteodystrophy and osteomalacia

   (9) Seizures

   (10) Coma

c) Prevention:

   (1) Adequately treated water used for dialysate preparation

   (2) Substitute non-aluminum based medications for those containing aluminum

   (3) Serum aluminum chelation with desferroxamine mesylate based on aluminum lab values

d) Treatment:

   (1) Same as prevention.

C. Dialysate Related Complications

Those complications which result from problems with the delivery of dialysate during dialysis.

1. Hemolysis

  a) Etiology:

    (1) Hypotontic dialysate – requires two simultaneous errors

     (a) Failure to connect concentrate

     (b) Obstruction of the concentrate source

     (c) Faulty concentrate

     (d) Concentrate pump malfunction

     (e) Conductivity alarm monitor failure

     (f) Dialysate bypass mechanism failure

    (2) Overheated dialysate ($<43^0C$) – requires two simultaneous errors

     (a) Thermostat failure

     (b) Thermostat not set properly

     (c) Heater calibration error

     (d) Heater cycle malfunction

     (e) High temperature sensor not set properly

     (f) Dialysate temperature alarm monitor failure

     (g) Dialysate bypass mechanism failure

     (h) Overheated water used to prepare dialysate caused by temperature blending valve problem

    (3) Undetected pre-blood pump arterial pressure in excess of -250 mmHg

    (4) Chloramines, copper, or nitrates in the water used to prepare dialysate

    (5) Formaldehyde or bleach in the dialysate; formaldehyde in reprocessed dialyzers

    (6) Other nondialysate related causes include a rapid bolus of hypotonic solution, improper occlusion of the blood pump rollers, and kinks in blood tubing post blood pump

  b) Signs and symptoms:

    (1) Tightness in the chest and dyspnea.

    (2) Back pain.

    (3) Hypotension.

    (4) Cherry kool-aid appearance of the blood.

    (5) Pain and burning at the venous access site

    (6) Decrease in hematocrit

    (7) Hyperkalemia

    (8) Dysrhythmias.

    (9) Seizures

    (10) Cardiac arrest

    (11) Additional signs and symptoms for hypotonic dialysate include:

     (a) Warmth in the throat

     (b) Erratic blood pressure

     (c) Throbbing headache

     (d) Anxiety and restlessness

     (e) Nausea, vomiting, abdominal cramping, diarrhea

    (12) Additional signs and symptoms for hyperthermic dialysate include:

     (a) The patient complains of feeling hot.

     (b) The skin is hot and may feel dry.

     (c) Headache and delirium

     (d) Rapid, weak respiration

     (e) Initial increase in systolic blood pressure, then a decrease with CHF

     (f) Derangement of normal clotting mechanisms

     (g) Increased WBCs as a result of physiologic stress

(13) Lactic acidosis from anaerobic metabolism and hemolysis.

c) Prevention:

(1) Removal of copper piping in water distribution and dialysate preparation systems

(2) Carbon filtration in the water treatment system to remove chloramines

(3) Testing the carbon filters for chloramine levels prior to each patient shift

(4) Routine cleaning of concentrate containers, lines, and filters.

(5) Appropriate checks of temperature and conductivity prior to dialysis initiation including:

(a) Verify actual temperature and conductivity values.

Figure 4.7

Pressure Monitoring Devices

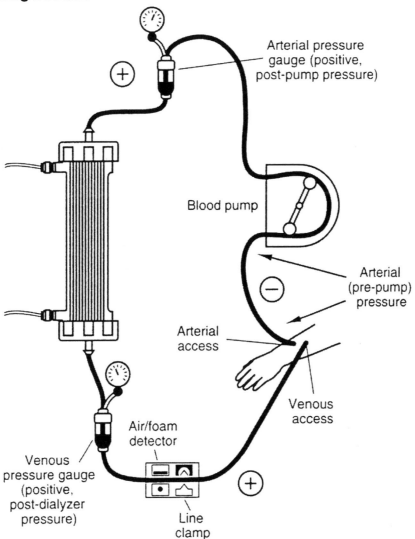

The extracorporeal circuit has gauges to measure
venous pressure and arterial pressure.

Reprinted with permission from AMGEN Core Curriculum, *p. 41, fig. 14*

(b) Verify alarm limits.

(c) Violate alarm limits to verify correct machine response.

(6) Monitor pre-blood pump arterial pressure and establish an alarm limit of <250 mmHg.

(7) Regular preventive maintenance of temperature and conductivity control systems, monitors, alarms, and bypass systems

(8) Verify removal of disinfectant solutions from water treatment systems, dialysis equipment, concentrate containers, and dialyzers.

(9) Shield dialysis equipment electrical components from the corrosive effects of concentrate and dialysate.

(10) Appropriate documentation for above activities.

d) Treatment:

(1) Discontinue dialysis.

(2) Immediately clamp the venous blood line and do not return the blood to the patient.

(3) Monitor vital signs, place on an ECG and observe for dysrhythmias, hypotension, and shortness of breath.

(4) Check patient's hematocrit and electrolytes as well as dialysate electrolytes.

(5) Administer oxygen.

(6) Replace volume and/or blood transfusion if symptoms are severe.

2. Crenation

a) Etiology:

(1) Hypertonic dialysate – requires two simultaneous errors

(a) Water supply diminished or shut off

(b) Faulty concentrate

(c) Proportioning unit not functioning properly

(d) Conductivity alarm monitor failure

(e) Dialysate bypass mechanism failure

(2) Rapid bolus of hypertonic saline for muscle cramps or hypotension

b) Signs and symptoms:

(1) Very dark red blood

(2) Hypernatremia

(3) Intracellular dehydration and hyperosmolality – contraction in cell size

(4) Gradient for calcium influx occurs

(5) Contracted or expanded extracellular volume

(6) Headache

(7) Nausea

c) Prevention:

(1) Routine cleaning of concentrate containers, lines, and filters

(2) Appropriate checks of conductivity prior to dialysis initiation including:

(a) Verify actual conductivity values

(b) Verify alarm limits

(c) Violate alarm limits to verify correct machine response

(3) Regular preventive maintenance of conductivity control systems, monitors, alarms, and bypass systems

(4) Hypertonic saline is best administered in 1:1 dilution with normal saline over 30 seconds

D. Pressures in the Extracorporeal Circuit

1. Pre-blood pump arterial pressure

a) Caused by the suction on the vascular access site by the blood pump.

b) The pressure range will be below 0mmHg, i.e., negative pressure.

c) The pressure typically should not be more negative than -250mmHg or hemolysis of RBCs may occur as well as air bubble formation pre-pump.

d) Increasing negative pressure may indicate:

(1) A flow problem with the access relative to the blood pump flow rate setting

(2) The arterial needle has infiltrated the access vessel

(3) The arterial needle is poorly positioned within the access vessel.

(4) The arterial needle is clotted.

(5) Kinking of the arterial blood tubing between the access and the arterial monitor

(6) Hypotension.

(7) Increased blood viscosity due to ultrafiltration.

(8) Decreased cardiac output due to plasma volume reduction.

e) Decreasing negative pressure may indicate:

   (1) Separation of the blood tubing from the access

   (2) An opened saline administration line

   (3) Any opening within the arterial blood tubing which allows air to enter

   (4) A decrease in the blood pump speed

2. Pre-dialyzer arterial pressure (post pump)

   a) An indicator of clotting within the dialyzer; it may also be used in conjunction with venous pressure to determine the mean dialyzer pressure.

   b) The pressure range will be above 0mmHg, e.g., positive pressure, and represent the greatest positive pressure within the extracorporeal circuit.

   c) Increasing pressure may indicate:

     (1) A clotted dialyzer or clotted venous drip chamber

     (2) A kink in the blood tubing between the monitor and distally to the patient

     (3) The venous needle has infiltrated the access vessel.

     (4) The venous needle is poorly positioned within the access vessel.

     (5) The venous needle is clotted.

     (6) Increased blood viscosity due to ultrafiltration

     (7) An increase in the blood pump speed

   d) Decreasing pressure may indicate:

     (1) A blood line separation or leak between the monitor and distally to the patient

     (2) Kinking of the blood tubing between the blood pump and the monitor

     (3) A decrease in the blood pump speed.

3. Venous pressure

   a) Indicates the resistance to blood flow back to the patient

   b) The pressure will be greater than 0mmHg, e.g., positive pressure, but will be less than the pre-dialyzer arterial pressure.

   c) Increasing pressure may indicate:

     (1) Kinking of the blood tubing between the monitor and distally to the patient

     (2) The venous drip chamber is clotted.

     (3) The venous needle has infiltrated the access vessel.

     (4) The venous needle is poorly positioned within the access vessel.

     (5) The venous needle is clotted.

     (6) Increased blood viscosity due to ultrafiltration.

     (7) An increase in the blood pump speed

     (8) Venous stenosis of the access

   d) Decreasing pressure may indicate:

     (1) Blood tubing separation at the venous access

     (2) Kinking in the blood tubing proximal to the monitor

     (3) The dialyzer is clotting.

     (4) A decrease in the blood pump speed

4. Mean dialyzer pressure

   a) The pressure at the arterial inlet is greater than the pressure at the venous outlet of the dialyzer.

   b) Monitoring venous pressure only causes a slight under-estimation of blood-side pressure.

   c) Adding venous pressure to the pre-dialyzer arterial pressure and dividing by 2 indicates the average pressure within the dialyzer blood compartment.

E. Treatment Factors and their Impact on Dialyzer Clearance

1. Clearance

   a) Defined as the amount of blood completely cleared of solute in a given period of time, typically expressed in ml/min.

   b) Clearance is calculated as:

   $Qb[(Cbi - Cbo)/Cbi] + Qf(Cbo/Cbi)$

   c) Where:

     (1) Qb = blood flow rate

     (2) Cbi = urea concentration at the dialyzer inlet

     (3) Cbo = urea concentration at the dialyzer outlet

     (4) Qf = ultrafiltration rate

2. Blood flow rate

   a) Small molecule clearance, e.g., urea, is determined by the number of open channels within the dialyzer and the flow rate through those channels.

b) Urea clearance does not increase in direct proportion to increases in the blood flow rate.

c) Larger weight molecules are much less influenced by the blood flow rate.

3. Ultrafiltration rate

a) Solutes are removed by convective forces, also known as solute drag, as result of the removal of plasma water through ultrafiltration.

b) Provides only a small portion of the total clearance.

(1) Affects large molecules more so than small ones

4. Dialysate flow rate

a) Dialysate flow rate will influence urea clearance to a degree.

b) Increasing dialysate flow from 500ml/min to 800ml/min using a high efficiency dialyzer and a Qb of at least 350ml/min will increase urea clearance 5-10%.

5. Anticoagulation

a) Insufficient anticoagulation will increase the amount of clotting within the dialyzer reducing its surface area by plugging fibers and/or coating membrane surfaces.

b) Reduced dialyzer surface area will reduce the dialyzer's clearance.

6. Treatment time

a) Determines the total solute which can be removed at a given clearance.

b) If a four-hour treatment is shortened by just 5 minutes each treatment, the patient can loose the equivalent of one treatment every 4 months.

7. Access recirculation

a) Two types of recirculation occur during dialysis: access recirculation and cardiopulmonary recirculation

b) Both cause a reduction in effective urea clearance by decreasing urea concentration in the dialyzer inflow line

c) Access recirculation may be caused by needle placement or access problems such as stenosis

d) Cardiopulmonary recirculation is caused by using an arteriovenous graft or fistula where arterial blood instead of venous blood is drawn into the extracorporeal circuit

F. Heparinization and Clotting Times

1. Properties and actions

a) Anionic mucopolysaccharide complex of varying molecular weight

b) Extracted from pork intestinal mucosa and beef lung

c) Bonds with circulating antithrombin III inactivating the coagulation factors

d) Activity is dependent upon the molecular weight of the heparin used.

e) Lot to lot variability of heparin activity can be as much as 10%

f) Patient response to heparin varies from patient to patient, as well as, within a single patient over time.

(1) The amount required to achieve a target level of anticoagulation varies three-fold from patient to patient.

(2) Heparin removal varies fourfold with half-lifes ranging from 30-120 minutes from patient to patient.

g) Removed by the reticuloendothelial system; metabolized in the liver.

h) Used in dialysis to prevent blood clotting in the extracorporeal circuit.

2. Assessing intradialytic anticoagulation

a) Clot times:

(1) APTT – activated partial thromboplastin time.

(2) ACT – activated clot time.

(3) PT – prothrombin time.

(4) LWCT – Lee-White clot time.

b) Changes in extracorporeal circuit pressures:

(1) Clotting within the dialyzer will cause an increase in the pre-dialyzer arterial pressure as resistance to blood flow increases.

(2) The venous pressure will decrease as clotting occurs within the dialyzer causing a widening in the pressure difference between pre-dialyzer arterial pressure and venous pressure.

(3) If clotting occurs within the venous drip chamber, venous and pre-dialyzer arterial pressure will both increase.

c) Visual inspection of the extracorporeal circuit for inadequate anticoagulation:

Figure 4.8

Heparin Infusion Line

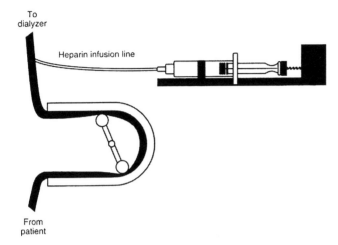

Reprinted with permission from AMGEN *Core Curriculum, p. 44, fig. 16*

(1) The blood may become darker in color.

(2) The dialyzer may develop streaking of the fibers.

(3) Clots may be observed in the drip chambers.

(4) If significant clotting occurs, the blood may begin to "teeter" between the venous line segment and the drip chamber as resistance to flow increases.

d) At termination of treatment:

(1) Additional normal saline rinseback may be required to return the patient's blood due to clotting.

(2) Clotting may be observed in the dialyzer fibers and headers, as well as the drip chambers.

(3) Dialyzer volume drops will be observed in reuse due to inadequate anticoagulation.

(4) Large quantities of blood may be rinsed out of the dialyzer during reuse due to inadequate anticoagulation.

(5) Dialyzer fiber streaking may be evident after reuse due to inadequate anticoagulation.

(6) The patient's access will require additional time to clot post treatment, generally more than 15 minutes, assuming proper site holding technique due to excess anticoagulation.

3. Complications of heparin therapy

a) Prolonged vascular site bleeding

b) Ecchymosis

c) Nose bleeds

d) Worsening of G.I., retinal, and menstrual bleeding

e) Pericardial and pleural effusions, subdural hematoma, and retroperitoneal bleeding

f) Hematuria

g) Osteoporosis

h) Leukocytopenia

i) Inhibition of aldosterone biosynthesis

4. Factors which may require an increase in heparin

a) Patient related:

(1) Increased hematocrit

(2) Fever

(3) Thrombosis

(4) Undetected low grade gram-negative infection

(5) Diabetic nephropathy

(6) Myocardial infarction

(7) Cancer

(8) Acute and chronic liver disease

(9) Fulminant hepatic diseases

(10) Long-term anticoagulant treatment.

(11) Estrogen therapy in patients with prostatic cancer

b) Treatment related:

(1) Reduced blood flow rate

(2) Increased treatment time

(3) Dialyzer

(4) Presence of clotting

(5) Intradialytic blood or lipid infusion

c) Medications:

(1) Digitalis

(2) Tetracycline

(3) Nicotine

(4) Antihistamines

5. Factors which may require a decrease in heparin

a) Patient related:

(1) Decreased hematocrit

    (2) Active bleeding

    (3) Recent surgery

  b) Treatment related:

    (1) Increased blood flow rate.

    (2) Decreased treatment time.

  c) Dialyzer:

    (1) Frequent saline rinses.

    (2) Medications:

      (a) Aspirin.

      (b) Ibuprofen.

      (c) Coumadin.

      (d) Dextran.

      (e) Persantine.

      (f) Phenylbutazone.

      (g) Indomethacin.

      (h) Hydroxychloroquine.

6. Patient risk factors

  a) Moderate risk of bleeding:

    (1) Recent surgery

    (2) History of G.I. or other bleeding

    (3) Prolonged vascular site bleeding

  b) High risk of bleeding:

    (1) Pericarditis

    (2) Any active bleeding

    (3) Recent surgery with bleeding complications or which bleeding would be dangerous

    (4) Thrombocytopenia

    (5) Coagulopathy

7. Heparinization methods

  a) Systemic heparinization – heparin is administered to the patient:

    (1) Routine systemic heparinization:

      (a) Administered to patients with no risk of bleeding

      (b) Intradialytic clot times are maintained at 1.5 to 2.0 times the baseline clot time.

      (c) Takeoff clot times should be 1.4 times the baseline clot time.

      (d) Commonly administered using a predialysis loading bolus 3-5 minutes pre-dialysis and then followed by a continuous infusion into the arterial blood tubing until the last one hour of the treatment

      (e) Intermittent boluses may be used intradialytically instead of an infusion.

    (2) Controlled, or tight, systemic heparinization:

      (a) Administered to patients with one or more bleeding risks.

      (b) Intradialytic clot times are maintained at 1.25 to 1.4 times the baseline clot time.

      (c) Takeoff clot times should be 1.25 to 1.4 times the baseline clot time.

      (d) Administered using a predialysis loading bolus 3-5 minutes pre-dialysis and then followed by a continuous infusion until the last one hour of the treatment

      (e) Intermittent boluses are not recommended.

  b) Regional heparinization

    (1) Heparin is infused pre-dialyzer and protamine is infused post-dialyzer as an antagonist to heparin.

    (2) Allows anticoagulation of the extracorporeal circuit without significant increases to the patient's clot time.

    (3) Used in patients where systemic heparinization is contraindicated.

    (4) Not widely used because:

      (a) Difficulty in balancing the infusion rates of heparin and protamine

      (b) Rebound anticoagulation from the dissociation of the heparin-protamine complex

      (c) Protamine side effects including flushing, bradycardia, hypotension, and dyspnea.

      (d) Simpler, safer, and more effective techniques are available.

  c) Regional citrate dialysis

    (1) Trisodium citrate is infused pre-dialyzer which complexes the extracorporeal blood ionized calcium and inhibits the clotting cascade.

    (2) A zero calcium dialysate is used

    (3) Calcium chloride is infused post-dialyzer to restore serum calcium.

    (4) About one-third of the infused citrate is dialyzed off and the other two-thirds is quickly metabolized by the patient.

(5) The disadvantages of citrate include:

    (a) The use of two infusions.

    (b) Frequent monitoring of serum calcium.

    (c) Complications may include hypocalcemia and citrate toxicity which includes nausea, paesthesias, muscle cramps, and tetany.

    (d) Citrate metabolism generates bicarbonate which could be dangerous for patients who are at risk for alkalemia.

d) Heparin-free dialysis

    (1) Uses a blood flow rate greater than 300 ml/min and intermittent normal saline flushes through the dialyzer

    (2) The extra normal saline must be calculated into the patient's weight loss goal.

    (3) Labor intensive

G. Charting

1. Documentation basics

    a) The patient's full name should be documented on every page in his/her chart.

    b) All entries must be legible and in ink.

    c) All entries must be timed and followed by the writer's name and title.

    d) Ditto marks, erasures, and correction fluid are not acceptable.

    e) Corrections should be made by drawing a single line through the error, writing the word "error" directly above with the writer's initials, and documenting the correct entry next to the error.

    f) All lines on a form should be filled; if not, draw a single line through the blank lines to prevent charting by someone else.

2. Chart information:

    a) All observations of the patient's condition, machine status, and course of care should be noted.

    b) Patient comments relevant to their condition and care should be noted.

    c) The effects and results of all treatments and procedures should be noted.

III. Discontinuation of Dialysis

A. Termination of Treatment

1. Heparin infusion or intermittent boluses should be terminated before the end of treatment based upon clotting times or patient prescription.

2. Patient and machine parameters are taken and documented.

3. TMP is turned off.

4. Post-dialysis blood samples may be taken at this time by reducing the blood pump speed usually to 100 ml/min or less and waiting a pre-determined time interval before drawing a sample from the arterial bloodline injection port. Some facilities choose instead to draw samples several minutes after termination of treatment to allow an equilibration of urea and other chemicals in the blood.

5. Blood is returned to the patient from the extracorporeal circuit using normal saline.

    a) The blood pump is usually used to return the blood.

    b) Extracorporeal circuit monitors should be used until the patient is disconnected from the circuit.

B. Removing the Needles

1. Check the patient's blood pressure before removing needles in case additional saline is required because of low standing pressures.

2. Remove one needle at a time.

    a) Untape the needle.

    b) Remove the needle at the same angle as it was inserted to avoid extending the incision.

    c) Do not apply any pressure until the needle is completely withdrawn from the skin.

    d) Apply moderate, direct pressure over the site where the needle entered the access not the insertion site of the skin. Palpate the access above and below the site for a thrill. Too little pressure may lead to prolonged bleeding or hematoma formation from oozing. Excessive pressure may lead to clotting of the access.

    e) Continue to apply pressure for five to ten minutes. Prematurely removing pressure to observe for clotting may extend the time needed to achieve hemostasis.

f) Fistula clamps may be used at times; however, it may be difficult to apply the correct pressure.

3. Clean and dress the site when bleeding is stopped. Ensure the dressing does not restrict flow through the access.

C. *Maintaining Catheter Patency*

1. Before removing the bloodlines, clean the catheter ports using sterile gauze saturated with povidone-iodine or chlorhexidine gluconate.

2. Flush both catheter lumens with normal saline.

3. Instill heparin into each lumen.

   a) Heparin use varies, but 5,000 and 10,000 units/ml heparin are most common.

Figure 4.9

Extracorporeal Circuit

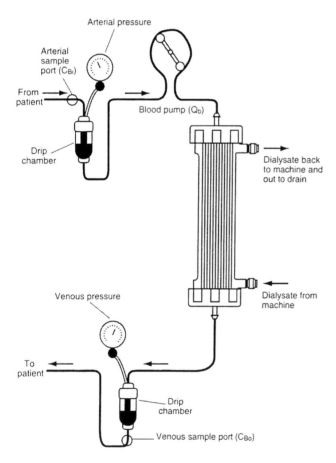

Reprinted with permission from AMGEN *Core Curriculum, p. 13, fig. 3*

---

b) the amount of heparin should be equal to or just slightly greater than the lumen volume.

4. Label the catheter.

   a) DO NOT FLUSH.

   b) _____ units heparin/lumen.

   c) Date and initials of staff member.

D. *Post-assessment of the Patient*

1. Vital signs and other physical assessments are performed and compared to pre-dialysis values including:

   a) Sitting and standing blood pressure

   b) Pulse.

   c) Temperature.

   d) Heart and lung sounds.

   e) Edema.

2. Weight is compared to the target weight.

3. Condition of the access is evaluated including any problems encountered achieving hemostasis.

4. Patient symptoms and overall condition are evaluated.

   a) Patient complaints or statements of well-being

   b) Behavior and mental status

E. *Documentation*

1. The time treatment was stopped.

2. The amount of saline used to return the blood.

3. Any complications encountered during takeoff.

4. Post-dialysis assessment.

5. Any blood loss including appearance of clot formation in the dialyzer and drip chambers.

6. Any special instructions given to the patient for home.

7. The time and method of departure from the facility.

F. *Dismantling the Delivery System*

1. Disconnect the concentrate lines from the concentrate and rinse per manufacturer recommendations.

2. Prepare the dialyzer for reuse.

   a) Ensure the dialyzer is completely filled with saline; any air will speed clotting of the residual blood.

b) Some facilities will fill the dialyzer with heparinized saline to further slow clotting.

c) If the bloodlines are to be reused, ensure they are treated like the dialyzer.

d) The dialyzer should be reprocessed within 10 -15 minutes to minimize volume loss unless it can be refrigerated.

3. Remove any non-disposables such as clamps and disinfect.

4. Discard the bloodlines and other biohazardous supplies into the biohazardous waste. All other disposables may be discarded into regular trash.

5. Clean and disinfect the outside of the machine with an approved disinfectant such as 1:100 dilution of household bleach (sodium hypochlorite) prior to the next treatment or if being pulled for maintenance/repair.

a) The surfaces should be scrubbed; simply wetting the surfaces will not provide adequate disinfection.

b) Special attention should be given to knobs and other surfaces likely touched and contaminated.

G. The Delivery System Hydraulic Flow Path

Must be cleaned and disinfected on a regular basis based on manufacturer recommendations.

1. Bicarbonate systems should be rinsed with an acetic acid solution such as vinegar to remove any carbonate precipitate buildup.

2. The delivery system should be disinfected either chemically or by heat to kill bacteria which may cause sepsis or pyrogenic reactions.

a) Chemicals, including sodium hypochlorite, peracetic acid, formaldehyde, and gluteraldehyde, may be used for disinfection.

b) Chemical disinfection includes a chemical fill where treated water and the chemical are mixed to a pre-determined concentration, circulated through the machine, and then rinsed with treated water only to reduce the disinfectant to safe levels.

c) The delivery system effluent must be tested prior to the next treatment to ensure safe residual levels. disinfection and residual test results should be documented.

d) Heat disinfection is an available alternative to chemical disinfection on some systems.

(1) Treated water is heated to 85°- 95° C and recirculated for a specified time.

(2) The heated water is drained and replaced with normal temperature water at some point after disinfection is complete.

(3) As heat disinfection does not kill spores or viruses, a periodic chemical disinfection is still required.

IV. Machine Troubleshooting

A. Alarm Actions

1. The machine should go into the dialysate bypass mode for:

a) High or low temperature

b) High or low conductivity

c) Most machines will come out of bypass modes automatically when the parameter is back in appropriate range

2. The blood pump should stop for any extracorporeal alarm

a) Blood leak

b) Venous pressure, low or high

c) Arterial pressure, low or high

d) Air in blood

e) Extracorporeal alarms on most machines require the operator to press a reset button to start the blood pump after alarm situation is cleared

3. All of the above alarms should be evident by an audible alarm and a visual indicator

B. Power Source Problems

1. Verify that power cord is securely in the outlet

2. Check/reset GFI outlet if applicable

3. Check circuit breakers in machine and electric panel

4. Plug into a different outlet

5. Inspect power cord for damage

C. Water Supply Problems

1. Assure water treatment system is on

2. Assure that water supply valve is open

3. Inspect water line of kinks and occlusions

4. Check drain line for kinks and occlusions

5. Check any inline filters.

Figure 4.10

Conductivity Monitor

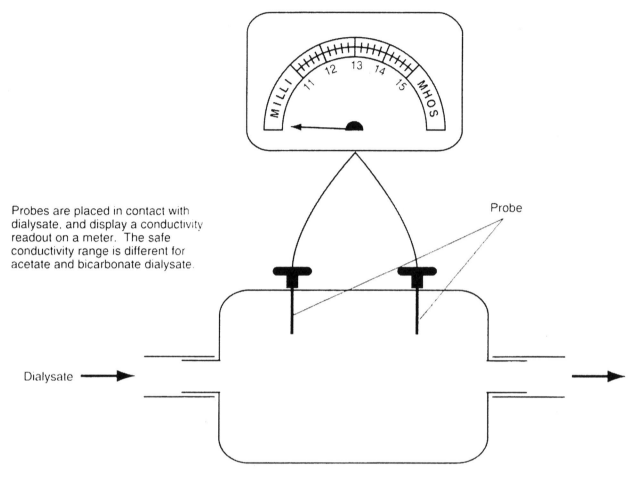

Probes are placed in contact with dialysate, and display a conductivity readout on a meter. The safe conductivity range is different for acetate and bicarbonate dialysate.

Probe

Dialysate

Reprinted with permission from AMGEN *Core Curriculum, p. 23, fig. 10*

D. Machine Monitors

1. Arterial pressure (between the patient and the blood pump) operation:
   An electronic pressure transducer measures the blood pressure within the extracorporeal circuit.
   a) Upper and lower limits are set either by the machine or the operator.
   b) The pressure is displayed by either a video screen, LED readout, meter, or gauge.
   c) Conditions which cause an alarm
      (1) See pressures in the extracorporeal circuit

d) Alarm response
   (1) The blood pump will stop.
   (2) An audible alarm will sound.
   (3) A visual alarm will be displayed.
   (4) Ultrafiltration will cease in ultrafiltration controlled machines.

2. Arterial pressure (between the blood pump and the dialyzer)
   a) Operation
      (1) An electronic pressure transducer measures the blood pressure within the extracorporeal circuit.
      (2) Upper and lower limits are set either by the machine or the operator.

(3) The pressure is displayed by either a video screen, LED readout, meter, or gauge.

b) Conditions which cause an alarm

(1) See pressures in the extracorporeal circuit.

c) Alarm response

(1) The blood pump will stop.

(2) An audible alarm will sound.

(3) A visual alarm will be displayed.

(4) Ultrafiltration will cease in ultrafiltration controlled machines.

3. Venous pressure

a) Operation

(1) An electronic pressure transducer measures the blood pressure within the extracorporeal circuit

(2) Upper and lower limits are set either by the machine or the operator

(3) The pressure is displayed by either a video screen, LED readout, meter, or gauge

b) Conditions which cause an alarm

(1) See pressures in the extracorporeal circuit

c) Alarm response

(1) The blood pump will stop.

(2) An audible alarm will sound.

(3) A visual alarm will be displayed.

(4) Ultrafiltration will cease in ultrafiltration controlled machines.

4. Dialysate pressure

a) Operation

(1) Measures the pressure using an electronic pressure transducer either as a passive monitor or, in some systems, as part of the ultrafiltration control system.

(2) Some systems incorporate the dialysate pressure with the venous pressure to display a TMP instead of dialyste pressure only.

(3) Systems have upper and lower limits which are set by the machine or set and adjusted by the operator.

(4) The pressure is measured in millimeters of mercury (mmHg).

b) Conditions which cause an alarm

(1) Malfunction of the negative pressure pump or volumetric control pump depending upon the system

(2) Obstructed blood side transducer

(3) Attempting fluid loss goals not consistent with the dialyzer's KUF and length of treatment

(4) Power supply failure

c) Alarm response

(1) An audible alarm will sound.

(2) A visual alarm will be displayed.

(3) In some systems, the blood pump and ultrafiltration pump will shut off, while in others, the dialysate flow and ultrafiltration pump will shut off.

5. Air-in-blood detector

a) Operation

(1) Detects air bubbles and/or foam in the venous blood line.

(2) Should be the last component in the extracorporeal circuit prior to the patient.

(3) New dialysis equipment uses an ultrasonic detection device located on or below the venous drip chamber.

b) Sound waves are transmitted through the blood which sense changes in density.

c) Some older systems used a photoelectric cell which was much less sensitive than ultrasonic detectors.

(1) Light is transmitted through the blood and changes in light transmission are detected due to refraction of light as it passes through air.

d) The system may be set manually or automatically depending on the manufacturer.

e) The alarm should be checked before each dialysis procedure.

f) Conditions which cause an alarm:

(1) Air, foam or microbubbles.

(2) Alarm response

(3) The blood pump shuts off.

(a) A venous clamp is activated just below the detector.

(b) The operator must intervene to correct and clear the alarm.

6. Dialysate conductivity

a) Operation

(1) Measures the electrical conductance of the dialysate by passing a small electrical current between two probes within the dialysate flow path before the dialyzer.

(2) Conductance relates to the ion concentration of the dialysate; sodium is the greatest contributor to conductivity.

(3) The conductivity is expressed as millimhos, or millisiemans.

(4) The upper and lower limits are generally set by the manufacturer but some systems may be set manually.

b) Conditions which cause an alarm

(1) Low conductivity may be caused by:

    (a) Loss of concentrate, e.g., empty concentrate container. If performing bicarbonate dialysis, it may be the loss of one or both concentrates.

    (b) Improperly prepared or incorrect concentrate

    (c) Plugged or kinked concentrate line

    (d) Plugged concentrate filter

    (e) Malfunctioning conductivity control system

(2) High conductivity may be caused by:

    (a) Inadequate water flow

    (b) Improperly prepared or incorrect concentrate

    (c) malfunctioning conductivity control system.

c) Alarm response

(1) The system bypasses dialysate flow away from the dialyzer

(2) An audible alarm sounds.

(3) A visual alarm is displayed.

7. Dialysate temperature

a) Operation

(1) A thermistor within the dialysate flow path before the dialyzer monitors dialysate temperature

(2) The alarm range is preset by the manufacturer.

b) Conditions which cause an alarm

(1) Malfunction of the heater control system

(2) Abnormally high or low incoming water temperature

c) Alarm response

(1) The system bypasses dialysate flow away from the dialyzer

(2) An audible alarm sounds.

(3) A visual alarm is displayed.

8. Dialysate flow

a) Operation

(1) Measures and indicates the dialysate flow rate either directly via a flow meter or indirectly via a digital display

(2) Some machines have a preset flow rate while others can be manually set by the operator including turning off dialysate flow.

(3) The flow rate is displayed in milliliters per minute (ml/min) and ranges from 0 to 1000 ml/min.

b) Conditions which cause an alarm

(1) Low water pressure

(2) Dialysate pump failure

(3) Obstruction in the dialysate flow path

(4) Power failure

c) Alarm response

(1) An audible alarm sounds.

(2) A visual alarm is displayed.

9. Blood leak

a) Operation

(1) A photoelectric cell within the dialysate flow path after the dialyzer detects changes in light transmission of the detector caused by blood entering the flow path.

(2) The sensitivity of the detector may be preset by the manufacturer but usually is adjustable by the operator.

(3) The detector may have multiple sensitivity settings which can be set manually.

(4) Air entering the dialysate flow path may cause a false alarm situation.

(5) Blood leaks should be verified by the operator with a Hemastix test of the dialysate after the dialyzer.

b) Conditions which cause an alarm

(1) Dialyzer membrane leak.

(2) Air in the dialysate flow path.

(3) Dirty or fouled light source or photoelectric cell.

(4) Malfunction of the detector system.

c) Alarm response

(1) The blood pump stops.

(2) An audible alarm sounds.

(3) A visual alarm is displayed.

(4) In some systems, ultrafiltration is stopped.

Suggested Readings

AMGEN, Inc. (1992), *Core Curriculum for Dialysis Technicians.* Wisconsin: Medical Media Publishing, Inc.

Daugirdas, John T. and Ing, Todd S., Editors (1993), *Handbook of Dialysis,* Second Edition. Little, Brown and Co.

Gutch, C.F., Stoner, Martha H, and Corea, Anna L.(1993) *Review of Hemodialysis for Nurses and Dialysis Personnel,* Fifth Edition, Mosby.

Lancaster, Larry E, Editor (1991), *Core Curriculum for Nephrology Nursing,* Second Edition, American Nephrology Nurses Association.

Man, N. K., Zingraff, J., and Jungers, P. (1995) *Long-term Hemodialysis,* Kluwer Academic Publishers.

Nissenson, et al, editors (1993), *Dialysis Therapy,* St. Louis, Mosby Year Book, Inc.

Chapter 5
Heparin Therapy for Hemodialysis Patients

Contributing Authors:
Philip Andrysiak, BS, MBA, CHT

Chapter Outline

I. Introduction

II. Anticoagulation Clotting Cascade

III. Anticoagulation Methodology

IV. Anticoagulation Tests

V. Principles of Anticoagulation

VI. Discussion

I. Introduction

    A. The first CQI response is to measure the current situation

    B. The importance of proper heparinization:

        1. Should be communicated to the staff

        2. Should be of primary importance to all staff

        3. Will provide the patient with more efficient treatments

    C. Improved heparinization protocols can improve hemodialyzer reuse and the patients URR

    D. Adequate heparinization prevents the hemodialyzer from clotting without giving the patient high doses of heparin

    E. Because of CLIA regulations clotting tests are not routinely done

    F. Heparin is single most dangerous medication used in dialysis

    G. Too little heparin and the dilaysis circuit clots which provides and inefficient treatment

    H. Different dialyzers will have clot either more or less with the same amount of heparin. This depends on the type of membrane.

    I. Different medications and patient conditions can either prolong or retard the anti-coagulation effect of heparin

    J. Heparin will vary between lot to lot and between brands

        1. When changing heparin brands reevaluate the patients anti-coagulation status

    K. Higher blood flow rates reduce the risk of clotting the dialyzer

    L. Longer treatment times require more heparin, usually in an increased infusion rate

II. **Anticoagulation Clotting Cascade**

    A. Heparin activates anitithrombin which inhibits prothrombin to thrombin formation

    B. Heparin is a medication and blood interaction, not medication dialyzer membrane interaction

    C. It takes approximately five minutes for heparin to activate antithrombin

III. **Anticoagulation Methodology**

    A. Systemic

        1. Heparinization of the blood circuit and patient

    B. Regional

        1. Heparinization of only the blood circuit

    C. Baseline

        1. Clotting time before heparin is administered

    D. Controlled

    Heparinization at 1.5 to 2.0 times baseline

    E. Tight

        1. Heparinization at 1.25 to 1.5 times baseline

IV. **Anticoagulation Tests**

    A. Whole blood clotting time

        1. Whole blood is placed in a test tub at 37° C and rotated every 30 seconds until it clots

        2. Measures fibrinogen to fibrin time

        3. Predialysis results are in the 3 to 6 minutes range

        4. During hemodialysis results are in the 15 to 20 minutes range

    B. Whole blood activated clotting time

        1. Same as whole blood clotting time except an activator is added to speed up clotting process

        2. Measures fibrinogen to fibrin time

        3. Predialysis results are in the 90 to 140 seconds range

        4. During hemodialysis results are in the 200 to 240 seconds range

Figure 5.1

Heparin Model©

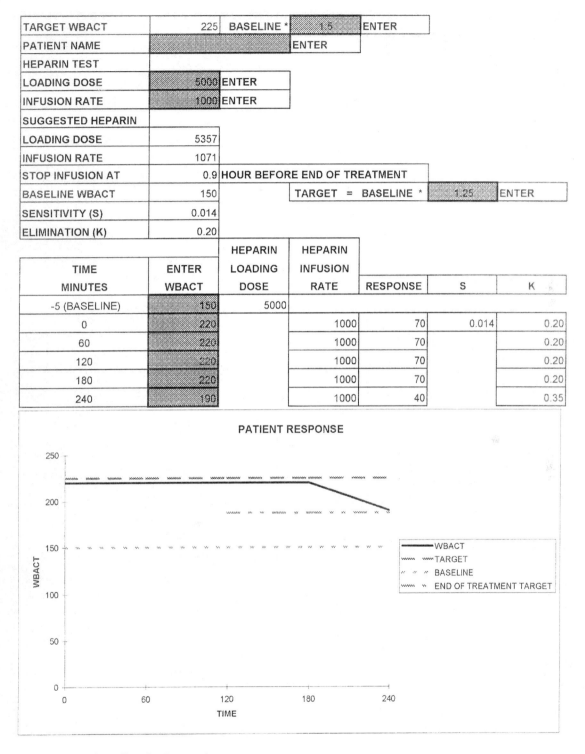

C. Whole blood partial thromboplastin time

1. Measures activity of prothrombin

2. Predialysis results are in the 60 to 85 seconds range

3. During hemodialysis results are in the 110 to 160 seconds range

V. Principles of Anticoagulation

A. Computerized Model

1. Patient sensitivity[1]

   a) Patient specific response to heparin

   b) Can be measured by giving a specific heparin dose and measuring the patient response

   c) This is a dose response calculation

   d) Example:

      (1) Administer 1,000U heparin

      (2) The ACT changes from a baseline of 100 to 150

      (3) Divide the amount of heparin administered by the change in ACT

      (4) 50/1000 = .05

2. Patient metabolism

   a) Can also be measured but the calculations are more complex

3. Heparin decay

   a) Heparin decay at the end of treatment can also be measured but the formula is very complex

4. A computer model utilizing the above formulas is available[2]

B. Heparinization based on patient weight

1. 100 units per kilogram body weight[3]

   a) This includes loading dose and total infusion dose

C. Heparinization based on Dr. Ward Formula[4]

1. Initial Bolus=1600+10x(Wgt-76)-300xF_{DB}-100xF_{SM} IU

   a) Where:

      (1) Wgt=Kilograms

      (2) FDB=1 for diabetics

      (3) FDB=0 for non diabetics

      (4) FSM=1 for smokers

      (5) FSM=0 for non smokers

2. Infusion Rate=1800 IU/hour

Figure 5.2

Heparin Dose 100µ/Kg

Kilograms	Pounds	Total Heparin Dose
64	140.8	6,400
65	143.0	6,500
66	145.2	6,600
67	147.4	6,700
68	149.6	6,800
69	151.8	6,900
70	154.0	7,000
71	156.2	7,100
72	158.4	7,200
73	160.6	7,300
74	162.8	7,400
75	165.0	7,500
76	167.2	7,600
77	169.4	7,700
78	171.6	7,800
79	173.8	7,900
80	176.0	8,000
81	178.2	8,100
82	180.4	8,200
83	182.6	8,300
84	184.8	8,400
85	187.0	8,500
86	189.2	8,600
87	191.4	8,700
88	193.6	8,800
89	195.8	8,900
90	198.0	9,000
91	200.2	9,100
92	202.4	9,200
93	204.6	9,300
94	206.8	9,400
95	209.0	9,500
96	211.2	9,600
97	213.4	9,700
98	215.6	9,800
99	217.8	9,900
100	220.0	10,000
101	222.2	10,100
102	224.4	10,200
103	226.6	10,300
104	228.8	10,400
105	231.0	10,500
106	233.2	10,600
107	235.4	10,700
108	237.6	10,800
109	239.8	10,900

Source: Physician Desk Reference

Figure 5.3

Heparin Dose: Non-Diabetic and Smoker vs. Diabetic and Smoker

Kilograms	Pounds	Infusion Rate	Initial Bolus	Kilograms	Pounds	Infusion Rate	Initial Bolus
64	140.8	1,800	1,380	64	140.8	1,800	1,080
65	143.0	1,800	1,390	65	143.0	1,800	1,090
66	145.2	1,800	1,400	66	145.2	1,800	1,100
67	147.4	1,800	1,410	67	147.4	1,800	1,110
68	149.6	1,800	1,420	68	149.6	1,800	1,120
69	151.8	1,800	1,430	69	151.8	1,800	1,130
70	154.0	1,800	1,440	70	154.0	1,800	1,140
71	156.2	1,800	1,450	71	156.2	1,800	1,150
72	158.4	1,800	1,460	72	158.4	1,800	1,160
73	160.6	1,800	1,470	73	160.6	1,800	1,170
74	162.8	1,800	1,480	74	162.8	1,800	1,180
75	165.0	1,800	1,490	75	165.0	1,800	1,190
76	167.2	1,800	1,500	76	167.2	1,800	1,200
77	169.4	1,800	1,510	77	169.4	1,800	1,210
78	171.6	1,800	1,520	78	171.6	1,800	1,220
79	173.8	1,800	1,530	79	173.8	1,800	1,230
80	176.0	1,800	1,540	80	176.0	1,800	1,240
81	178.2	1,800	1,550	81	178.2	1,800	1,250
82	180.4	1,800	1,560	82	180.4	1,800	1,260
83	182.6	1,800	1,570	83	182.6	1,800	1,270
84	184.8	1,800	1,580	84	184.8	1,800	1,280
85	187.0	1,800	1,590	85	187.0	1,800	1,290
86	189.2	1,800	1,600	86	189.2	1,800	1,300
87	191.4	1,800	1,610	87	191.4	1,800	1,310
88	193.6	1,800	1,620	88	193.6	1,800	1,320
89	195.8	1,800	1,630	89	195.8	1,800	1,330
90	198.0	1,800	1,640	90	198.0	1,800	1,340
91	200.2	1,800	1,650	91	200.2	1,800	1,350
92	202.4	1,800	1,660	92	202.4	1,800	1,360
93	204.6	1,800	1,670	93	204.6	1,800	1,370
94	206.8	1,800	1,680	94	206.8	1,800	1,380
95	209.0	1,800	1,690	95	209.0	1,800	1,390
96	211.2	1,800	1,700	96	211.2	1,800	1,400
97	213.4	1,800	1,710	97	213.4	1,800	1,410
98	215.6	1,800	1,720	98	215.6	1,800	1,420
99	217.8	1,800	1,730	99	217.8	1,800	1,430
100	220.0	1,800	1,740	100	220.0	1,800	1,440
101	222.2	1,800	1,750	101	222.2	1,800	1,450
102	224.4	1,800	1,760	102	224.4	1,800	1,460
103	226.6	1,800	1,770	103	226.6	1,800	1,470
104	228.8	1,800	1,780	104	228.8	1,800	1,480
105	231.0	1,800	1,790	105	231.0	1,800	1,490
106	233.2	1,800	1,800	106	233.2	1,800	1,500
107	235.4	1,800	1,810	107	235.4	1,800	1,510
108	237.6	1,800	1,820	108	237.6	1,800	1,520
109	239.8	1,800	1,830	109	239.8	1,800	1,530

Source: Physician Desk Reference

Figure 5.4

Heparin Dose: Non-Diabetic and Non-Smoker vs. Diabetic and Non-Smoker

Kilograms	Pounds	Infusion Rate	Initial Bolus	Kilograms	Pounds	Infusion Rate	Initial Bolus
64	140.8	1,800	1,480	64	140.8	1,800	1,180
65	143.0	1,800	1,490	65	143.0	1,800	1,190
66	145.2	1,800	1,500	66	145.2	1,800	1,200
67	147.4	1,800	1,510	67	147.4	1,800	1,210
68	149.6	1,800	1,520	68	149.6	1,800	1,220
69	151.8	1,800	1,530	69	151.8	1,800	1,230
70	154.0	1,800	1,540	70	154.0	1,800	1,240
71	156.2	1,800	1,550	71	156.2	1,800	1,250
72	158.4	1,800	1,560	72	158.4	1,800	1,260
73	160.6	1,800	1,570	73	160.6	1,800	1,270
74	162.8	1,800	1,580	74	162.8	1,800	1,280
75	165.0	1,800	1,590	75	165.0	1,800	1,290
76	167.2	1,800	1,600	76	167.2	1,800	1,300
77	169.4	1,800	1,610	77	169.4	1,800	1,310
78	171.6	1,800	1,620	78	171.6	1,800	1,320
79	173.8	1,800	1,630	79	173.8	1,800	1,330
80	176.0	1,800	1,640	80	176.0	1,800	1,340
81	178.2	1,800	1,650	81	178.2	1,800	1,350
82	180.4	1,800	1,660	82	180.4	1,800	1,360
83	182.6	1,800	1,670	83	182.6	1,800	1,370
84	184.8	1,800	1,680	84	184.8	1,800	1,380
85	187.0	1,800	1,690	85	187.0	1,800	1,390
86	189.2	1,800	1,700	86	189.2	1,800	1,400
87	191.4	1,800	1,710	87	191.4	1,800	1,410
88	193.6	1,800	1,720	88	193.6	1,800	1,420
89	195.8	1,800	1,730	89	195.8	1,800	1,430
90	198.0	1,800	1,740	90	198.0	1,800	1,440
91	200.2	1,800	1,750	91	200.2	1,800	1,450
92	202.4	1,800	1,760	92	202.4	1,800	1,460
93	204.6	1,800	1,770	93	204.6	1,800	1,470
94	206.8	1,800	1,780	94	206.8	1,800	1,480
95	209.0	1,800	1,790	95	209.0	1,800	1,490
96	211.2	1,800	1,800	96	211.2	1,800	1,500
97	213.4	1,800	1,810	97	213.4	1,800	1,510
98	215.6	1,800	1,820	98	215.6	1,800	1,520
99	217.8	1,800	1,830	99	217.8	1,800	1,530
100	220.0	1,800	1,840	100	220.0	1,800	1,540
101	222.2	1,800	1,850	101	222.2	1,800	1,550
102	224.4	1,800	1,860	102	224.4	1,800	1,560
103	226.6	1,800	1,870	103	226.6	1,800	1,570
104	228.8	1,800	1,880	104	228.8	1,800	1,580
105	231.0	1,800	1,890	105	231.0	1,800	1,590
106	233.2	1,800	1,900	106	233.2	1,800	1,600
107	235.4	1,800	1,910	107	235.4	1,800	1,610
108	237.6	1,800	1,920	108	237.6	1,800	1,620
109	239.8	1,800	1,930	109	239.8	1,800	1,630

Source: Physician Desk Reference

VI. Discussion

A. *Heavier patients require substantially more heparin.*

B. *It takes heparin 5 minutes to work so it is extremely important to wait 5 minutes before you connect the patient.*

C. *If you do not wait 5 minutes before patient connection part of the hemodialyzer clots at the very beginning of treatment and the whole treatment becomes sub optimal.*

D. *Computer model is the most accurate.*

E. *See worksheets for heparin dose based on patient weight.*

F. *See worksheets for heparin dose based on Dr. Ward Formula.*

G. *The CQI protocol calls for first measuring the current situation, making a change, and then analyzing the result.*

H. *Too little heparin will eventually clot the dialysis circuit*

I. *Pick a heparin protocol to use and then follow it*

  1. Heparin protocols are a starting point and should not be used to replace good clinical judgement

J. *If a large number of patients are clotting their dialysis circuit check to see if you are using the same brand*

K. *Heparin potency can also change between lot numbers*

L. *If possible become CLIA certified so that you can perform anti-coagulation testing*

M. *If you have access to a laboratory PTT can be substituted for ACT*

  1. Make sure laboratory is set up to test in the range for a heparinized dialysis patient

N. *If the heparin therapy is improved you should see improved hemodialyzer reuse and higher URR's.*

Notes

1. Nissenson and Fine, *Dialysis Therapy,* Second Edition, St. Louis, Mosby Year Book, Inc.

2. Contact the author, Philip Andrysiak, via the NANT office for the computer model

3. Physician Desk Reference

4. *Artificial Organs,* June 1997, Volume 21, Number 6

References

Carbone, Vera (1995). *Heparin and Dialyzer Membranes during Hemodialysis: A Literature Review, ANNA Journal,* Volume 22, Number 3

Burrows-Hudson, S., Vlchek, D. (1989). *Monitoring Anti-coagulation is a QA Issue, Nephrology News and Issues,* March

Ward, Richard A. (1995). *Heparinization for Routine Hemodialysis, Advances in Renal Replacement Therapy,* Volume 2, No. 4, October

Wei, S.S., Ellis, P.W., et al (1994). *Effects of Heparin Modeling on Delivered Hemodialysis Therapy, American Journal of Kidney Diseases,* Volume 23, Number 3, March

Chapter 6

Therapeutic Renal Nutrition

Contributing Authors:

Fern G. Reyes, MPH, RD, LD

Lori Fedje, RD, LD

Chapter Outline

I. Therapeutic Renal Nutrition

A. Role of the Renal Dietitian

B. Renal Diet Considerations

C. Adequacy of Dialysis

D. Special Considerations for Specific Patient Population

A. Role of the Renal Dietitian

1. Overall goal is to promote nutritional intake to ensure the patients optimal health.

2. Assess patient's nutritional needs which include:
   a) Dietary interviews and diaries;
   b) Dietary restrictions/food preferences;
   c) Anthropometric measurements;
   d) Biochemical evaluation;
   e) Medical history;
   f) Subjective global assessment (SGA)- *nutrition-related physical assessment.*

3. Develop and individualize meal plans based on the nutritional assessment.

4. Educate patients on the renal meal plan.
   a) Teach what foods and amounts are appropriate.
   b) Involve family members and caregivers or extended-care facility.

5. Monitor nutritional status as indicated; provide recommendations, suggestions, solutions, or plan of action (includes education plan).

6. Renal Dietitians are registered with the American Dietetic Association (ADA).
   a) The ADA recognizes renal nutrition as a specialized area of practice.
   b) The ADA offers certification in renal nutrition for dietitians who meet certain criteria.

B. Renal Diet Considerations

1. Calories
   a) Provides the energy needed for the body to function.
   b) Carbohydrates, protein, and fats provide the total caloric needs of the renal patient.
      (1) The function of carbohydrate and fat are to spare protein.
      (2) Complex carbohydrates are stressed whenever possible to provide extra fiber for aiding in constipation.
      (3) A high-fiber diet may aid in control of serum lipid concentration.
      (4) Inclusion of monounsaturated and polyunsaturated fats are encouraged to help reduce or avoid lipid abnormalities.
   c) Requirements:
      (1) The general energy requirements is 35 calories/kg of body weight/day for those who are less than 60 years of age and 30 to 35 calories/kg body weight/day for 60 years or older.
      (2) Caloric requirements for underweight and overweight individuals are to be adjusted using the <95% and >115% of standard body weight.
      (3) Carbohydrates should supply about 45% of the total calorie intake.
      (4) Emphasize use of consistent carbohydrates in meal plan.
      (5) The percentage of calories from fat should be from 30-40% of total energy intake. The ratio of polyunsaturated to saturated fat should be 1:1.
      (6) Cholesterol intake should be limited to <300 mg/day.
   d) Sufficient calories are essential to meet energy requirements and to prevent malnutrition.

2. Protein
   a) Essential for creation and repair of body tissues.
   b) Necessary for acid-base balance.
   c) Used to create amino acids for metabolic functions, e.g., enzyme formation and to support the immune system that help maintain resistance to disease.
   d) Requirements:
      (1) 1.2 gm/kg body weight.
      (2) Protein needs are increased during periods of growth, pregnancy, lactation, illness, infection, and surgery.
   e) The renal meal plan should be at least 50% from high biological value (HBV) protein (animal protein). Sources include: eggs, milk products, beef, pork, fish, and poultry. The meal plans for patients with special needs and preferences, e.g., vegetarian, religion, are individualized.

3. Malnutrition
   a) Malnutrition may become a problem with hemodialysis patients. Research shows about 10% to 70% suffer from malnutrition.
   b) Low serum albumin, blood urea nitrogen (BUN) and serum cholesterol levels are indicators of poor nutrition.
      (1) Keep in mind low serum albumin levels can also be due to chronic inflammation (from dialysis procedure) and infection. In these cases, treatment may or may not respond to diet changes.

c) The causes of malnutrition can be attributed to one or multiple factors:

(1) Anorexia, inappropriate or poor intake;

(2) Metabolic acidosis;

(3) Illnesses other than kidney failure;

(4) Drug-nutrient interactions;

(5) GI losses with vomiting/diarrhea;

(6) Loss of protein and amino acids secondary to dialysis;

(7) Inadequate dialysis treatment;

(8) Hospitalizations and surgeries;

(9) Excessive dietary restrictions.

d) Careful attention of the changes in dry weight and listening to patient comments about eating habits can help alert dialysis staff (physician, nurse, dialysis technician, dietitian, and social worker) if a patient is eating enough.

e) Approaches to the treatment of malnutrition could be one or combination of the following:

(1) Increase the amount of food the patient eats;

(2) Initiate use of oral nutritional supplements.

(a) There are products especially designed for renal patients. These products are high calorie and high protein with reduced amounts of sodium, potassium, and phosphorus.

(b) As with the diet plan, selecting nutritional supplements for dialysis patients is individualized. Patient acceptance must be considered for better compliance and overall improvement in nutritional status.

(3) Nutrition support via:

(a) Tube feeding;

(b) Intradialytic parenteral nutrition (IDPN); or

(c) Total parenteral nutrition (TPN).

f) Improving appetite:

(1) Periodic review of patient's dietary plan, considering preference.

(2) Try small, frequent meals.

(3) Ensure patient is having adequate dialysis.

(4) Resolve other medical problems (i.e., relating to gastrointestinal)

(5) Attention must be given to oral hygiene to prevent breath odor and bad taste in the mouth.

(6) Control other noxious stimuli during meals.

g) Close follow-up of the patient's overall nutrition status is important. Communication among the dialysis staff can help with early detection and treatment of malnutrition.

4. Fluid Balance

a) Water is necessary for all life and metabolic functions, gives structure and form to the body, and acts as a transport medium for nutrients and wastes.

b) Renal patients are generally restricted to fluid intakes due to little or no urine output.

c) Fluid status needs are assessed based on:

(1) Urinary output;

(2) Serum sodium;

(3) Clinical volume status to include evaluation of proteinurea and serum Albumin level;

(4) Presence of edema;

(5) Medical history (CHF, HTN);

(6) Biochemical data;

(7) Medications;

(8) Insensible loss for normal body functions, e.g., breathing, stool, perspiration.

d) The general guideline of fluid restriction is two to four cups (500 to 1000 mL) of fluid per day plus the volume of urine produced in 24 hours.

(1) The physician usually prescribes the patient's fluid allowance and is individualized.

e) Acceptable *interdialytic* (between dialysis treatments) weight gain is usually 1.5 to 2.2 kg (3 to 5 lbs.) per day.

f) Fluid is anything that is liquid in room temperature, e.g., ice, gelatin, soda pop, soup, ice cream, popsicles, as well as fluids taken with medications.

g) Controlling fluid intake can be challenging for the dialysis patient. The following are techniques a patient can do to keep fluid intakes at a minimum:

(1) Suck on ice chips, chill foods and fluids to increase sense of fluid satisfaction;

(2) Use spray mouth wash, sports gum, rinse mouth with cold water or diluted mouth wash to relieve dryness;

(3) Add small amount of lemon juice to drinking water or to ice cubes;

(4) Use small cups for fluids;

(5) For diabetic patients, blood sugar control will help reduce thirst;

(6) Take medications with mealtime liquids whenever possible. Applesauce can also be used to take with medications.

(7) Drink to thirst only. Don't drink from habit or to be social;

(8) Limit sodium (salt) intake;

(9) Snack on ice-cold or frozen fruits (grapes, strawberries, blueberries) and vegetables when thirsty.

5. Sodium

a) Necessary for: conduction of nerve impulses, control of muscle contraction, acid-base regulation and cell wall permeability. Major cation of extracellular fluid—functions in regulation of extracellular fluid volume.

b) Sodium balance needs in renal failure patients are individualized.

c) Sodium status is monitored by the following parameters:

(1) Urinary output;

(2) Urinary sodium excretion;

(3) Clinical signs of edema, along with serum Albumin and urinary protein losses;

(4) Blood pressure;

(5) Medications.

d) It is important for dialysis patients to restrict sodium intake when:

(1) Signs of edema are present in the face, hands, or feet;

(2) Decreased urine output;

(3) Presence of hypertension;

(4) Rapid weight gain.

e) The recommended sodium restriction is generally 2 to 3 grams (87 to 130 mEq per day).

(1) All foods contain small amounts of naturally occurring sodium. This sodium cannot be eliminated from the diet.

(2) High sodium food sources include canned goods, table and cooking salt, salt substitutes (which may contain sodium as well as potassium), preserved meats (cold cuts, hot dogs), and processed foods.

6. Potassium

a) Necessary for: aid in maintaining electrolytes, acid-base regulation, neuromuscular action, transmission of cardiac electrical impulses, conversion of glucose to glycogen in the liver. Major cation of intracellular fluid.

b) Potassium balance is closely monitored by the following parameters:

(1) Urinary output;

(2) Serum potassium;

(3) Urinary potassium excretion;

(4) Blood glucose control;

(5) Medications (anti-hypertensive agents, diuretics);

(6) Etiology of renal disease;

(7) Any superimposed catabolic process;

(8) Acid-base status;

(9) Potassium loss via GI tract (i.e., gastrointestinal bleeding)

c) The general potassium dietary recommendation is 2 to 3 grams (51 to 77 mEq) per day but individualized.

d) Patients need to be aware of the following:

(1) Potassium overload can cause sudden death;

(2) Symptoms of hyperkalemia include muscle weakness, abnormal heart rhythms, and cardiac arrest;

(3) High potassium foods should be avoided to achieve potassium balance. Potassium is found in large amounts in bananas, orange juice, dried fruit, tomato sauce, spinach and potatoes. Most salt substitutes also contain potassium and should be avoided

(4) Appropriate portion sizes are important as low potassium foods can add to potassium overload. For example, an apple is considered a low potassium food but eating more than what is allowed on the meal plan could cause hyperkalemia.

7. Phosphorus

a) Necessary for building and maintenance of bones, energy transfer within cells, activation of normal neuromuscular function, fat transport, acid-base balance.

b) Renal insufficiency leads to an increase in phosphorus level and in calcium/phosphorus product as well as high parathyroid hormone (PTH) levels and bone damage.

c) Phosphate binding agents are often used in combination with dietary therapy to maintain normal serum phosphorus levels.

    (1) Most phosphorus binders contain calcium. When using aluminum base phosphate binders, aluminum levels should be monitored to avoid aluminum toxicity.

d) Patients must be counseled as to timing of ingestion of medications.

    (1) Phosphate binders are generally taken with meals and snacks to reduce phosphorus absorption. This will allow the phosphorus in foods to combine in the gut and be eliminated in the patient's stool.

    (2) Phosphate binders may inhibit the effectiveness of other medications when taken at the same time, such as with iron. Therefore, iron supplementation should not be taken at the same time as binders.

    (3) Phosphorus binders may also cause constipation in which a stool softener may be prescribed.

e) The general phosphorus dietary restriction is less than 17 mg per kg of body weight per day (800 to 1,200 mg/day).

    (1) Phosphorus is found in large amounts in milk, cheese, nuts, dried beans and peas, and cola drinks.

8. Calcium

a) Necessary for: creation and maintenance of bones and teeth, activation of enzymes, blood coagulation, permeability of cell membranes, transmission of nerve impulses, contraction of muscle fibers.

b) Renal failure patients have less ability to absorb and use calcium properly.

c) Calcium supplementation and active forms of vitamin D are usually prescribed to help improve calcium absorption.

d) Calcium balance can be achieved if:

    (1) Serum phosphorus is controlled;

    (2) Adequate intake is provided and supplementation may be used and taken between meals to ensure adequate elemental calcium absorption.

9. Vitamin/Mineral

a) Vitamin deficiency can occur in the dialysis patient due to:

    (1) Low intakes;

    (2) Loss of water soluble vitamins with dialysis;

    (3) Lack of kidney function to convert vitamin D to its active form.

b) Vitamin supplementation is recommended and dependent on the degree of renal function.

    (1) Water soluble vitamins that are especially designed for dialysis patients are provided. Patients should receive a maximum of 60-100 mg of Vitamin C, 800-1,000 mg of folic acid, and the recommended daily allowance (RDA) for the B-complex vitamins.

    (2) Fat soluble vitamins (A, E, and K) are not regularly supplemented due to side effects and possible toxic levels from lack of kidney function. However, the active form of oral or IV Vitamin D (Calcitriol, Paricalcitriol) is used to treat renal osteodystrophy when indicated to maintain calcium. Calcitriol works to suppress parathyroid hormone, and raise calcium levels to avoid bone loss and treat renal osteodystrophy.

    (3) Trace mineral (zinc, magnesium) supplementation is individualized with regard to what type and dose of each trace mineral preparation is prescribed.

10. Iron

a) People who have kidney disease often develop a low blood count (anemia). One of the causes is the kidneys not making enough of a hormone called erythropoietin (EPO). This hormone helps to make red blood cells.

b) Anemia can also be caused by:

    (1) Having too little iron in the body;

    (2) Having too little vitamin B12 or folic acid;

    (3) Having a bleeding problem;

    (4) Having an infection or inflammation;

    (5) Inadequate dialysis;

    (6) Blood loss due to blood testing.

c) Iron profiles are evaluated frequently, and if the levels are below normal, iron therapy is prescribed.

    (1) Dietary sources of iron rarely can maintain iron levels.

d) Treatment of anemia are in the following forms:

   (1) EPO. EPO can be injected subcutaneously or given during dialysis treatment.

   (2) Iron supplements. Iron can be intravenous (IV) or taken orally. Maintenance IV iron is commonly given.

e) The goals to treat anemia are:

   (1) Serum ferritin levels should be at least 100 ng/mL but not greater than 800 ng/mL.

   (2) Hematocrit (Hct) level should increase to at least 33 to 36 percent.

   (3) Transferrin Saturation (TSAT) level should be at least 20%.

C. Adequacy of Dialysis

a) Research has shown getting the optimal amount of dialysis treatment is important to improve overall health; help patients live longer and improve quality of life on dialysis.

b) The dialysis care team measures the "delivered dose" of dialysis. This measurement tells how well the patient's dialysis treatment is removing urea from the blood.

c) Two methods utilized to assess adequacy of dialysis are:

   (1) Kinetic modeling.

   (2) Urea reduction ratio (URR).

d) DOQI recommends formal kinetic modeling which looks at all aspects of the dialysis treatment and calculates the Kt/V based on the size of the patient and residual renal function (K= clearance, t= time, V= volume). The DOQI standard is for Kt/V is 1.2 (single pool).

D. Special Considerations for Specific Patient Population

1. Pediatric ESRD Patient

a) Recommended daily energy nutrient intake for pediatric patients are calculated based on the RDA level for chronological age.

b) Recommended dietary protein is based on the RDA level for chronological age and an additional increment of 0.4 grams/kg/d.

c) Fluid needs are calculated based on patient's weight, urine output, and modality of dialysis treatment.

   (1) If edema or hypertension is present, fluid limits are based on insensible losses plus urine output.

d) Laboratory values differ between children and adults. The following chemistries related to renal disease have different ranges in children:

   (1) Serum Albumin;

   (2) Alkaline Phosphatase;

   (3) Blood Urea Nitrogen;

   (4) Serum Cholesterol;

   (5) Serum Creatinine;

   (6) Ferritin;

   (7) Glucose;

   (8) Hematocrit;

   (9) Hemoglobin;

   (10) Iron;

   (11) Mean Corpuscular Volume (MCV); and

   (12) Phosphorus.

e) High energy and protein requirements are hard to meet due to acid-base imbalance, growth, poor dietary intake, bone disease, dialysis, and anorexia.

f) Intellectual, social, and emotional growth can be affected due to chronic nature of disease and frequent hospitalization.

g) Food can become a source of power and control conflicts between parent and child.

h) Renal osteodystrophy is greater in infants, children, and adolescents.

   (1) Maintenance of calcium and phosphorus balance is critical to bone growth.

   (2) Renal osteodystrophy contributes to growth retardation.

   (3) Dosage of oral or IV active vitamin D is dependent on serum calcium, phosphorus, alkaline phosphatase, and PTH levels.

   (4) Phosphate binder of choice is calcium carbonate, as it provides additional supplementation while decreasing serum phosphates.

i) Malnutrition is the most common nutritional disorder in children with renal disease.

   (1) Failure to thrive is the term used to describe mild or moderate undernutrition.

   (2) Nutrition support via oral nutritional supplements, tube feeding, or intravenous feeding are used to treat malnutrition.

   (3) Biochemical data (electrolyte levels) and anthropometric measurements (response to growth) determine formula selection, concentrations and feedings.

j) The concepts of urea kinetic modeling are the same for children as they are for adults but there is a need for special consideration for interpretation and application of urea kinetic calculation.

    (1) Target Kt/V is at least 1.4.

k) Diet considerations:

    (1) Infants should be fed formula rather than breast milk, so that constituents and fluid amounts can be regulated.

    (2) Formula can be fortified with additional carbohydrates and oils to meet energy requirements.

    (3) Vitamin and mineral requirements should achieve 100% of the Dietary Reference Intakes or RDA.

    (4) Solid foods are introduced as usual, but must consider that strained prepared foods are still about 75% water.

    (5) Avoid overemphasizing diet as child grows. May turn into a power struggle or point of manipulation.

l) Recombinant Human Growth Hormone (hGH) may be used for children with growth problems.

2. Adolescent ESRD patient:

  a) Need for independence increases decision-making by adolescent.

  b) Compliance may be a problem at this stage due to peer pressure.

  c) Bone growth may stop which may lead to short stature.

  d) Diet considerations:

    (1) Allow for occasional dietary indiscretions without punishment.

    (2) Encourage adolescent to take control over intake and to become knowledgeable about the reason for restrictions.

    (3) Assess need for additional supplements of iron and folic acid where menses are heavy in adolescent females.

  e) Target Kt/V is at least 1.4.

3. The Diabetic ESRD patient

  a) Goals are similar to other ESRD patients, plus adequate control of blood sugar and complications secondary to the diabetic disease process.

b) Complications, e.g., retinopathy and neuropathy can alter ability to prepare food.

c) Uncontrolled blood glucose levels can increase thirst that contributes to weight gain.

d) ESRD decreased tissue sensitivity to insulin and a reduction in insulin breakdown by the kidney, therefore, insulin requirements may need to be adjusted.

e) Hyperglycemia causes potassium shifting from intracellular to extracellular fluids. Therefore, high blood glucose can lead to hyperkalemia.

f) Recommended treatments for hypoglycemic reaction:

    (1) Use glucose tablets; or

    (2) Plain table sugar; or

    (3) Use lemon-lime soda; or

    (4) Use juice (apple or cranberry; avoid high potassium juices).

g) Diet considerations:

    (1) Consistent carbohydrate diabetic meal plans are used for metabolic control in acute care settings. These meal plans are based on a consistent carbohydrate control for each meal rather than specific calorie levels for each meal.

    (2) Use small, frequent meals to enhance appetite.

h) Monitor for constipation and need for GI motility medication.

Figure 6.1

Abnormal Lab Values

Imbalance	Lab Values	Etiology	Clinical S/S	Treatment

Hyperkalemia	K > 5.5mEq/L
	Notify MD when
	> 6.0mEq/L
	
	May note:
	Hyperglycemia,
	acidosis
		1. Decreased renal excretion
		2. Translocation from cells
		   - acidosis
		   - hyperglycemia
		   - hemolysis
		   - tissue damage
		   - GI bleeding
		3. Excessive intake
		   - IV infusions
		   - dietary ingestion
			CNS: Confusion
			Neuromuscular:
			Muscular weakness,
			paresthesia, paralysis
			Cardiovascular:
			Arrythmias, elevated
			T-wave on EKG, arrest
			GI: Nausea/vomiting
			diarrhea
				1. Kayexalate 15-30gm
				2. $NaHCO_3$
				3. IV dextrose and insulin
				4. Decrease dietary intake
				5. Lower dialysate (K)
				6. Dialysis

Hypokalemia	< 3.5mEq/L
	
	May note: Alkalosis
		1. Increased intracellular shift
		   - alkolosis
		   - IV dextrose & insulin
		2. Decreased K intake
		   - dietary deficiency
		3. GI loss of K
		   - vomiting
		   - diarrhea
		   - laxative abuse
		4. Increased renal loss
		5. Increased integumentary loss
		   - excessive perspiration
			CNS: Drowsy,
			confused, coma
			Neuromuscular:
			Muscle weakness and
			cramps, paresthesias,
			paralysis
			Cardiovascular:
			Cardiac arrythmias,
			depressed T-wave on
			EKG, digoxin toxicity
			GI: Nausea/vomiting,
			anorexia
				1. Increased dietary intake
				2. K supplements
				   - K-lor
				   - K-lite
				3. Raise dialysate (K)

Hypernatremia	Na > 147mEq/L
	(these lab values are
	highly dilutional)
	
	May note:
	Hyperchloremia
		1. Water loss
		   - decreased
		   - vomiting
		   - diarrhea
		   - fever
		   - hyperventilation
		   - excessive perspiration
		2. Na retention
		   - excessive Na intake
		   - excessive NaCl infusion
		   - renal dysfunction
		   - corticosteriods
			CNA: Lethargy,
			irritability, seizures
			Neuromuscular:
			Tremors, muscular
			rigidity
			Cardiovascular:
			Tachycardia
			Integumentary: Dry
			mucous membranes,
			flushed dry skin,
			elevated temperature,
				1. Replace fluid loss if indicated
				2. Restrict Na if indicated

Hypocalcemia	Total Ca > 9mg % Ionized Ca < 3.5mEq/L	1. Hypoparathyroidism 2. Post para-thyroidectomy 3. Renal dysfunction 4. Hyperphosphatemia 5. Vitamin D deficiency 6. Inadequate dietary intake 7. Excessive administration of citrated blood 8. Alkalosis 9. Osteomalacia 10. Osteodystrophy	**CNS:** Seizures, depression, psychoses **Neuromuscular:** Paresthesia, muscle cramps, tetany, hyperreflexia **Cardiovascular:** Arrest **GI:** Cramps, nausea and vomiting, diarrhea **Integumentary:** Circumoral paresthesia, cataracts, keratitis, dry skin, brittle nails, alopecia **Skeletal:** Pathologic fractures	1. Lower dialysate (Ca) 2. Adjust Ca supplement, PO_4 binders, vitamin D supplements needed 3. $NaHCO_4$

Reprinted with permission of Legacy Health System, Portland Oregon.

Figure 6.1 (continued)

Imbalance	Lab Values	Etiology	Clinical S/S	Treatment
Hyperphos-phatemia	PO_4 >6.0mg % May see hypocalcemia	1. Renal dysfunction 2. Hypoparathyroidism 3. Excessive PO_4 intake	**CNS:** Seizures, depression, psychoses **Neuromuscular:** Paresthesia, muscle cramps, tetany, hyperreflexia **Cardiovascular:** Arrest **GI:** Nausea/vomiting, diarrhea **Integumentary:** Circumoral, paresthesia, cataracts, keratitis, dry skin, brittle nails, alopecia, soft tissue calcification **Skeletal:** Pathologic fractures	1. Restrict PO_4 intake 2. Increase PO_4 binders
Hypophos-phatemia	PO_4 >3.6mg % May see hypercalcemia	1. Hyperparathyroidism 2. PO_4 binding drugs 3. Starvation	**CNS:** Lethargy **Neuromuscular:** Muscle weakness **GI:** Anorexia **Skeletal:** Mild bone pain	1. Increase dietary intake 2. Decrease PO_4 binders 3. Regulate Ca and vitamin D supplements
Elevated Alkaline Phosphatase	Alk Phos >250mU/ml	1. Liver, bone, kidney, and intestinal disease 2. Renal osteodystrophy	S/S of Ca/PO_4 imbalance	1. Correct Ca/PO_4 imbalance
Positive Hepatitis Surface/Core Antigen	HAA reactive	1. Hepatitis B	S/S of hepatitis B	1. Isolate patient & machine 2. Isolation for stool and blood
Metabolic Acidosis	Serum CO_2 <15mEq/L pH <7.35 May see hyperkalemia	1. Renal dysfunction - decreased H excretion - decreased HCO_3 reabsorption - decreased $H2PO_4$ and NH_4 formation 2. Hyperkalemia	**CNS:** Headache, drowsiness, confusion, coma, seizures **Neuromuscular:** Fatigue **Cardiovascular:** arrythmias **Respirations:** Deep and fast **GI:** Anorexia, nausea, vomiting **Integumentary:** Tissue hypoxia	1. IV $NaHCO_3$ 2. Bicarbonate dialysate 3. Oral $NaHCO_3$
Hypoalbuminemia	Albumin >3.5g/dl	1. Inadequate high biologic value protein 2. Nephrotic syndrome 3. Liver disease 4. Peritoneal dialysis	**GI:** Weight loss **Integumentary:** Third space fluid, muscle wasting **Cardiovascular:** Hypotension	1. Increase dietary intake of complete protein 2. Infuse albumin 3. Nutritional support
Uremia	BUN > 80mg % Creatinine >10mg %	1. Renal dysfunction 2. Excessive protein 3. GI bleeding	See "Body Systems Affected by Uremia"	1. Increase dialysis time 2. Decrease protein intake
Low BUN	BUN >60mg % May see hypo-albuminemia	1. Inadequate protein intake	1. Decreased muscle mass 2. Weight loss	1. Increase complete protein intake 2. Nutritional supplementation

Reprinted with permission of Legacy Health System, Portland Oregon.

References

Fedje L, Moore L, McNeely M: A role for oral nutrition supplements in the malnutrition of renal disease. *JRN* 6:198-202, 1996.

Hakim R, Levin N: Malnutrition in hemodialysis patients. *Am J Kidney Dis* 21:125-137, 1993.

Kopple, JD: Effect of nutrition on morbidity and mortality in maintenance dialysis patients. *Am J Kidney Dis* 24:1002-1009, 1994.

Kopple JD, Massry SG (Eds): *Nutritional Management of Renal Disease*. Baltimore , MD, Williams and Wilkins, 1997.

Lowrie EG, Lew NL: Death risk in hemodialysis patients: The predictive value of commonly measured variables and an evaluation of death rate differences between facilities. *Am J Kidney Dis* 15:458-482, 1990.

McCann L, Nelson P, Spinozzi N, et al (Eds*): Pocket Guide to Nutrition Assessment of the Renal Patient* (2nd Ed). New York, NY, National Kidney Foundation, 1998.

McCann L: Subjective global assessment as it pertains to the nutritional status of dialysis patients. *Dial Transplant* 25:190-202, 1996.

Mitch WE, Klahr S (Eds): *Nutrition and the Kidney* (2nd Ed). Boston, MA, Little Brown, 1993.

NKF-DOQI clinical practice guidelines for hemodialysis adequacy. *Am J Kidney Dis* 30:S15-S66, 1997.

NKF-DOQI clinical practice guidelines for nutrition in chronic renal failure. *Am J Kidney Dis* 35:(6)S2, 2000.

NKF-DOQI clinical practice guidelines for the treatment of anemia of chronic renal failure. *Am J Kidney Dis* 30:S192-S240, 1997.

Stover J (Ed): *A Clinical Guide to Nutrition Care in End-stage Renal Disease* (2nd Ed). The American Dietetic Association, 1994.

Wilkens KG, Schiro KB (Eds): *Suggested Guidelines for Nutrition Care of Renal Patients,* (2nd Ed). The American Dietetic Association, 1992.

Chapter 7
Water Treatment System (WTS)

Contributing Author:
Philip M. Varughese, BS, CHT

Chapter Outline

I. Purpose of Water Treatment System

A. Water plays a very important role in the hemodialysis process. Besides being one of the most aggressive polar solvents, water is also termed the universal solvent because it will, to a certain extent, dissolve anything to which it is exposed. Water serves as a solvent medium for both the preparation of dialysate and the establishment of healthy physiological balance.

B. The average dialysis patient is exposed to 400 - 500 liters of water per week. The various contaminants found in tap water and in concentrate used in dialysate preparation may enter the blood stream via the thin, non-selective, semi-permeable membrane. The non-selective diffusion of small molecule toxins across the membrane exposes these patients to the hazards of the chemical contaminants in the water used for dialysis treatment.

C. Dialysis patients have compromised urinary excretion and therefore are less able to excrete toxic substances in their urine. This diminished capacity, combined with the extensive exposure to water, places dialysis patients at a much greater risk to water-borne contaminants than the normal population.

D. The EPA passed the Safe Drinking Acts of 1974 and 1994 which regulate and control the standards of drinking water. In compliance with these regulations, municipal water treatment facilities add chemicals that can contaminate and foul water treatment systems (WTS). The chemicals can be harmful to patients unless they are removed and the water is monitored on a regular basis. Although the treatment of municipal water by dialysis centers produces a safer and higher quality of water, malfunction of purification systems or human oversight can elicit additional hazards.

E. Concerns about the safety of dialysis water have arisen due to the increase in dialyzer reuse and bicarbonate dialysate. Fortunately, the ongoing advancement of reverse osmosis membrane technology has significantly improved the quality of dialysis water.

II. Contaminants Found in the Water

There are five major groups of contaminants:

A. Suspended material: sediment, suspended solids, sands, grit; can cause turbidity and colloid formation.

Suspended matters are expressed quantitatively in parts per million (ppm) by weight or milligram per liter (mg/l). The Silt Density Index (SDI) test is commonly used in dialysis units to measure the level of suspended solids in the feed water that tends to foul the water treatment system.

B. Inorganic materials: non-carbon based impurities.

e.g. calcium, magnesium, potassium, sodium, sulfates, nitrates, iron, copper, aluminum, manganese and fluoride.

Includes also trace elements, e.g. arsenic, barium, cadmium, lead, mercury, selenium, tin and zinc.

C. Organic materials: contain the element carbon; includes domestic waste, decayed plant animal waste, pesticides, herbicides and chloramine. Found in both plants and animals.

D. Microbiological contaminants: (bacteria, endotoxins, virus, algae). can be classified as viable and nonviable. Viable organisms are those that have the ability to reproduce and proliferate. Nonviable organisms cannot reproduce or multiply. Most microbiological contaminants found in water systems are gram-negative bacteria.

E. Dissolved gases: hydrogen sulfide (rotten egg odor), carbon dioxide, radon.

III. Signs and Symptoms Resulting from Improperly Treated Water Used for Dialysis

Contaminant	Toxic effects
Aluminum	Anemia
	Dialysis dementia
	Osteomalacia
	Bone diseases
Chloramine	Hemolysis
	Anemia
	Methemoglobinemia
Fluoride	Osteomalacia
	Osteoporosis
Calcium/Magnesium	Muscle Weakness
	Nausea and Vomiting
Copper	Hemolysis
	Liver damage
Zinc	Anemia
Nitrates	Methemoglobinemia
	Hypotension
Microbial/endotoxin	Pyrogenic reaction
	Infection
Sulfates	Nausea, Vomiting
	Metabolic acidosis

IV. Chemical Contaminants in Water with Documented Toxicity:

A. Aluminum Sulphate (Alum) is a flocculent added to water by the municipal supplier. Alum coagulates suspended materials for filtration. Exposure of the hemodialysis patient to high levels of aluminum in the water used for hemodialysis can result in a progressive, often fatal, syndrome of neurological deterioration and encephalopathy. Aluminum has also been associated with bone diseases such as osteomalacia, and osteodystrophy characterized by progressive bone pain, myopathy, and generalized weakness.

B. Chloramine is used as a bactericidal agent in municipal water treatment. They are powerful oxidants which denature hemoglobin by direct oxidation. Exposure to chloramine in the hemodialysis setting has been associated with hemolysis, hemolytic anemia and methemoglobinemia, a condition on which hemoglobin is unable to carry oxygen. Chloramine is produced by reacting chlorine with ammonia. Chlorine used for disinfection reacts with organic matter to form trihalomethanes which can cause cancer; therefore the less reactive chloramine is the agent most commonly used.

C. Fluoride is often added to the water supply during municipal treatment because of its efficacy in prevention of cavities in teeth. It has been suggested that even the recommended level of 4.0mg/l maximum in drinking water and 0.2 mg/l in dialysate water may lead to osteomalacia and bone disease in dialysis patients. Prolonged exposure may cause bone disease.

D. Copper: Leaching of copper in acidic water may result in symptoms such as chills, nausea, and headache as well as liver damage and hemolysis.

E. Zinc: The use of galvanized iron in the water treatment or distribution system can result in high zinc concentrations in the water used for dialysate preparation. The toxic consequences of zinc exposure include nausea, vomiting, fever, and anemia.

F. Nitrate: The use of fertilizers in both rural and urban settings can contribute to nitrate contamination. Methemoglobinemia, cyanosis, hypotension, and hemolytic anemia have also been reported due to nitrate contamination.

G. Calcium/Magnesium: The presence of calcium and magnesium ions is responsible for hard water. The use of hard water for hemodialysis has resulted in hard water syndrome characterized by nausea, vomiting, muscular weakness, skin flushing, and hypertension or hypotension. Hard water can also contribute to the formation of mineral deposits, and scaling on pipes and RO membranes.

H. Microbiological Contamination: The purest water is most susceptible to bacterial growth. It is crucial to maintain bacterial growth at the minimum concentration set by AAMI standards. A high level of gram negative bacteria can result in pyrogenic reaction. Dead bacteria leave behind endotoxins, which induce pyrogenic toxicities including fever, chills, shaking, and hypotension.

I. Endotoxin, a bacterial lipopolysaccharide, is released from bacterial cell walls when the organism dies. They are large molecules (100,000 daltons) and because of their size, they cannot pass through the dialyzer membrane under normal circumstances. However, a large volume of endotoxins in the dialysate can stimulate production of a pyrogenic substance called interleukin-1.

V. Essential Components of the Water Treatment System:

Distribution System *(See Figure 7.1)*

In early years, dialysis centers used tap water to prepare dialysate. However the use of tap water was found to complicate the dialysis process by inducing a variety of medical complications, including hard water syndrome, aluminum dementia, fluoride and chloramine poisoning and toxicities mentioned in the preceding section. Since the publication of AAMI guidelines, nearly all dialysis centers have incorporated the use of some water purification equipment in order to insure that they meet AAMI regulations/standards. The water system technology has progressed from the simple installation of a water filter to a more advanced and effective system which incorporates prefilters, softeners, carbon filters, reverse osmosis deionization and ultrafiltration components.

A. Temperature Blending Valve

The temperature blending valve is used to mix hot and cold incoming water to provide the desired water temperature in a reverse osmosis unit. This blending should be carefully monitored with a temperature gauge, to maintain at 72°F to 80°F. For optimum performance, water temperature should be maintained at 77°F. R.O membranes work most effectively at this temperature. Colder temperatures

will reduce the permeate flow of the R.O. system. Water that is too hot (>100°F) may damage R.O membranes and cause hemolysis if the hemodialysis machine does not alarm for high temperature.

B. Pre-Filtration

Pre-filtration is used to protect the equipment from becoming inoperable due to mechanical plugging or fouling. Silt Density Index (SDI) can be used to measure performance ability of water to plug a 0.45 micron filter within any given time. For water purification, feed water SDI levels should be less than five. This will minimize membrane fouling and increase the required clearing interval. There are two basic mechanisms of filtration,

- depth filtration

- surfacefiltration

Depth filtration removes particles from water by mechanically trapping them in the top layer of the filter media. Surface filters trap and remove suspended particles on the surface.

1. Sand Filtration:

   a) Sand filtration is used to remove turbidity. Typical sand filters have an average filtration rate between 10 to 50 microns. Silt Density Index (SDI) can be used to measure performance ability of water to plug a 0.45 micron filter within a given time.

Figure 7.1

Water Treatment with Holding Tank

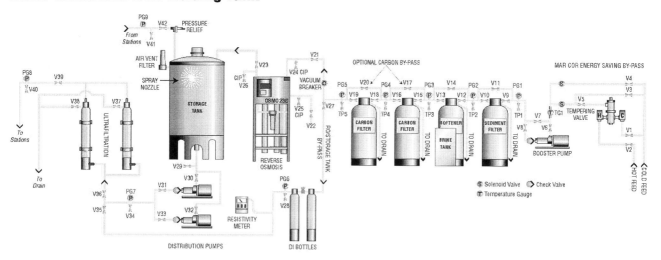

Reprinted courtesy of Mar Cor Services

Figure 7.2

Direct Feed System

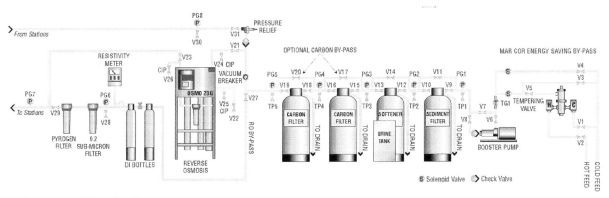

Reprinted courtesy of Mar Cor Services

2. Bed Filtration:
   a) Bed Filters are multimedia filters constructed of multiple layers that effectively remove particulate matter from water. The use of multiple layers enables the retention of increasingly small particles, therefore, the filtration process is spread throughout the bed and is used to its fullest extent.

3. Cartridge Filtration:
   a) Cartridge filters consist of a cylindrical cartridge with a central drainage core; they can be depth filtration, surface filtration, or

a combination of both. The materials of the filter element vary, but commonly include materials such as cotton, polypropylene and acrylics. The configuration of the filter element can also vary from woven string elements, pleated, bonded polymer meshes, etc.

4. Membrane Filtration:
   a) Membrane filters, which consist of a thin sheet of material perforated by small channels or pores, also operate by surface filtration. Ideally, the membrane will retain those materials whose size is greater than the pore size of the membrane, while allowing smaller particles to pass. Membranes are typically fabricated from a variety of polymers, including cellulose, nylon and acrylics.

C. Water Softeners

A water softener is an ion exchange device that is used to remove calcium, magnesium and other polyvalent cations from the feed water and exchange them for sodium. In the case of high calcium and high magnesium, a condition known as hardwater syndrome can result causing nausea and vomiting during dialysis. Hard water can foul R.O. membranes and distribution pipes.

A softener has four major components: resin tank, resin, brine tank to hold sodium chloride, and a valve or controller.

1. During ion exchange (softening), softeners retain calcium and magnesium while releasing sodium, and sodium levels increase in proportion to the amount of calcium and magnesium retained.

Figure 7.3

Schematic Representation of Softening

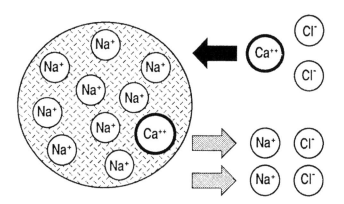

Calcium from calcium chloride being exchanged for sodium which forms sodium chloride

Source: NANT Water Treatment Manual, *p. 100, fig. 6.11.*

2. Resins beads in the softener tank are saturated with sodium chloride. The resin has a greater affinity for multivalent ions than it does for sodium. During the service cycle, the hard water is passed through the resin tank as calcium and magnesium ions adhere to the resin. When most of the sodium ions have been replaced by multivalent ions, the resin is exhausted and must be regenerated.

3. During a regeneration cycle, a concentrated solution of brine (NaCl) is passed through the

exhausted cation resin. The high concentration of sodium ions forces the resin to release the calcium, magnesium, and other positively charged contaminants and replace them with sodium ions.

4. Hardness is used to describe the total concentration of calcium and magnesium, expressed as mg/l of calcium carbonate or as the equivalent concentration of calcium carbonate in grains. (*Grains per gallon and parts per million as calcium carbonate are two common ways to do*

Figure 7.4

Water Softener

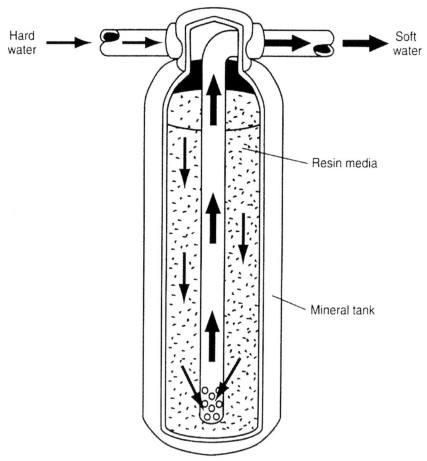

Inside a portable water softener, such as this one, "hard water" mineral ions (calcium and magnesium which form scale) are traded for sodium chloride ions in a process called ion exchange. A bed of resin media beads attracts and holds calcium and magnesium ions, and releases sodium ions into the water. The water that results is called "soft."

Reprinted with permission from AMGEN *Core Curriculum, p. 25, fig. 8.*

---

so in the water treatment industry). Grains per gallon expressed as calcium carbonate can be converted into metric units (mg/l) by multiplying the former by 17.1 and it can be converted into mEq/l by multiplying by 0.342. Soft water contains less than 1 grain per gallon or 17.1 parts per million of hardness expressed as calcium carbonate.

Since the primary purpose of a softener is to remove calcium and magnesium, daily monitoring for hardness breaks is necessary. Routine monitoring of the brine tank is critical since lack of brine indicates no regeneration will take place and routine checking of the softening timer is important. Checking the softening timer and valve function is critical in preventing regeneration during dialysis which may cause fatal hypernatremia.

D. Carbon Filtration

1. Carbon Filtration is commonly used to remove chlorine, Chloramine, undesirable organic contaminants, and odor from water. Granular activated carbon (GAC) is prepared by the pyrolysis of a variety of organic materials such as coal, wood, bones, nut shell or pulp waste. Exposing a carbon containing material to high temperatures in the absence of oxygen creates "activated carbon."

2. In dialysis, carbon adsorption is used to remove two kinds of contaminants: toxins, such as chloroform, and reactive agents such as hypochlorite. Free chlorine can combine with organic chemicals in the water to form carcinogenic compounds known as trihalomethanes. Activated carbon is a sorbent that attracts or retains substances by adsorption.

3. The presence of chloramine in dialysate may cause hemolytic anemia and methmpglobinemia, a condition which inhibits hemoglobin in the red cell from efficiently carrying oxygen.

4. To monitor the carbon beds, a protocol should be established to measure the total and free chlorine prior to each shift of patients to verify that the chlorine and chloramine levels fall below the 0.5 mg/l and 0.1 mg/l.

5. Carbon tanks must be placed in series with the first tank as the "working tank" and the second tank as the "polishing tank."

Figure 7.5

Permanent Softener

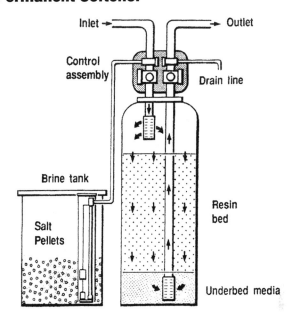

Source: NANT Water Treatment Manual, p. 104, fig. 6.13.

Carbon tanks should be sized to maintain a total empty bed contact time (EBCT) between 6 and 10 minutes.(3 to 5 minutes for each of the working and polishing tanks)

6. The FDA recommends that two tanks filled with GAC be used in series. Each tank should have an EBCT of 3-5 minutes. When the first GAC filter has a chloramine concentration in effluent sample>0.1 mg/l, it should be replaced within 72 hours. If the chloramine level in the effluent of the second tank exceeds 0.1mg/l, the water must not be used for dialysis.

7. The EBCT is used as a measure of how much contact time occurs between activated carbon, and water as the water flows through a bed of the particles.

   a) $EBCT = V_m/Q$
   where V_m is the volume of particles in the carbon tank and Q =Volumetric flow rate of the water.

   If carbon volume is expressed in cubic feet, water flow must be in cubic feet per minute.

   The required dimensions of a carbon bed can be estimated from the water flow and the recommended EBCT.

(1) The volume of carbon required (V, ft³) is calculated from

V= (Q x EBCT) / 7.48

where Q is the water flow rate (gal/min), and 7.48 is the number of gallons contained in one cubic foot of space(ft³)

8. The carbon tanks should be rotated with fresh carbon. This can be done by rotating the polishing tank (second tank) to the working tank (first tank) position, and installing new carbon in the polishing tank position. This is possible only when using portable exchange units or back washing systems with hoses set up for rotation.

9. It is desirable to rotate the tank periodically even if breakthrough is not detected. The polishing tank has a relatively low flow through it, and all the chlorine is removed in the working tank, creating potential for bacterial growth. As carbon continues to adsorb organic materials, the accumulation will create an enriched environment, serving as an excellent incubator for bacterial growth and build up. It is for this reason that carbon should be replaced as a routine course of system maintenance.

10. Back washing: The flow in the carbon tank is reversed periodically to "rebed" and clean the carbon and prevent water channeling. Backwashing will not regenerate carbon.

E. Reverse Osmosis

1. Reverse Osmosis (R.O.) is a form of water purification treatment which utilizes the rejection characteristics of ion exclusion membranes. R.O. applies the principles of high hydrostatic pressure across a semipermeable

Figure 7.6

Overview of Osmosis and Reverse Osmosis

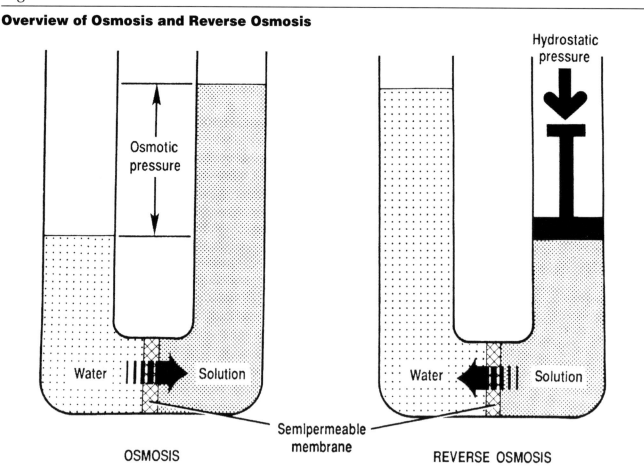

Source: NANT Water Treatment Manual, *p. 82, fig. 6.7.*

membrane to a solution to prepare a purified solvent. This process rejects 90 to 95% of univalent ions and 95-99% of divalent ions. This process rejects 99.9% of virus, bacteria and pyrogens. R.O. membranes repel ions and mechanically screen out biological contaminants. It is much more energy-efficient compared to distillation and the ion exchange system.

2. In normal osmosis, water molecules will flow from areas of higher water concentration to those of lesser water concentration in order to establish an ionic (osmotic pressure) equilibrium. On the other hand, in reverse osmosis, water flows from regions of low water concentration (high salt concentration) to regions of high water concentration (low salt concentration). *[See Chapter 14, Section VI, A., 3), c, page 196]*

In R.O. the hydraulic pressure overcomes the osmotic pressure, hence the name reverse osmosis.

3. R.O. Systems are composed of three major components, (a) R.O. membrane, (b) the pressure source and (c) the system control mechanisms.

a) A variety of R.O. membranes are available to accommodate varying water conditions and requirements. These membranes come in two major configurations.

 (1) hollow fiber membrane -where thousands of fibers are closely bundled in each housing; pressurized feed water flows slowly over the outside of the fibers and pure water permeates to the center.

 (2) spiral wound membrane- this design allows for optimum membrane surface area and fluid dynamics to produce a high permeate flow. This feature dramatically reduces fouling, thereby enhancing performance and membrane life.

 (3) R.O. membrane technology advanced greatly in the late 1970's, with the development of thin film composite (TFC) membranes which offered several advantages over the earlier used membranes. R.O. pre-treatment failure can cause the membrane to foul, scale or stop producing water at the required flow rate. R.O. membrane performance must be monitored daily. Percent rejection monitoring can be used as a tool to test the performance of the R.O. membrane. Percent rejection measures the product total dissolved solute (TDS)

Figure 7.7

Schematic Representation of Ion Exchange

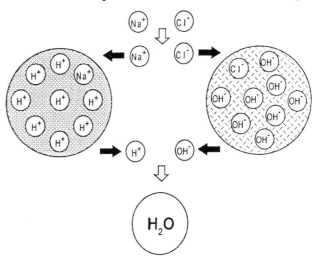

Source: NANT Water Treatment Manual, *p. 109, fig. 6.15.*

Figure 7.8

Portable Mixed Bed Deionizer

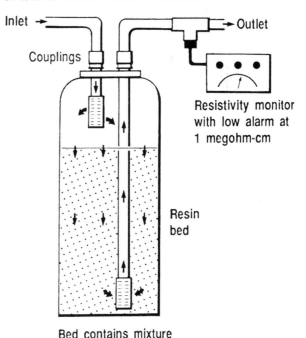

Source: NANT Water Treatment Manual, *p. 110, fig. 16.6.*

against the feed water T.D.S. Because the ion exclusion rate of a membrane is a function of the feed water ion concentration, it is important to monitor changes within the feed water to understand the impact of the final product. Minimum rejection levels should be established to avoid exceeding the AAMI standards. Monitoring a downward trend on percentage rejection should be an indicator for membrane cleaning or replacement to avoid potential problems.

b) The pressure source is the second major component. This pressure source drives water through the R.O. membrane. For R.O. to function effectively in the water purification process, the pressure must exceed the natural osmotic pressure that exists in the feed water. The higher the salt concentration in the water, the more hydrostatic pressure is necessary to drive reverse osmosis. For example, regular tap water membranes may require pressure between 30 to 300 psi, while brine or sea water membranes require pressures as high as 800 psi.

c) The R.O. system control mechanisms can vary from a very simple on and off switch to a microprocessor controlled unit. Standard control packages contain pre-treatment

Figure 7.9

Advantages and Disadvantages of R.O. Membranes

Type of R.O Membrane	Advantages	Disadvantages
Cellulose Acetate	Have been around a long time Softener sometimes not required Moderate chlorine tolerance (1-5ppm)	pH excursions outside 5-7 will destroy membranes Low flux Not very cleanable Moderate to low rejection
Thin Film Composite	Moderately good flux (15-25) High rejection Somewhat cleanable fouling Wide pH operating range Softener sometimes not required	Pressure limited (225) Not resistant to silt Virtually no chlorine tolerance
Polysulfone/ High Flux	Very high flux Can be run at 400 psi Very cleanable (pH2-12) Resistant to silt fouling Wide pH operating range (3-11) High rejection Chlorine sanitizable (100 ppm)	Must use softener

Figure 7.10

Typical Configuration of Deionizers

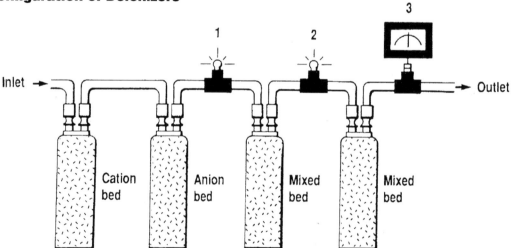

Typical configuration for deionizers used as primary purification. (1) "Light" type resistivity indicator is lit at greater than 50 000 ohm-cm. (2) "Light" type resistivity indicator is lit at greater than 1 megohm-cm. (3) Temperature compensated resistivity monitor produces audible and visible alarm at less than 1 megohm-cm.

Source: NANT Water Treatment Manual, *p. 112, fig.16.18.*

component interfacing, conductivity monitors and pressure and temperature monitors. There is also a monitor to measure the quality of product water as well as the rejection rate. Proper installation of audio and visual alarms is mandatory to alert staff in case of malfunction. The components of the R.O. system should be compatible with disinfectant agents. It is critical to realize that areas of dead space or stagnation will facilitate bacterial growth and disinfection will be difficult.

F. Deionization

1. Deionization (DI) is a process that exchanges ions in a solution. Like water softeners, deionizers also work by the ion-exchange principles. However, deionizers remove all types of cations and anions, whereas in the softening process, hardness ions (calcium and magnesium) are removed and replaced with sodium ions.

a) A cation resin is necessary to remove positively charged ions and an anion resin is essential in removing negatively charged ions. In a DI tank, hydrochloric acid (HCl) and sodium hydroxide (NaOH) are used as regeneration chemicals.

Figure 7.11

FDA-Recommended Features of Water Purification System

Component/System	Feature
Reverse Osmosis	• A Total Dissolved Solids (TDS) indicator should be provided for product quality as well as percent rejection. • The TDS alarm should be temperature compensated. • Whenever the product quality alarm is activated, there should be an audible and visible alarm in the treatment area and permeate flow should divert to drain. • All water contact materials should be appropriate for this use and should pass a leachables test.
Deionization	• A temperature compensated, resistivity monitoring alarm with audio and visual alarms should be provided to indicate bed exhaustion. Resistivity should be >1meg/cm and the conductivity should be <1 microsiemen/cm. • Ultrafilters or submicron filters should be provided on the product water output line for removal of bacteria and endotoxins. • If used for primary purification, flow should divert to drain in the event of bed exhaustion, and an alarm should be seen and heard in the patient care area. • Deionization should only be used when carbon filters are installed for pretreatment (to prevent formation of nitrosamines). • All water contact materials should be appropriate for this use and should pass a leachables test. • Do not use industrial or process resin. • Divert waterflow to drain if resistivity <1meg ohm/cm
Carbon Filters	• There should be a 6 minute empty-bed contact time (EBCT) for chlorine removal and a 10-minute EBCT for chloramine removal. • Two tanks should be installed in series (i.e. worker/polisher configuration), and after every shift, chlorine/chloramine should be monitored using the sample valve in between the tanks. • Media iodine number ≥900.
Water Softeners	• Regeneration lockouts should be included. Use pellet salt designed for softeners and check hardness before dialysis. • Recommend regeneration timers be visible.
Complete System	• Product water must meet all applicable industry and government standards and should pass a leachables test. • Failure analysis of the complete system must demonstrate safe operation in the event of a single component failure. • Each component of the system must be labeled with the name and address of the supplier. • The user must be supplied with clear and adequate instructions for startup, monitoring, maintenance, and troubleshooting of the system.
Sediment Filters	• Remove particulates down to 5 microns. • Use opaque housing to prevent algae growth.
Ultrafilters (UF)	• Remove bacteria and endotoxins. • Cross flow recommended • Use opaque housing to prevent algae growth.
Ultraviolet (UV)	• Destroys bacteria, potential to release endrotoxins. • Online monitor for radiant energy output. • Follow with UF
Storage Tanks	• Conical or bowl shaped bottom; 0.2 micron hydrophobic air vent fitter • Easy access for effective disinfection.

Figure 7.12

Hemodialysis water quality: Chemical contaminant levels[a]

Maximum allowable chemical contaminant levels in water used to prepare dialysate and concentrates and to reprocess dialyzers for multiple use.

Contaminant	Maximum Concentration (mg/L)[b]
Calcium	2 (0.1 mEq/L)
Magnesium	4 (0.3 mEq/L)
Potassium	8 (0.2 mEq/L)
Sodium	70 (3.0 mEq/L)
Antimony	0.006
Arsenic	0.005
Barium	0.10
Beryllium	0.0004
Cadmium	0.001
Chromium	0.014
Cyanide	0.02
Lead	0.005
Mercury	0.0002
Selenium	0.09
Silver	0.005
Aluminum	0.01
Chloramines	0.10
Free chlorine	0.50
Copper	0.10
Fluoride	0.20
Nitrate (as N)	2.00
Sulfate	100.00
Thallium	0.002
Zinc	0.10

[a] The physician has the ultimate responsibility for ensuring the quality of water used for dialysis.

[b] Unless otherwise noted.

Source: NANT Water Treatment Manual, Appendix E, Table B.1

b) Cation deionization resins release hydrogen (H^+) in exchange for cations such as, sodium (Na^+), potassium (K^+), and magnesium (Mg^{2+}). Anion resin exchanges hydroxide (OH^-) ions for anions such as bicarbonate (HCO_3^-), chloride (Cl^-), and sulfate (SO_4^-). The resulting process leaves only H^+ and OH^-, which will combine to form water (H_2O).

c) Deionizer efficacy is monitored by measuring the resistivity of the effluent. As resistivity varies with temperature, resistivity monitors must be temperature compensated to measure the resistivity units known as ohms-cm. The higher the purity of the water, the higher the resistance to passage of electrical current. AAMI standards specify that product water should have a specific resistivity of >1mΩ-cm at 25°C, ultrapure water is measured at 18.3 mΩ-cm at 25°C. This translates to an ionic quality level of around 0.020ppm. Audible and visual alarms must be used and placed between the worker and polishing DI units, in case of malfunction or tank exhaustion.

d) There are two basic forms of deionization,
   (1) two bed and
   (2) mixed bed.
      (a) Two bed-dual bed deionizers have separate tanks for cation and anion resins.
      (b) In mixed bed deionizers, the two resins are blended together in a single tank. The mixed bed system produces better quality than the dual-bed or two bed system, but it is more expensive.

e) DI does not remove bacteria, pyrogen, colloids or particulate material. DI may in fact become a breeding ground for bacteria due to the low flow rate. Therefore, ultrafiltration is required following the deionization of a system.

f) DI system must be monitored closely to prevent contaminants from passing through. When the DI system is exhausted, previously adsorbed ions can be released into the effluent, causing ion related toxicities. Reports of fluoride, aluminum and copper intoxication have all appeared as consequences of unrecognized DI exhaustion.

g) DI resin must be regenerated by a water treatment vendor specializing in dialysis.

h) It is recommended that DI tanks be installed in recirculation loops to prevent stagnation and minimize microbial growth.

VI. AAMI Standards

See figure 7.12

VII. Monitoring of the System

A. Consistency and testing frequency are two key factors in every monitoring program. Monitoring requires collection and review of data on a continual basis. Not only does monitoring provide useful information on quality of water coming in and leaving the treatment system, it also monitors the performance of the individual components in the system and alerts the user to any changes that occur within the system.

Monitoring can be divided into three areas:
1. Feed water quality
2. Product water quality
3. Individual components.

1. Feed water:

   The composition of the available feed water sets the basis for the design of a water purification system. Therefore, any major changes in the feed water composition will most likely necessitate a change in the water treatment system.

2. Product water:

   The final determinant in the effectiveness of any water treatment system is the quality of the product water and whether or not it meets the acceptable standards. Conductivity and resistance monitors serve as a day to day monitor of chemical contamination. Water product analysis should be performed on a regular basis as per unit protocol or when warranted by certain circumstances.

3. Individual components:

   a) A crucial aspect of monitoring is the use of logs to record values of the parameters of each of the components in the system. Monitoring logs are frequently the only written record of the performance of the water treatment system. It also assures compliance with AAMI standards. Because of the importance it may assume in certain circumstances, log maintenance and any reports of standards deviation should be clearly delineated.

   b) Water treatment monitoring logs should be simple and straightforward and easy to follow. All necessary monitoring parameters should be recorded, so they can later be used for trend analysis.

   c) The person documenting the readings should be aware of the acceptable ranges and properly trained to act upon any deviations in an appropriate and safe manner. It is highly recommended that log maintenance and the individual's knowledge be audited and validated periodically.

   On line and off line monitoring requires that components and functions be checked and recorded as per the protocol.

   d) Filters:

   Daily monitoring and recording the pressure drop (DP) across all system components, use Opaque housing and filters should be replaced as necessary. Regular recording of pressures will allow changes in equipment performance to be easily assessed.

   e) Carbon Adsorption Tank:

   AAMI recommends testing the chlorine/chloramine level with every patient shift. If

Figure 7.13

Factors Influencing Microbial and Endotoxin Contamination of Dialysis Water Treatment Devices

Device	Principle of Operation	Contamination Potential
Softener ion exchange	Exchanges calcium and magnesium cations for sodium ions. Protect against scaling of RO system	Reservoir for bacteria and endotoxins
Carbon Tank	Removes organics, chlorine and chloramine	Reservoir for bacteria and endotoxins
Deionizer	Removes all types of cations and anions	Reservoir for bacteria and endotoxins
Reverse Osmosis	Removes ions (univalent and divalent), bacteria and endotoxins	Can become colonized by bacteria
Ultraviolet light	Kills some bacteria; no chemical residual	UV-resistant bacteria can develop; does not remove endotoxins and may cause high endotoxin levels if bacteria are present

carbon tanks are used in series configuration, monitor chlorine/chloramine levels between the two beds. The first carbon (worker) tank should be replaced if any chlorine/chloramine is detected in the water sample.

f) Reverse Osmosis:

There are two important measures of R.O. performance:

(1) Percent rejection:

Percent rejection is a measure of the ability of the R.O. membrane to remove ionic contaminants.

Percent rejection = (1-Product water concentration/ Feed water concentration) x100

(2) Product water recovery: is the difference of the feed water flow rates and reject flow rates. In hemodialysis, most R.O. units operate with recoveries in the range of 30-50%.

However, in monitoring recovery, it is important to also monitor temperature of the feed water and the pressure difference across the R.O. membrane, since decreases in either of these will decrease the product water flow rate and the recovery.

g) Ion Exchange:

(1) Softener - In general, the hardness of effluent water from a softener should not exceed 10mg/l of calcium carbonate and the timer should be checked daily.

(2) Deionizer - Resistance is measured in units of ohm-centimeters. It indicates the concentration of ions in the water. In hemodialysis, the minimum specific resistance for product water from a deionizer is 1 million ohm-centimeters, or 1 megohm-cm (.500ppm). Because deionizers can produce dangerous effluents when exhausted, resistance should be monitored continuously, and both audible and visible alarms should activate if the resistance decreases below 1 megohm-cm.

VIII. Sample Collection

A. Sampling is an important technique in monitoring the quality of purified water

B. Samples should only be taken from designated areas.

C. There should be proper disinfection of the port before any sample collection.

D. Samples for determining the hardness of water leaving a softener is best collected at the end of the day as opposed to in the morning. This time is suggested because most softeners are regenerated during the night and expected to produce soft water in the morning, whereas their capacity may be expended by the end of the day if they are undersized.

E. Meticulous care must be taken to avoid sample contamination, particularly for samples for microbiological testing. Colony count measures the amount of living bacteria in the water.

1. Clean the surface of the outlet to the sampling port with bactericidal agent.

2. Open the sampling valve and allow at least one liter of water to run to waste.

3. Collect a clean catch sample in a sterile container and close the valve.

a) Samples for microbiological testing should be processed within 60 minutes or stored in a refrigerator and processed within 24 hours. According to the AAMI guidelines, tryptic soy agar is recommended to culture water samples for 48 hours at 37°C. The sample should be placed in the agar with a pipette rather than a calibrated loop, since the loop will only allow for a small sample that will not meet test sensitivity needed in culturing dialysis fluids. Blood agar and standard plate count agar were used previously, but these media were later found to be ineffective in culturing microorganisms associated with bicarbonate concentrate based fluids.

b) The LAL (Limulus Amebocyte Lysate) assay measures endotoxins in endotoxin units/ml (EU/ml). Endotoxins are the toxic compounds released by living bacteria and the decomposition of dead bacteria. 1 nanogram/ml is equal to 5 endotoxin units/ml (EU/ml). The current thought by the AAMI committee members is that the total viable count of microorganisms per ml be lowered from 200 CFU /ml to 100 and to set action limits at 50 CFU /ml. All dialysis water will be required to have an endotoxin concentration of < 5 EU/ml with an action level of 2EU/ml.

IX. Disinfection

A. The primary microbial contaminants of dialysis fluids are naturally occurring water bacteria. These include gram-negative bacteria and non-tuberculous mycobacteria. These bacteria can survive and multiply in water containing little organic matter, such as DI or R.O. treated water. They pose a significant health risk to dialysis patients because of the endotoxins created by the dead bacteria -lipopolysaccharide (LPS), endotoxin is lipid A, which is a piece of the outer membrane LPS of gram-negative bacteria. LipidA/endotoxin is very toxic and is released when the bacterial cell undergoes lysis (destruction).

B. Disinfection strategies for the HD system are targeted at gram-negative bacteria. Bacteria are colorless and colorful stains have been developed to visualize them. The Gram stain separates organisms in to 2 groups; gram-positive bugs and gram-negative bugs. When the slide is studied under a microscope, cells that absorb the crystal violet stain (a blue dye) and hold onto it will appear blue. These are called gram-positive organisms. However, if the alcohol washes off the crystal violet, these cells will absorb the safranin and appear red. These are called gram-negative organisms.

C. Although bacteria may be inactivated by exposure to chemical germicides, bacterial endotoxins may remain in the WTS. Though endotoxins are produced by bacteria, they can persist despite the absence of bacteria. Although nontuberculous mycobacterium does not produce endotoxins, it is more resistant to chemical germicides than gram negative bacteria. They have been responsible for many patients' infections as a result of an inadequately disinfected dialyzer.

D. Sterilization is a procedure that leads to the total destruction of microorganisms, including highly resistant bacteria spores.

E. Disinfection is defined as a process that eliminates most recognizable bacterial organisms but not necessarily the more resistant microorganisms. Disinfection processes can be either high-level or low-level (Sanitization) depending on germicidal activity. High-level Disinfection inactivates all microorganisms except bacterial spores. Low-level Disinfection inactivates many, but not all, microorganisms and reduces the bacterial population to a level considered safe, but will produce endotoxin.

F. Endotoxins can cause pyrogenic reactions that elicit symptoms including chills, fever, hypotension, headache, nausea, vomiting and leukopenia followed by leukocytosis. The symptoms usually begin 30-60 minutes into the dialysis treatment and unless they are very severe, stop shortly after the treatment.

G. Disinfectants:

1. Chlorine, formaldehyde, glutaraldehyde, ozone, peracetic acid, Ultraviolet light.

   Components that require disinfection:
   a) The R.O. system
   b) The distribution system
   c) The system for mixing concentrate
   d) The dialysis machines

2. Recommended disinfectants:
   a) Sodium hypochlorite, household bleach, is widely used to sanitize water purification systems and some types of R.O. membranes. 500ppm of chlorine efficiently kill almost all microorganisms, with 2 hours of contact time. (1part chlorine bleach in 100 parts water will give 500ppm). Chlorine is easy to rinse out of WTS. It is not compatible with ion exchange and most R.O. membranes.
   b) Formalin 4% is very effective to disinfect the WTS and membranes. Its is very stable and effective against a wide range of bacteria. However, because of health concerns and government regulations, this is not a widely used disinfectant.
   c) Peroxyacetic Acid (mincare) 1.0% (10,000ppm) is used to disinfect WTS and membranes. (1part with 100 parts of water). Recirculate and maintain a minimum contact time minimum of 1 hour.

3. Ultraviolet sterilization:

   UV sterilization is another form of disinfection to kill water bacteria. Water exposed to ultraviolet light will result in deactivation of DNA structure of bacteria and ultimate destruction. The water must be free of suspended solids in order for the UV rays to penetrate the water. Properly functioning UV systems are simple and reliable in significantly reducing the amount of bacteria. However, the dead bacteria can release LPS and endotoxins.

4. Ozone

Ozone (O_3) is a strong oxidizing agent and is twice as powerful an oxidant as chlorine. It is necessary to keep 1 ppm ozone residual maintained for 10 minutes in the WTS or 0.5 ppm for 20 minutes. The system can then be drained and refilled with RO water and recirculated. Ozone breaks down quickly and cannot be stored, so it must be added into water on a continuous basis. Ultraviolet can also be used to breakdown the ozone to oxygen. Water temperature, pressure and pH affect ozone concentration. Ozone destroys bacteria, viruses, cysts, and destroys endotoxins.

Suggested Readings

1. *AAMI Standards and Recommended Practices,* Volume 3, 1998 Edition

2. Amgen, Inc.(1992), *Core Curriculum for Dialysis Technicians*, Wisconsin: Medical Media Publishing, Inc.

3. Ameriwater 1998. *Water Technology Solutions,*

4. David M. Ward, *Water Disasters-pitfalls and precautions;* Contemporary Dialysis and Nephrology , December 1999.

5. Daugirdas, JT and Ing, TS, editors (1994), *Handbook of Dialysis,* Boston: Little, Brown and Co

6. Leuhmann, D.A.,et.al, (1989), *A Manual on Water Treatment for Hemodialysis*, National Association of Nephrology Technologists

7. Nuhad Ismail, Bryan N. Becker and Raymond M.Hakim; *Water Treatment for Hemodialysis,* American Journal of Nephrology 1996;16:60-72

Chapter 8
Medications

Contributing Author:

Joan Arslanian, MS, MPA, MSN, RN, CS, FNP, CNN

Chapter Outline

I. Medications Commonly Used by Patients with Renal Failure

A. Analgesics

B. Antacids and Phosphate Binders

C. Antianemic Drugs

D. Anticoagulants

E. Antihypertensives

F. Antimicrobials

G. Antipruritics

H. Cardiovascular Drugs

I. Chelating Agents

J. Electrolytes

K. Hypolipidemic Agents

L. Laxatives and Cathartics

M. Local Anesthetics

N. Potassium Ion Exchange Resin

O. Thrombolytic Agents

P. Vitamins

II. Common Complications during Dialysis and Their Management with Medications

A. Hypotension

B. Muscle Cramps

C. Nausea and Vomiting

D. Headache

E. Fever/Chills

F. Angina

G. Pruritis

III. Dialysis and Its Affect on Drug Therapy

I. Medications Commonly Used by Patients with Renal Failure

A. Analgesics

1. Overview

   a) Analgesics are medications used to relieve or control pain.

   b) Analgesics can be both narcotic and non-narcotic.

   c) Non-narcotic

      (1) Used for mild to moderate pain of the skeletal muscles and joints

      (2) Act on the peripheral nervous system at pain receptor sites

      (3) Most lower an elevated body temperature, thus having an antipyretic effect.

      (4) Some such as aspirin, have anti-inflammatory and anticoagulant effects as well. (Hemodialysis patient should not take aspirin unless specifically ordered by a physician.)

   d) Narcotic

      (1) Used for moderate to severe pain in the smooth muscles, organs, and bones

      (2) Act mostly in the central nervous system

      (3) Not only suppress pain impulses but can suppress respiration and coughing

2. Examples

   a) Non-narcotic

      (1) Acetaminophen (Tylenol)

      (2) Acetylsalicylic acid (aspirin)

      (3) Ibuprofen's (Motrin, Nuprin, Advil)

   b) Narcotic

      (1) Morphine

      (2) Codeine

      (3) Meperidine (Demerol)

      (4) Oxycodone (Percocet, Percodan)

   c) Route of Administration

      (1) PO

      (2) IV

      (3) IM

   d) Common Side Effects

      (1) Non-narcotic

         (a) Aspirin – gastric discomfort, tinnitus, vertigo, deafness, increased bleeding

         (b) Ibuprofens – gastric discomfort

         (c) Tylenol – high dosages can cause liver toxicity

      (2) Narcotic

         (a) Respiratory distress, orthostatic hypotension, drowsiness, mental cloudiness, constipation, papillary constriction, and withdrawal symptoms

   e) Considerations

      (1) Vital signs should be monitored closely.

      (2) The smallest effective dose should be administered to alleviate pain.

      (3) Most non-narcotic analgesics, except for acetaminophen, are removed by dialysis and should be avoided when managing pain in renal patients.

      (4) Most narcotics require no dosage adjustment and are not removed by dialysis.

B. Antacids and Phosphate Binders

1. Overview

   a) Systemic and non-systemic antacids

   b) Systemic antacids used to assist in treating metabolic acidosis

   c) Non-systemic antacids used to decrease the gastrointestinal effects of renal failure and to bind phosphorus in the intestinal tract

   d) The phosphorus in foods binds to the antacids, which prevents the phosphorus from crossing the intestinal wall. The bound phosphorus is excreted in the stool.

   e) Antacids are effective as phosphate binders only if they are taken with or immediately after meals.

   f) Calcium supplements increase the serum calcium levels and decrease the serum phosphorus level.

   g) Long-term use of antacids containing aluminum can cause dialysis dementia and aluminum bone disease.

   h) Antacids containing magnesium salts are contraindicated in patients with renal disease because of the risk of hypermagnesemia.

2. Examples

   a) Non-systemic

      (1) Aluminum hydroxide gel (Amphojel, Alternagel, Alutab)

      (2) Basic aluminum carbonate (Basaljel)

(3) Calcium carbonate (Oscal, Tums)

(4) Calcium acetate (PhosLo)

(5) Sevelamer hydrochloride (Renagel)

3. Route of Administration

a) PO

4. Common Side Effects

a) Aluminum containing antacids – constipation, intestinal obstruction, aluminum intoxication, hypophosphatemia, osteomalacia

b) Calcium containing antacids – nausea, loss of appetite, constipation, cramping, continuous headache, muscle pain or twitching, and/or confusion

5. Considerations

a) Serum calcium and phosphorus levels should be monitored frequently.

b) Stool softeners are often prescribed to avoid problems with constipation.

c) Medication needs to be taken with meals in order to bind phosphorus.

d) Other medications should be taken 1 hour before or 3 hours after Renagel to prevent possible binding that could alter the therapeutic effects of other drugs.

C. Antianemic Drugs

1. Anemia Overview

a) Anemia is a condition in which there is a deficiency in the number of RBCs or in the hemoglobin level within those cells.

b) Hemoglobin is a complex substance consisting of a large protein (globin) and an iron containing chemical referred to as heme.

c) The hemoglobin is contained inside the RBCs. Its function is to combine with oxygen in the lungs and transport it to all tissues of the body, where it is exchanged for carbon dioxide (which is transported back to the lungs where it can be excreted).

d) A lack of either RBCs or hemoglobin may result in an inadequate supply of oxygen to various tissues.

e) New RBCs have to be constantly formed. They are produced in the bone marrow, with both vitamin B12 and folic acid playing an important role in their formation. A sufficient amount of iron is also necessary for the formation and maturation of RBCs.

2. Iron Preparations

a) Overview

(1) These medications are usually a complex of iron and another substance and are normally taken by mouth.

(2) The amount absorbed from the GI tract depends on the dose administered; the largest dose that can be tolerated without causing side effects is given. Under certain conditions, iron compounds must be given parenterally particularly when there is some disorder limiting the amount of drug absorbed from the intestine or when the patient is unable to tolerate oral iron.

(3) Iron is an essential mineral normally supplied in the diet.

(4) Iron salts and other preparations supply additional iron to meet the needs of the patient.

(5) Iron is absorbed from the GI tract through the mucosal cells where it combines with the protein transferrin. This complex is transported in the body to bone marrow where iron is incorporated into hemoglobin.

(6) How well iron is absorbed depends on the iron salts taken and on the degree of iron deficiency.

(7) Under normal circumstances, iron is well conserved by the body although small amounts are lost through shedding of skin, hair, and nails and in feces, perspiration, urine, breast milk, and during menstruation.

b) Uses

(1) Prophylaxis and treatment of iron deficiency anemia

(2) Patients receiving Epoetin alfa (Epogen) therapy (Failure to give iron supplements either IV or PO can impair the response Epoetin has hematologically.)

c) Examples

(1) Ferrous sulfate (PO)

(2) Ferrous gluconate (PO)

(3) Iron dextran (IV, IM)

(4) Ferric gluconate (IV)

(5) Iron sucrose (IV)

d) Common side effects

(1) Constipation, nausea, abdominal cramps, anorexia, vomiting and diarrhea

e) Considerations

(1) Administered PO, IV, IM

(2) Eggs and milk inhibit absorption of iron. Also coffee and tea taken with a meal or one hour after may significantly inhibit absorption of dietary iron.

(3) Ingestion of calcium and iron supplements with food can decrease iron absorption.

(4) Iron absorption is not decreased if calcium carbonate is used and it is taken between meals.

(5) Patient may complain of indigestion, change in stool color (black and tarry or dark green), and constipation.

3. Folic Acid

   a) Overview

   (1) Folic acid is necessary for normal production of RBCs and for synthesis of nucleoproteins. Synthetic folic acid is absorbed from the GI tract and stored in the liver.

   b) Uses

   (1) Prophylaxis and treatment of folic acid deficiency

   c) Common Side Effects

   (1) Allergies

   d) Administration

   (1) PO, IM, IV, deep SC

4. Epoetin alfa – recombinant (Epogen)

   a) Overview – erythropoietin

   (1) Erythropoietin (EPO) is a glycoprotein produced by the kidney that stimulates red blood cell production in response to decreased oxygen to body tissues (hypoxia).

   (2) Specifically, EPO stimulates the division and differentiation of committed red blood cell progenitors (parent cell destined to become circulating red blood cells) in the bone marrow.

   (3) Epoetin alfa will elevate or maintain the red blood cell level, decreasing the need for blood transfusions.

   b) Side Effects in Chronic Renal Failure Patients

   (1) Headache; athralgias (joint pain); nausea; edema; fatigue; diarrhea; vomiting; chest pain; injection site skin reaction; weakness; dizziness; seizures; thromboses (clots); and allergic reactions

   c) Administration of

   (1) Both intravenously (IV push) or subcutaneously (SQ)

   d) Considerations

   (1) Blood pressure may rise in CRF patients receiving EPO during the early phase of treatment when the hematocrit (HCT) is rising.

   (2) The dose of Epoetin alfa should be reduced when the target hematocrit range (33% to 36%) is reached.

   (3) It is recommended that the dose of EPO be decreased if the HCT increase exceeds 4 points in any two week period.

   (4) A rise in HCT may cause increase vascular access clotting.

   (5) Patients may require increased heparinization during EPO therapy to prevent clotting of the dialyzer.

   (6) Patients iron stores should be evaluated during EPO therapy. Transferrin saturation (serum iron, multiplied by 100 divided by total iron binding capacity – TIBC) should be ≥ 20% and ferritin (the iron-apoferritin complex that is one of the chief forms in which iron is stored in the body) should be ≥ 100mg/dl. Iron supplements may be needed to increase and maintain transferrin saturation to support EPO-stimulated erythorpoiesis.

   (7) If the patient does not respond to or maintain a response, the following situations should be considered and evaluated:

   (a) Iron deficiency

   (b) Underlying infections, inflammatory or malignant processes

   (c) Occult blood loss

   (d) Underlying hematologic (blood) disease

   (e) Folic acid or Vitamin B12 deficiency

   (f) Hemolysis

   (g) Aluminum toxicity

   (8) EPO therapy may also have possible long-term hazards – hypertensive cardiovascular disease, electrolyte abnormalities, and decreased dialysis effectiveness.

5. Darbepoetin alfa (Aransep)

a) Overview

(1) Indicated for the treatment of anemia associated with chronic renal failure (CRF) including patients on or not on dialysis.

(2) Longer serum half-life than Epoetin alfa (3 time longer terminal half-life) and greater biological activity than epoetin alfa.

(3) Achieves and maintains target hemoglobin levels with less frequent dosing than epoetin alfa.

b) Side effects

(1)_Infection

(2) Hypertension

(3) Hypotension

(4) Myalgia

(5) Headache

(6) Diarrhea

c) Administration

(1) Both intravenous (IV) or subcutaneous (SQ)

d) Considerations

(1) Refer to 4. d.

Figure 8.1

Coagulation Pathway

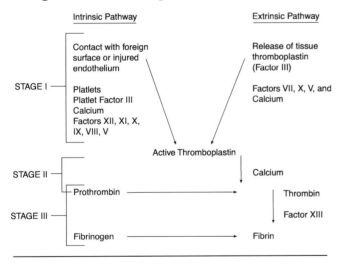

D. Anticoagulants

1. Blood Coagulation

a) Blood coagulation is a mechanism that results in the formation of a stable fibrin clot. The process is dependent upon a number of reactions involving interaction of clotting factors, platelets, and tissue materials. The coagulation process that generates thrombin consists of two pathways – the extrinsic and the intrinsic systems.

b) The extrinsic system is initiated by the activation of clotting Factor VII, and the release of tissue thromboplastin. The intrinsic system is triggered by the activation of clotting Factor XII, following its contact with a foreign surface or damaged endothelium. Both systems involve a number of reactions that transform various plasma factors to their active forms, ultimately producing thrombin. Thrombin plays a key role in coagulation – it speeds up the conversion of fibrinogen to fibrin. Thrombin also activates clotting Factor XIII (necessary for stabilizing the fibrin into an insoluble clot) as well as activating other blood clotting factors. If thrombin is not formed, or its function is impeded, coagulation is inhibited.

c) The coagulation pathway can be summarized as follows. (see Figure 8.1)

(1) Thromboplastin and other blood clotting factors help convert the protein prothrombin to thrombin.

(2) Thrombin mediates the formation of soluble fibrinogen to soluble fibrin.

(3) Soluble fibrin is converted to insoluble fibrin by activated fibrin-stabilizing factor. The insoluble fibrin forms a clot, trapping blood cells and platelets.

d) Drugs: Two types of drugs are used in preventing blood coagulation, heparin and the Vitamin K antagonists. Their mechanisms of action differ as to their clinical uses.

2. Warfarin Sodium: Oral anticoagulant

a) Examples

(1) Coumadin

(2) Panwarfin

b) Action

(1) Interferes with the synthesis of Vitamin K – dependent clotting factors resulting in depletion of clotting factors VII, IX, X, and II

(2) Has no direct effect on an established thrombus although therapy may prevent further extension of a formed clot as well as secondary thromboembolic problems

(3) Peak activity – 1.5 to 3 days

c) Uses

(1) To prevent blood from clotting in the patient's access

(2) Prophylaxis and treatment of venous thrombosis and pulmonary embolism

(3) Prophylaxis and treatment of atrial fibrillation with embolization

d) Adverse Effects

(1) The principle untoward reaction is hemorrhage. Therefore it is important to monitor the anticoagulant effect. Minor bleeding may be treated by withdrawal of the drug and administration of oral vitamin K. Severe bleeding requires greater doses of vitamin K given intravenously. Symptoms of hemorrhage include headache, paralysis, pain in the joints, abdomen, or chest; difficulty in breathing or swallowing; SOB, unexplained swelling and shock.

(2) Symptoms of overdose: Early symptoms include melena (black, tarry stools), petechiae (small, purplish, hemorrhage spots on the skin), microscopic hematuria (blood in the urine), oozing from superficial injuries (e.g., nicks from shaving, excessive bruising, bleeding from gums after brushing teeth), excessive menstrual bleeding.

e) Drug Interactions

(1) A number of drug interactions potentiate the anticoagulant effects of Warfarin, e.g., acetaminophen, nonsteroidal anti inflammatory agents (Motrin, Advil) increases the anticoagulant effects.

f) Monitoring

(1) Determination of PT, PTT, INR

(2) Desired range for patients will vary.

3. Anticoagulation During Dialysis

a) Purpose: To prevent blood clotting in the extracorporeal circuit, without loss of membrane efficiency, while avoiding anticoagulation bleeding complications in the patient.

b) Indications for anticoagulation

(1) Blood characteristics

(a) Uremia decreases platelet adhesiveness; dialysis can reverse this.

(b) Tendency to clot when in contact with foreign surfaces

(c) Platelet damage leads to coagulation of platelets, the release of platelet factor 3, and the accelerating activity of blood coagulation factors

(2) Dialyzer/membrane characteristics

(a) A foreign surface

(b) Cooler surface fosters fibrin formation

c) Agents and approaches to anticoagulation

(1) Heparin

(a) A systemic anticoagulant that is effective immediately

(b) Structure of heparin

(i) chemically, heparin is classified as a sulfated mucopolysaccharide (very high sulfuric acid content)

(ii) molecular weights range from 6,000 to 20,000

(iii) strongly acid, because of the number of sulfates

(iv) neutralized by strong basic compounds such as protamine, causing it to lose its anticoagulant properties

(c) Source of Heparin

(i) lung tissue of beef (bovine heparin)

(ii) intestinal mucosa of hogs (porcine heparin)

(iii) common concentration for hemodialysis is 1000 USP units per milliliter

(iv) milligram for milligram, pork intestinal heparin is more potent on the average than beef lung heparin

(v) potency stated on the label is accurate within $\pm$ 10% of the stated label value. For example, if in heparin with a stated label potency of 1000 USP units, the activity of the heparin in a particular vial may range from

900 USP units to 1100 USP units per ml. This is one of the variables which must be considered in the effective heparinization of hemodialysis patients.

(d) Effects of Heparin on Coagulation and Hemostasis

  (i) Deactivation of thrombin – it blocks the action of thrombin on fibrinogen.

  (ii) It retards the generation of thromboplastin and the conversion of prothrombin to thrombin.

  (iii) Reduction of platelet adhesiveness – it appears to prevent platelet agglutination in the intrinsic pathway.

(e) Variables to consider

  (i) Patient – related variables

    a. Past experience with heparin

    b. Clotting profile
      i. baseline clotting time
      ii. heparin sensitivity
      iii. heparin metabolic and elimination rates

    c. Platelet count

    d. Several states of health (particularly in respect to the risk of serious bleeding)

    e. Weight

    f. Type of access

    g. Certain medical conditions
      i. fever
      ii. infection
      iii. thrombophlebitis
      iv. infections with thrombosing tendency
      v. myocardial infarction
      vi. cancer
      vii. liver disease
      viii. coagulopathy

    h. Use of drugs such as
      i. aspirin or other antiplatelet agents
      ii. warfarin and other anticoagulants
      iii. digitalis
      iv. tetracyclines
      v. nicotine
      vi antihistamines

  (ii) Technical variables

    a. Variations of +/– 10% of stated label potency

    b. Types of dialyzer
      i. dialyzer design and flow geometry

    c. Type of dialyzer membrane

    d. Duration of dialysis

    e. Blood flow rates

    f. Dialysate/blood pH

    g. Occurrence of fibrin in the extracorporeal circuit

(f) Methods of Heparin Administration

  (i) Systemic

    a. Both patient and the extra-corporeal circuit are heparinized

    b. Continuous – heparin is delivered at a constant rate with an infusion pump which is connected to the inflow (arterial) blood line.

    c. Intermittent – injection of heparin on a periodic basis (usually hourly) after the loading dose has been given.

  (ii) Regional

    a. Heparinize only the blood circuit by pre-dialyzer infusion of heparin and simultaneous post dialyzer administration of protamine (strongly basic and acts by combining chemically with the strongly acid heparin to form a stable compound with no anticoagulant properties) to neutralize the heparin before it reaches the patient.

    b. Used for individuals with increased risk of hemorrhage, such as trauma or post-surgical patients

    c. Used primarily during acute dialysis

    d. Problems with heparin rebound after regional heparinization, a rebound state of anticoagulation may occur up to 10 hours later. This can lead to bleeding problems after dialysis.

e. Protamine can act as an anti-coagulant if more is given than is needed to neutralize heparin.

f. Protamine side effects include hypotension, bradycardia, dyspnea, bleeding tenderness, and hypersensitivity reactions.

(iii) Low dose or "tight" heparinization

a. Systemic administration (using either continuous or intermittent methods) of the minimal amount of heparin necessary to prevent clot formation in the dialyzer and lines and requires frequent heparin monitoring during the dialysis session.

b. This technique allows for dialysis of patients who have an increased risk of bleeding without having to use regional anticoagulation.

c. More practical method for managing the patient who is at risk for bleeding.

(iv) Heparin free

a. Method of choice in:
- Actively bleeding patients
- Patients with an increased risk of bleeding
- Pericarditis
- Coagulopathy
- Thrombocytopenia

b. Blood lines and dialyzer are primed with heparinized saline. The primary saline is then discarded.

c. Blood flow rates set as high as possible (minimum 250ml/min).

d. The dialyzer is rinsed with normal saline (100-200 cc's) periodically throughout the treatment (usually every 1/2 hour or 1 hour) to check for clotting in the extracorporeal circuit. The additional saline given during the treatment is included as part of the total fluid to be removed during treatment when calculating UFR.

(g) Heparin Dose and Administration

(i) Loading dose

a. Given before dialysis in order to bring the patient's baseline clotting time up above the level at which dialyzer clotting occurs (@ 1.5 to 2x the baseline)

b. Given directly to the patient via the venous fistula needle prior to onset of dialysis

c. Or can be injected into the injection port on the arterial blood line as dialysis is initiated (before the blood reaches the dialyzer)

(ii) Maintenance dose

a. Administered during dialysis to maintain the elevated clotting time 1.5 to 2 times the baseline clotting time) either by continuous infusion or by intermittent injection into the arterial blood line

(iii) Determining loading and maintenance doses

a. Use of a common, empirically determined dosage schedule for all patients

b. A standard amount/kg of body weight

c. Kinetic modeling – can calculate a loading maintenance dose based on individual assessment of heparin activity in each patient. Provides for more efficient and safe use of heparin.

(h) Complications of Heparin Therapy

(i) Under heparinization

a. Clotting of the dialyzer (first check for – late doses, omitted doses and insufficient dose)

b. Fibrin rings or clots in the drip chambers (check if blood pump was off for needle adjustment, lower than normal blood flow, higher than normal pressure)

c. Increasing pressure differential

d. Drop in clotting time

e. Poor rinseback

f. Progressively lower hematocrits

(ii) Over heparinization

    a. Report or evidence of bleeding

    b. Ecchymoses

    c. Prolonged post dialysis bleeding

    d. Internal bleeding, for example, GI, retinal, intracranial, subdural hematoma, hemorrhagic pericardial and pleural effusions

    e. Osteoporosis

(i) Monitoring Heparin Effect: Measuring the effect of heparin on a patient's coagulation system

    (i) Response (sensitivity)

        a. The response or degree of sensitivity of patients to a given heparin dose

        b. Loading doses must be tailored to meet an individual patient's response to heparin

    (ii) Elimination Rate

        a. Metabolism or elimination rate of heparin differs from patient to patient with the result that clotting times decrease at varying rates among heparinized patients

    (iii) Effective Heparin Therapy – Objectives

        a. To elevate the patients clotting time using an appropriate loading dose

        b. To maintain the level throughout the dialysis

        c. To discontinue the administration of heparin so that the clotting time returns to normal before the patient leaves the unit

(j) Methods of Monitoring Heparin Activity

    (i) Modified Lee-White Clotting Time Method (MLWCT) based on contact activation

    (ii) Activated Partial Thromboplastin Time (APTT)

    (iii) Whole Blood Clotting Time (WBACT) – based on contact activation. Example: Hemochron

    (iv) Whole Blood Partial Thromboplastin Time (WBPTT)

    (v) Thrombin Clotting Time (TCT)

(k) Heparin Modeling: In order to determine an effective heparinization regime for a patient, three key parameters must be defined:

    (i) The patient's normal or baseline clotting time

    (ii) Sensitivity to heparin – measures the patient's response to heparin as determined by the prolongation in clotting time above baseline per unit of heparin administered

    (iii) The patient's elimination rate constant (k) is an individualized proportionality constant, the value of which depends on the rate of hepatic heparin metabolism and can be calculated from three or more serial clotting time measurements

d) Trisodium citrate forms a complex with calcium in the blood, obstructing the normal clotting pathway

    (1) A calcium free dialysate is used to allow the citrate to bind with calcium in the blood

    (2) Calcium chloride is reinfused post dialyzer, to prevent hypocalcemia and reverse anticoagulation

    (3) Hypertonic sodium citrate can be removed by decreasing the sodium level in dialysate

    (4) Advantage: may reduce morbidity associated with bleeding complications

    (5) Disadvantage: cumbersome, expensive, may cause hypo or hyper calcemia

e) Prostacycline – inhibits platelet activation

    (1) A prostaglandin with anticoagulation properties

    (2) Administered in similar fashion as heparin

    (3) Can be given alone or in combination with heparin

    (4) Advantage: alternate form of anticoagulation

    (5) Disadvantage: side effects include flushing, headache, vasodilation leading to hypotension, expensive, dialyzer efficiency is reduced when used with heparin

f) Low molecular weight heparin, Fragmin – has less antithrombin activity than regular preparations, and is associated with fewer side effects than regular, higher, molecular weight preparations

(1) Advantages

    (a) Reduced risk of bleeding complication

    (b) Longer half life may allow single bolus administration

    (c) Alternate form of anticoagulation

(2) Disadvantages

    (a) Limited experience

    (b) Cost

E. Antihypertensives

1. Hypertension – introduction

  a) Hypertension is a condition in which the blood pressure is elevated.

  b) Most causes of hypertension are of unknown etiology and result from a generalized increase in resistance to flow in the peripheral vessels (arterioles). This is known as primary or essential hypertension.

  c) Primary (essential) hypertension can precede, exacerbate and even cause renal disease

  d) Hypertension usually appears as a secondary development of renal disease.

  e) Most cases of hypertension in ESRD are believed to be volume dependent.

  f) In many individuals with ESRD and hypertension, the blood pressure will normalize without antihypertensive medication. Fluid removal by ultrafiltration during hemodialysis and adherence to fluid restricted diet, can control the blood pressure. Antihypertensive medications may have to be started when there is further deterioration in GFR as renal failure progresses.

  g) A small group of patients with non-volume dependent hypertension, which is unresponsive to ultrafiltration and conventional antihypertensive medications and is believed to be caused by an increased secretion of renin.

2. Definition

  a) Post dialysis diastolic B/P > 90mmHg when the patient is believed to be at their dry weight.

3. Purpose of Antihypertensive Medications

  a) In order to manage a patient's blood pressure, antihypertensives (medications used to lower the B/P) are prescribed.

  b) Most medications used to treat hypertension lower blood pressure by relaxing the constricted arterioles leading to a decrease in the resistance to peripheral blood flow. These drugs relax arteriolar smooth muscle, or by acting on the centers in the brain that control blood pressure.

4. Indications for drug therapy for hypertension in dialysis patients

  a) Drug therapy mandatory

    (1) At dry weight post dialysis, with a diastolic B/P > 99mmHg

    (2) At dry weight post dialysis, with a diastolic B/P = 90-99mmHg and patient is anemic, to receive EPO, or patient has an enlarged left ventricle

    (3) Drug therapy recommended when:

        (a) Patient is at dry weight post dialysis, with a diastolic B/P = 90-99mmHg and the patient is already on EPO and is not anemic, and left ventricle is not enlarged

        (b) Post dialysis diastolic B/P < 90mmHg, and the patient has an enlarged left ventricle

5. Examples of commonly prescribed antihypertensive medications:

  a) Clonidine (Catepres®)

  b) Hydralazine (Apresoline®)

  c) Atenolol (Tenormin®)

  d) Diltiazem (Cardizem®)

  e) Metroprolol (Lopressor®)

  f) Nifedipine (Procardia®)

  g) Propanolol (Inderal®)

  h) Captopril (Capoten®)

  i) Prazosin (Minipress®)

  j) Enalapril (Vasotec®)

  k) Labetalol (Normadyne®)

  l) Amlodipine (Norvasc®)

  m) Nadolol (Corgard®)

  n) Timolol (Blocadren®)

  o) Terazosin (Hytrin®)

  p) Candesartan (Atacand®)

  q) Losartan (Cozaar®)

6. Considerations

  a) The patient should be taught and encouraged to learn to take his/her own blood pressure at home. Blood pressures ideally should be monitored prior to taking blood pressure medication.

b) Most blood pressure medications are not removed by dialysis and patients may experience drops in their blood pressure during dialysis.

c) Most physicians recommend that the patient not take his/her blood pressure medication prior to dialysis, but wait and take it after treatment.

d) Patients will often have separate instructions for taking their blood pressure medication on DD (dialysis days) and non-dialysis days (NDD).

e) Weakness, dizziness and sometimes fainting may occur with rapid changes of positions from supine to standing. Patient should be advised to rise slowly from a lying or sitting position and to dangle legs for several minutes before standing to minimize the occurrence of orthostatic hypotension.

F. Antimicrobials

1. Overview

   a) Antimicrobial drugs are effective in the treatment of infections because of their selective toxicity – the ability to kill an invading organism without harming the cells of the host.

   b) Selection of the most appropriate antimicrobial drug depends on:

      (1) The identity of the organism and its sensitivity to a particular drug.

         (a) Characterization of the organism is essential to the selection of the proper drug.

         (b) It is essential to obtain a sample culture of the organism prior to initiating treatment if possible.

      (2) The site of the infection

         (a) Effective levels of the antibiotic must reach the infection site, any changes that diminishes access of the drug, e.g., poor blood flow access of the drug to the infected area may alter the effectiveness of the treatment.

         (b) Antimicrobial drugs can be divided into those that are bacteriostatic – they arrest the multiplication and further development of the infectious agent or bactericidal – eradicate all microorganisms.

         (c) Some antimicrobials halt the growth of or eradicate many different microorganisms and are termed broad spectrum antibiotics. Others affect only certain specific organisms and are termed narrow spectrum antibiotics.

         (d) Certain antimicrobial agents have marked side effects some of the more serious of which are neurotoxicity, including ototoxicity, and nephrotoxicity.

      (3) The safety of the agent

         (a) Many antibiotics are not specific and are reserved for life threatening infections because of the drug's potential for serious toxicity.

      (4) Patient factors (status of the patient)

         (a) Poor kidney function (10% or less of normal) causes accumulation of antibiotics that are ordinarily eliminated by the kidney. This may lead to serious adverse effects that can be controlled by adjusting the dose or the dosage schedule of the antibiotic.

         (b) Elimination of infecting organisms from the body depends on an intact immune system. Antibacterial drugs decrease the microbial population, or inhibit further bacterial growth, but the patient's defenses must ultimately eliminate the invading organisms. Immunocompromised patients have weakened immune defenses and higher than usual doses of bacterial agents are required to eliminate the infective organism.

         (c) Antibiotics that concentrate in the liver (for example, erythromycin, tetracycline) are contraindicated in treating patients with liver disease.

         (d) Patients with renal failure have an increased susceptibility to infection. Patients frequently require the intervention of antimicrobial medications in order to combat infections.

2. Examples

   a) Aminoglycosides (e.g., gentamicin, tobramycin, streptomycin)

      (1) Administered IM and IV

      (2) Broad spectrum antibiotics

(3) Primarily used for the treatment of serious gram-negative (e.g., pseundomonas, E. coli, proteus, klebsiella, enterobacter) infections causing bone and joint infections, septicemia, skin and soft tissue infections, respiratory tract infections, post operative infections, intraabdominal infections (including peritonitis), urinary tract infections

(4) Common side effects

  (a) Ototoxicity

  (b) Neurotoxicity

  (c) Nausea and vomiting

  (d) Diarrhea

  (e) Increased salivation

  (f) Anorexia

  (g) Weight loss

b) Cephalosporins (e.g., cefazolin (Ancef), cefoxitin, cephalothin (Keflin))

(1) Administered IV, IM

(2) Broad spectrum antibiotics

(3) Effective against infections of the biliary tract, GI tract, GU system, bones, joints, upper and lower respiratory tract, skin, and skin structures. Also gynecologic infections, meningitis, osteomyelitis, endocarditis, intra-abdominal infections, peritonitis, otitis media, gonorrhea, septicemia, and prophylaxis prior to surgery.

(4) Infections caused by organisms such as gram-positive cocci, e.g., staph aureus, staph epidermis, and streptococcus pneumoniae; gram negative bacteria, e.g., hemophilus influenzae, some enterobacter aerogenes, and neisseria species

(5) Common side effects: rashes, urticaria, pruritis, fever, chills, nausea and vomiting, diarrhea, abdominal cramps or pain, heart burn, anorexia and sore mouth

c) Penicillins (e.g., ampicillin, carbenicillin, nafcillin)

(1) Administered PO, IM, SC

  (a) Depending on the penicillin, these drugs are effective against one or more of the following organisms: gram positive organisms, e.g., Beta-hemolytic streptococci, staph aureus, streptococci. Gram negative

organisms, e.g., Enterobacter species, E. coli, Haemophilus influenzae, klebsiella, serratia species. Anaerobic organisms, e.g., clostridium species, Bacteriodes species.

(2) Common side effects: Hypersensitivity reactions: skin rashes, hives, pruritis, wheezing, anaphylaxis, fever, diarrhea, abdominal cramps, or pain, neurotoxicity; and electrolyte imbalance

d) Quinolones (e.g. ciprofloxacin, (Cipro®), levofloxacin, (Levaquin®))

(1) Administered PO and IV

(2) Broad spectrum antibiotics

(3) Used to treat susceptible infections, including respiratory tract, skin structures, UTI's, sinusitis, pneumonia and prostatitis.

(4) Common side effects , GI upset, headache, convulsions, anxiety, rash, photosensitivity and abdominal pain.

e) Tetracyclines (e.g., doxycycline, tetracycline)

(1) Administered PO, topical, IV, IM

(2) Used mainly for infections caused by Rickettsia, Chlamydia, and Mycoplasma

(3) Common side effects: Nausea and vomiting, thirst, diarrhea, anorexia, sore throat, flatulence, epigastric distress, bulky loose stools

f) Macrolides (e.g., erythromycin)

(1) Administered PO, topical

(2) Uses: Upper respiratory tract infections due to Streptococcus pyrogenes, streptococcus pneumoniae, and haemophilus influenzae; mild to moderate lower respiratory tract infections due to S. pyrogenes and staph pneumoniae. Respiratory tract infections due to mycoplasma pneumoniae; pertusis (whooping cough) caused by bordetella pertusis; corynebacterium diphtheriae, used to eliminate the carrier state; Legionnaire's disease due to Legionella pneumophilia; an alternative for patients allergic to penicillin in the treatment of syphilis caused by Treponema pallidum; an alternative to tetracycline in the treatment of urethral, endocervical, rectal or epididymal infections due to Chlamydia.

(3) Common side effects: Nausea, vomiting, diarrhea, cramping, abdominal pain, anorexia, and heart burn

g) Others

  (1) Vancomycin

    (a) Administered PO or IV

    (b) Bactericidal

    (c) Used in the treatment of severe staphylococcal and streptococcal infections in patients who have not responded to penicillins or cephalosporins, or have resistant infections.

    (d) Common side effects: Ototoxicity; red neck syndrome – chills, erythema of neck and back, fever, paresthesias; urticaria, rashes; drug fever, hypersensitivity; anaphylaxis.

3. Considerations

a) The bacteriologic sensitivity of the infectious organism to the anti-infective (especially the antibiotic) should be tested by the lab before initiation of therapy and during treatment.

b) If the anti-infective is mainly excreted by the kidneys, there should be a reduced dosage in patients with renal dysfunction.

c) Serum drug levels should be monitored throughout therapy to ensure that the patient is receiving the appropriate dose of medication.

d) Serum electrolyte levels may be increased by the electrolyte composition (especially sodium and potassium) of the drug.

e) The patient needs to be monitored closely for signs of superinfections (drug therapy, particularly with broad spectrum antimicrobials, can lead to alternations of the normal microbial flora of the upper respiratory, intestinal and genito-urinary tracts, permitting the overgrowth of opportunistic organisms, especially fungi.) These infections can involve resistant organisms and are often difficult to treat.

G. *Antipruritics:* Histamine H1 Receptor Antagonists (histamine – a substance in the body found wherever tissues are damaged)

1. Overview

a) Antihistamines, or H1 blockers, compete with histamine for receptor sites, thus preventing a histamine response.

b) When the effects of histamine are blocked, the pruritis that is associated with renal failure is decreased.

2. Examples

a) Diphenhydramine (Benadryl)

b) Trimeprazine (Temaril)

c) Hydroxyzine (Atarax) (Antihistamine action)

3. Route of Administration

a) PO

b) IV

c) IM

4. Common Side Effects

a) Drowsiness, dizziness, fatigue, and disturbed coordination

b) Skin rashes, dry mouth, blurred vision and wheezing

5. Considerations

a) May result in sedation and depression of central nervous system (CNS)

b) Monitor vital signs

c) Medication should be taken with food

H. *Cardiovascular Drugs:* Three groups of drugs, cardiac glycosides, the antianginals, and the antidysrhythmics (a dysrhythmia is an abnormal disordered, or disturbed rhythm) regulate heart contraction, heart rate and rhythm and blood flow to the heart muscle.

1. Cardiac Glycosides

a) Digitalis

  (1) Effective in treating congestive heart failure

  (2) Used to correct atrial fibrillation (cardiac dysrhythmia with rapid uncoordinated contractions of atrial heart muscle) and atrial flutter (cardiac dysrhythmia with rapid contractions of 200-300 beats per minute.)

  (3) Digitalis preparations have three effects on heart muscle.

    (a) increases heart muscle contraction

    (b) decreases heart rate

    (c) decreases conduction of the heart cells

  (4) In patients with a failing heart, cardiac glyco-sides increase myocardial contraction, which increases circulation and tissue perfusion.

  (5) Therapeutic serum levels:

    (a) Digoxin – 0.5-2.0 ng/ml

    (b) Digitoxin – 10-35 ng/ml

(6) Route of Administration

    (a) Digoxin – PO, IV

    (b) Digitoxin – PO

(7) Side effects

    (a) Overdose or accumulation of digoxin causes digitalis toxicity. Signs and symptoms of digitalis toxicity include anorexia, diarrhea, nausea and vomiting, bradycardia (pulse rate below 65), and tachycardia (pulse rate above 120), cardiac dysrhythmias, headaches, malaise; blurred vision, visual illusions (white, green, yellow halos around objects), and confusion.

(8) Considerations

    (a) Serum digoxin levels above 2.0 ng/ml and a serum digitoxin level above 35 ng/ml are indicative of digitalis toxicity.

    (b) Patients that use digitalis preparations are at the highest risk of arrhythmias, partly from the drug itself, and also due to underlying heart disease.

    (c) Electrolyte shifts during hemodialysis should be minimized, ensuring that the serum potassium does not fall below 3.5 mEq/liter.

    (d) Dialysate potassium may need to be increased to 3.0-3.5 mEq/liter; restricting dietary potassium to avoid predialysis hyperkalemia.

b) Antianginal Drugs

  (1) Overview

    (a) Used to treat angina pectoris (acute chest pain from inadequate blood flow due to plaque occlusion in the coronary arteries).

    (b) With decreased blood flow, there is a decrease in oxygen to the myocardium that causes pain.

    (c) Angina pain is frequently described by the patient as tightness, pressure in the center of the chest, and pain radiating down the left arm. Referred pain felt in the neck and left arm commonly occurs with severe angina pectoris.

    (d) Anginal attacks may lead to heart attack.

    (e) Anginal pain usually lasts for only a few minutes.

    (f) Antianginal drugs increase blood flow either by increasing oxygen supply or by decreasing oxygen demand by the heart muscle. Three types of antianginals are the nitrates, beta blockers, and calcium channel blockers.

(2) Nitrates

    (a) Nitroglycerin given sublingually (under the tongue)

    (b) the sublingual tablet is given for cardiac pain, and repeated every 5 minutes for a total of 3 doses.

    (c) Examples

      (i) nitroglycerin (Nitrostat)

      (ii) isosorbide (Isordil)

    (d) Route of Administration

      (i) sublingual

      (ii) topical – ointment, transdermal patch

      (iii) IV

    (e) Side effects

      (i) headaches, dizziness, faintness, nausea

(3) Beta Blockers

    (a) Decrease the heart (pulse) rate

    (b) Used as antianginal, antiarrhythmic and antihypertensive drugs

    (c) Effective as antianginals by decreasing the heart rate and myocardial contractility they reduce the need for oxygen consumption and therefore, the pain of angina.

    (d) Examples

      (i) propranolol (Inderal)

      (ii) atenolol (Tenormin)

      (iii) metroprolol (Lopressor)

    (e) Route of Administration

      (i) PO

    (f) Side Effects

      (i) Decrease in pulse rate and blood pressure

(g) Considerations

    (i) Monitor vital signs closely

    (ii) With discontinuation of use, the dosage should be tapered for a week or two to prevent a rebound effect (tachycardia and vasoconstriction)

(4) Calcium Channel Blockers

    (a) Decrease cardiac contractility and the workload of the heart, thus decreasing the need for oxygen.

    (b) Examples

        (i) Verapamil (Calan)

        (ii) Nifedipine (Procardia)

        (iii) Diltiazem (Cardizem)

    (c) Side Effects

        (i) Headache, hypotension, dizziness, and flushing of the skin

    (d) Considerations

        (i) Monitor vital signs. Hypotension is common.

(5) Antidysrhythmias

    (a) A cardiac dysrhythmia (arrhythmia) is defined as any deviation from the normal rate or pattern of the heart beat; this includes heart rates that are too slow, too fast, or irregular.

    (b) Cardiac dysrhythmias frequently follow a heart attack or can result from things like lack of oxygen to body tissues, increased carbon dioxide in the blood, or electrolyte imbalance.

    (c) Therapeutic effects of antidysrhythmics

        (i) slow conduction of cardiac tissue

        (ii) decreases excitability of the heart

    (d) Examples

        (i) Quinidine (Cardioquin, Duraquin)

        (ii) Procainamide (Pronestyl)

        (iii) disopyramide (Norpace)

    (e) Side Effects

        (i) Fatigue, headache, dizziness, hypotension, nausea and vomiting

    (f) Considerations

        (i) Vital signs should be checked

        (ii) Therapeutic serum drug levels should be checked

I. Chelating Agents

1. Overview

    a) Heavy metal chelating agents are used to treat aluminum and iron toxicity in chronic renal failure patients.

    b) Heavy metal chelators form complexes with the heavy metals, and prevent the metallic cations from further chemical reactions in the body.

    c) Chelating agents are water soluble, resist metabolic degradation, have the ability to penetrate metal storage sites, and are excreted by the kidney.

2. Examples

    a) Deferoxamine mesylate (Desferal)

    b) A heavy metal chelating agent that is used with renal failure patients

3. Uses

    a) Treatment of iron overload and aluminum intoxication in renal failure patients

    b) Administered intravenously during dialysis, forms metal-drug complexes that are dialyzable and removed by subsequent dialysis treatments.

4. Common Side Effects

    a) Rash, itching, anaphylaxis; abdominal discomfort, diarrhea; dysuria, blurred vision, leg cramps, fever, tachycardia, high frequency hearing loss; impaired peripheral, night or color vision, decreased visual acuity; hypotension, urticaria, erythema, if infused rapidly IV.

5. Route of Administration

    a) IM

    b) IV

6. Considerations

    a) For those patients who still urinate, medication may give urine a reddish color.

    b) Visual disturbances, such as changes in color vision or altered visual acuity may be related to drug therapy.

    c) Sudden hearing loss may also be drug related.

    d) When given intravenously, must be given slowly.

J. Electrolytes

1. Overview

   a) Patients may require replacement of various electrolytes at different points in time.

   b) The electrolyte requiring replacement in most renal patients is calcium.

   c) The absorption of dietary calcium form the intestinal tract is decreased in chronic renal failure.

   d) The replacement of calcium in renal failure patients is hampered by the lack of conversion of vitamin D to its active metabolites (1,25-dihydroxycholecalciferol).

   e) It is insufficient to administer calcium preparations alone.

   f) The active form of vitamin D must be also given in order for the calcium to be absorbed and utilized.

2. Calcium Supplements

   a) Inadequate calcium causes calcium to leave the bone in order to maintain normal serum calcium levels.

   b) Fractures may occur if calcium deficit persists because of calcium loss from the bones (bone demineralization).

   c) Calcium supplements are used to increase the amount of calcium in the blood and bones.

   d) When taken with meals, calcium supplements may also bind phosphorus (acts as a phosphate binder).

   e) Calcium salts also act as an acid. They have the ability to buffer the pH of the stomach contents.

   f) Route of Administration

      (1) PO

      (2) IV

   g) Common Side Effects

      (1) Nausea

      (2) Symptoms of high serum calcium levels – loss of appetite, constipation, cramping, continuous headache, muscle pain or twitching, and/or confusion. These symptoms need to be reported to the MD.

   h) Examples

      (1) Calcium carbonate (Os-Cal, Tums)

      (2) Calcium gluconate

      (3) Calcium lactate

3. Vitamin D

   a) Enhance the absorption of calcium from the gastrointestinal tract

   b) Also helpful in maintaining bone formation

   c) Dose depends on the serum calcium level

   d) Route of Administration

      (1) PO

      (2) IV

   e) Common Side Effects

      (1) Nausea, vomiting, loss of appetite, constipation, continuous headache, unusual tiredness, bone pain and itching.

   f) Examples

      (1) 1,25-dihydrocholecalciferol (e.g., Rocaltrol PO, Calcitriol (Calcijex) – IV)

      (2) Paricalcitriol (Zemplar) – IV

      (3) Doxercalciferol (Hectorol) - PO (soon to be available IV)

   g) Considerations

      (1) When administering vitamin D, serum calcium and phosphorous levels, the calcium/phosphrous product and PTH, should be measured frequently.

      (2) Intake of phosphate should be limited. Phosphate binders should be used to bind dietary phosphorus.

      (3) Calcium supplements should be taken approximately one hour after meals to promote absorption.

K. Hypolipidemic Agents

1. Overview

   a) Used to decrease hyperlipidemia, which in turn decreases atherosclerotic effects

   b) Main goal of treatment is to lower low density lipoprotein cholestrol.

   c) Four different types of hypolipidemic agents; bile sequestering agents, fibric acid derivatives, cholesterol synthesis inhibitors and nicotinic acid.

   d) Cholestrol synthesis inhibitor or HMG-CoA reductase inhibitors (Statins) are useful in treating patients with renal failure. These drugs decrease cholestrol, triglycerides and low density lipoprotein(LDL) , and increase high density lipoprotein (HDL).

   e) Benefits include a reduction in major coronary events and procedures, strokes and mortality.

2. Examples of HMG-CoA reductase inhibitors (Statins)

   a) Lovastain (Mevacor®)

   b) Pravastatin (Pravachol®)

   c) Simvastatin (Zocor®)

   d) Fluvastatin (Lescol®)

   e) Atorvastatin (Liptor®)

3. Common Side Effects

   a) Diarrhea

   b) Nausea

   c) Vomiting

   d) Leg cramps

   e) Myopathy

   f) Increased liver enzymes

4. Considerations

   a) Liver function tests should be monitored frequently.

   b) CPK levels monitored for myopathy.

L. Laxatives and Cathartics

1. Overview – Constipation

   a) Constipation – an accumulation of hard fecal material in the large intestine

   b) Causes of constipation are: Insufficient water intake; poor dietary habits; fecal impaction; bowel obstruction; chronic laxative use; neurologic disorder; ignoring the urge to have a bowel movement; lack of exercise; and selected drugs (e.g., certain antacids and phosphate binders)

2. Overview – Cathartics (stool softener) and Laxatives

   a) Used to eliminate fecal matter

   b) Laxatives promote a soft stool

   c) Cathartics result in a soft to watery stool with some cramping

   d) Frequently the dosage determines whether the drug acts as a laxative or cathartic

   e) Four types of laxatives:

      (1) Osmotics (saline)

      (2) Contact (stimulants or irritants)

      (3) Bulk forming

      (4) Emollients

   f) Frequently prescribed for renal failure patients because these patients are prone to constipation due to a restricted diet, limited fluid intake and regular ingestion of phosphate binders

   g) Bulk forming or contact laxatives are preferred to osmotic which contain magnesium, sodium and/or potassium

3. Uses

   a) Short term treatment of constipation

4. Examples

   a) Osmotic laxatives (hyperosmolar)

      (1) Includes salts or saline products

      (2) Hyperosmolar salts pull water into the colon and increase water in the feces to increase bulk, which stimulates peristalsis

      (3) Good renal function is needed to excrete only excess salts that is absorbed systemically

         (a) Lactulose: draws water into the intestines and promotes water and electrolyte retention; not absorbed

         (b) Glycerin: increases water in the feces in the large intestine; the increased water in the feces stimulates peristalsis and defecation

   b) Contact laxatives (stimulant or irritant)

      (1) Increase peristalsis by irritating sensory nerve endings in the intestinal mucosa

         (a) Bisacodyl (Dulcolax)

         (b) Senna (Senokot)

         (c) Castor Oil (Purgative)

   c) Bulk – Forming Laxative

      (1) Natural fibrous substances that promote large soft stools by absorbing water in the intestine, increasing fecal bulk and peristalsis

      (2) Psyllium colloid (Metamucil)

   d) Emollients

      (1) Stool softeners and lubricants used to prevent constipation

      (2) Work by promoting water accumulation in the intestine

      (3) Dioctyl sodium sulfosuccinate (Colace)

      (4) Dioctyl calcium sulfosuccinate (Surfak)

      (5) Docusate sodium with cusanthranol (Peri-colace)

5. Route of Administration

   a) PO

   b) Suppository (e.g., glycerin dulcolax)

6. Common Side Effects
   a) Contact Laxatives: nausea, abdominal cramps, weakness, and reddish brown urine
   b) Emollients: nausea, vomiting, diarrhea, and abdominal cramping

7. Considerations
   a) Patient should be instructed by dietitian on foods they can eat which are rich in fiber
   b) Encourage patients to adhere to a program of regular exercise
   c) Encourage patients to plan a regularly scheduled time for bowel movements
   d) These medications are excreted by non-renal mechanisms and are not removed by dialysis.

M. Local Anesthetics

1. Overview
   a) Local anesthetics block pain at the site where the drug is administered. Uses for local anesthetics include dental procedures, suturing of skin lacerations, venipuncture, short term (minor) surgery at a localized area, spinal anesthesia by blocking nerve impulses (nerve block) below the insertion of the anesthetic, and such diagnostic procedures as lumbar punctures and thoracentesis.
   b) Lidocaine hydrochloride (Xylocaine) was developed in the mid 1950s to replace procaine (Novocain), except for dental procedures.
   c) Lidocaine has a rapid onset and a long duration of action, is more stable in solution, and causes fewer hypersensitivity reactions than procaine.
   d) Since the introduction of lidocaine, many local anesthetics have been marketed.

2. Examples of Local Anesthetics used for venipuncture:
   a) Lidocaine hydrochloride (xylocaine)
      (1) Overview
         (a) A sterile, non-pyrogenic, isotonic solution containing 1% or 2% lidocaine hydrochloride and water for injection.
         (b) Lidocaine stabilizes the neuronal membrane and prevents the initiation of transmission of nerve impulses, thereby effecting local anesthesia.
         (c) The onset of action is approximately 2 to 5 minutes and the duration of action is relatively short (average approximately 1 hour).
      (2) Use
         (a) A drug injected under the skin (intradermally), which produces localized insensitivity to pain.
      (3) Route of Administration
         (a) Intradermal: injection of local anesthetic between the internal layers of the skin, over the area of the vessel selected for venipuncture; its effect is limited only to the immediate area where the injection is made.
      (4) Side Effects
         (a) Reactions due to over-dosage (increased plasma levels), inadvertent intravascular injection, hypersensitivity, or diminished tolerance to the drug involve the central nervous system and the cardiovascular system.
         (b) Reactions involving the Central Nervous System:
            (i) Excitation (may be transient) and/or depression
            (ii) Nervousness
            (iii) Dizziness
            (iv) Blurred vision or tremors may occur followed by drowsiness
            (v) Convulsions
            (vi) Unconsciousness
            (vii) Possible respiratory arrest
         (c) Reactions involving the Cardiovascular System:
            (i) Depression of the myocardium (muscular substance of the heart)
            (ii) Hypotension
            (iii) Bradycardia (abnormal slowness of the heart rate and pulse)
            (iv) Cardiac arrest
         (d) Allergic reactions:
            (i) Skin lesions of delayed onset
            (ii) Urticaria
            (iii) Edema
            (iv) or other manifestations of allergy
         (e) Considerations
            (i) Avoid intravascular injection. Before lidocaine is injected aspirate (pull back on the syringe plunger) to make sure the needle is not in a blood vessel.

(ii) The needle used for injection should be a small gauge, usually 25 or 27 gauge.

(iii) All lidocaine vials must be checked twice for correct medication, strength, and expiration date.

(iv) The anesthetic is slowly injected intradermally, under the skin in the tissue layers between the top of the blood vessel and the inner surface of the skin.

(v) As the anesthetic enters the intra-dermal skin layer the patient will feel a slight stinging or burning sensation. A "wheal" or small swelling about the size of a mosquito bite will appear.

(vi) After injection wait about 30 seconds to allow the anesthesia to take effect. When the injected area feels numb, good anesthesia has been achieved.

(5) Ethyl Chloride (chloroethane)

(a) Overview

(i) Ethyl Chloride is a vapocoolant intended for topical application to control pain associated with minor surgical procedures, e.g., lancing boils, or incision and drainage of small abscesses, venipuncture, athletic injuries, infections, and for treatment of myofascial pain, restricted motion, and muscle spasm.

(b) Route of Administration

(i) Topical

(c) Side Effects

(i) Cutaneous sensitization may occur, but is extremely rare.

(ii) Freezing can occasionally alter pigmentation.

(d) Considerations

(i) Inhalation of Ethyl Chloride should be avoided as it may produce narcotic and general anesthetic effects, and may produce deep anesthesia or fatal coma with respiratory or cardiac arrest.

(ii) Adjacent skin areas should be protected when used to produce local freezing of tissues.

(iii) The venipuncture site should be cleansed with a suitable antiseptic. Spray Ethyl Chloride for a few seconds to the point of frost-formation, when the tissue becomes white. Avoid prolonged spraying of skin beyond this state.

(iv) The anesthetic action of Ethyl Chloride rarely lasts more than a few seconds to a minute.

(v) Quickly swab the venipuncture site with antiseptic and promptly insert the cannula set.

(6) Emla Cream (Lidocaine 2.5% and prilocaine 2.5%)

(a) Overview

(i) Emla Cream applied to intact skin under occlusive dressing, provides dermal analgesia by the release of lidocaine and prilocaine from the cream into the epidermal and dermal layers of the skin and the accumulation of lidocaine and prilocaine in the vicinity of dermal pain receptors and nerve endings.

(ii) The onset, depth and duration of dermal analgesia provided by Emla Cream depends primarily on the duration of application.

(iii) To provide sufficient analgesia for venipuncture, Emla Cream should be applied under an occlusive dressing for at least one hour

(b) Use

(i) A topical anesthetic for use on normal intact skin for local analgesia.

(c) Route of Administration

(i) Topical

(ii) For minor procedures, e.g., venipuncture, apply 2.5 grams of Emla Cream (1/2 the 5 g tube) over 20 to 25 cm² of skin surface for at least one hour.

(d) Adverse Reactions

    (i) During or immediately after treatment with Emla Cream, the skin at the site of treatment may develop erythema or edema or may have abnormal sensation. Rare cases of hyperpigmentation have been reported.

    (ii) Allergic and anaphylactic reactions associated with lidocaine or prilocaine can occur. They are characterized by urticaria, angioedema, bronchospasm, and shock.

N. Potassium Ion Exchange Resin (sodium polystyrene sulfonate (Kayexalate))

1. Overview
   a) Sodium polystyrene sulfonate (kayexalate) is a resin that exchanges sodium ions for potassium ions primarily in the large intestine. Excess amounts of potassium (as well as calcium and magnesium) are removed in the feces.

2. Use
   a) Hyperkalemia

3. Route of Administration
   a) PO
   b) Enema

4. Common Side Effects
   a) Anorexia, nausea, vomiting, hypokalemia and hypocalcemia

5. Considerations
   a) For PO administration to prevent constipation, give the medication in water or sorbitol (a laxative)
   b) Several hours are required for the medication to alter potassium levels significantly.
   c) When given by enema, to be effective the drug must be kept in the colon as long as possible (3-4 hours).
   d) The patient must be monitored for hypokalemia (low potassium), hypocalcemia (low calcium), and hypernatremia (high sodium).

O. Thrombolytic Agents (Streptokinase, Activase - TPA, Alteplase)

1. Overview
   a) It converts plasminogen to the enzyme plasmin, which destroys the fibrin in the blood clot.
   b) Serum half-life is approximately 70 minutes.
   c) Most effective for clots less than seven days old.

2. Uses
   a) Restoration of patency to intravenous catheters, including central venous catheters (e.g., subclavian and internal jugular), obstructed by clotted blood or fibrin.

3. Contraindications
   a) Active internal bleeding.
   b) History of CVA.
   c) Recent (within 2 months) intracranial or intraspinal surgery.
   d) Recent trauma.

4. Side Effects
   a) Superficial bleeding, severe internal bleeding; rarely, skin rashes, bronchospasm; fever.

P. Vitamins

1. Overview
   a) Vitamins are organic chemicals that are necessary for normal metabolic functions and for tissue growth and healing.
   b) Dialysis patients may be at risk for deficiencies of certain water soluble vitamins because of poor nutritional intake, drug-nutrient interactions, altered vitamin metabolism, and loss through dialysis.

2. Multivitamins
   a) Used to replace any vitamins that are lost during dialysis.
   b) Most contain folic acid, Vitamin C and the B vitamins.

3. Examples
   a) Nephrocaps®
   b) Nerphrovite®
   c) Diatx®

4. Common Side Effects
   a) Occasional nausea

5. Route of Administration
   a) PO

6. Considerations
   a) Multivitamins are taken daily. On dialysis days they are usually taken after dialysis.
   b) Supplemental vitamin A should be avoided because of potential toxicity in renal failure patients.
   c) Vitamins should not be taken at the same time and antacids because the two bind together and reduce vitamin absorption.
   d) Folic Acid – see section on antianemic drugs.
   e) Vitamin D – see section on electrolytes.

II. Common Complications during Dialysis and Their Management with Medication

A. *Hypotension (the most common complication during hemodialysis)*

1. Common causes of:
   a) Hypovolemia – excessive decreases in blood volume
      (1) Fluctuations in the ultrafiltration rate
      (2) High ultrafiltration rate
      (3) Target weight set too low
      (4) Dialysis solution sodium level too low
   b) Lack of vasoconstriction
      (1) Autonomic neuropathy (e.g., diabetic)
      (2) Antihypertensive medications
   c) Related to cardiac factors
      (1) Cardiac output unusually dependent on cardiac filling
      (2) Failure to increase cardiac rate
         (a) Ingestion of beta-blockers
         (b) Anemic autonomic neuropathy
      (3) Inability to increase cardiac output for other reasons
         (a) Poor heart muscle contractility due to age, hypertension, etc.

2. Management of Hypotension with Medications
   a) Volume Replacement
      (1) The most common successful method of treating acute hypotension during dialysis is restoration of vascular volume by bolus administration of normal saline.
      (2) the average 70kg adult usually requires 100-200cc of normal saline (0.9% sodium chloride) or more to restore the blood pressure to normal.
      (3) When an average size adult who has not been taken below his dry weight requires more than 500cc volume replacement during a single hypotensive episode, the existence of a more serious problem, such as cardiac failure, should be considered.
      (4) Rarely, as much as 1000cc of normal saline is needed to restore the blood pressure when massive dehydration occurs, but this pertains mainly to large size individuals manifesting signs of circulatory shock.
   b) Colloids (a glue-like substance such as a protein or starch, whose particles or molecules when dispersed in a solvent to the greatest possible degree remain uniformly distributed and fail to form a true solution).
      (1) When albumin is infused intravenously, it has an immediate and relatively long-acting effect on the vascular refilling rate since it is contained within the vascular compartment.
      (2) Administration of albumin is a highly effective means of restoring blood volume and blood pressure.
      (3) Concentrates "salt poor" albumin should be given to fluid-overloaded patients.
      (4) Saline-diluted albumin preparations may be given for patients near their dry weight.
      (5) IV albumin preparations are expensive, and their use is usually reserved for patients who are truly hypoalbuminemic.
   c) Osmotic Solutions
      (1) Preservation of plasma osmolality during dialysis is necessary for maintenance for the vascular refilling rate.
      (2) Mannitol, a sugar alcohol, is used for elevation of plasma osmolality during acute hypotension. Often mannitol is most efficacious when given prophylactically – before rather than during or after a sudden drop in blood pressure occurs.
   d) Hypertonic sodium chloride
      (1) Another method of treating acute hypotension during dialysis.

(2) The amount and concentration used varies, e.g., 20-40 ml of 10% sodium chloride, 10-15 ml 23.5% sodium chloride.

(3) Hypertonic solutions act to transfer water osmotically into the blood compartment from surrounding tissues, helping to maintain the blood volume.

(4) Most important the total number of milliequivalents infused is important for restoration of plasma osmolality.

e) Hypertonic Dextrose

(1) Occasionally used for treatment of dialysis-induced hypotension.

(2) The modest blood pressure response versus the rapid changes in blood glucose levels following a bolus injection of concentrated dextrose must be taken into consideration.

f) Vasoactive drugs

(1) IV administration, via the venous blood line of vasopressor drugs, e.g., metaremitrolbitartrate (Aramine) has been shown to be effective in increasing blood pressure.

3. Medications

a) Antihypertensive medications are usually avoided on dialysis days.

b) Small oral doses of sympathomimetic drugs (drugs that stimulate the sympathetic nervous system and cause such things as the heart rate to increase and the blood vessels to constrict) are sometimes taken before dialysis prophlactically by hypotension prone patients who manifest evidence of autonomic dysfunction (autonomic nervous system is involuntary and controls and regulates the functioning of the heart, respiratory system, gastrointestinal system, and glands) during treatment. One such drug is midodrine.

4. Prevention of Hypotension during dialysis with the use of intravenous solutions.

a) When albumin is given to hypoalbuminemic hypotensive patients, it should be infused whenever possible, at the beginning of dialysis as a prophylactic measure.

b) It is also advisable to administer blood and osmotic solutions, e.g., mannitol before a severe drop in blood pressure occurs.

c) Continuous infusions of mannitol can help maintain the patient's blood pressure (e.g., 50cc vials containing 12.5 g mannitol, give 25cc or 6.25g q 1/2 hour up to last 1 hour of dialysis).

d) Early administration of albumin, osmotic solutions allows for ultrafiltration during dialysis and avoids over expansion of the vascular space which can occur post dialysis when colloids and/or osmotic solutes are administered late in the treatment.

e) Blood pressures can be also maintained for some patients by dripping in saline over the course of the entire treatment.

B. Muscle Cramps

1. Causes: The cause(s) of dialysis-related muscle cramps is uncertain. It is generally assumed, that it is intravascular hypovolemia and/or fall in plasma osmolality that are the primary factors leading to this complication.

2. Management of muscle cramps with medications. (The ideal method of management is using sodium and UF modeling.)

a) Acute management of dialysis-related muscle cramps is aimed at restoring blood volume and/or plasma osmolality.

b) The most common forms of treatment include:

(1) Administration of normal saline (50-500cc)

(2) Hypertonic sodium chloride

(a) 20-40 ml 10% sodium chloride

(b) 10-15 ml 23.5% sodium chloride

(3) Hypertonic glucose

(a) 50 ml 50% dextrose (D50W)

(4) Mannitol

(a) 50 ml 25% mannitol

C. Nausea and Vomiting

1. Causes

a) There are multiple causes of nausea and vomiting. Most episodes are probably related to hypotension.

2. Management of nausea and vomiting with medications

a) First, treat any associated hypotension

b) If nausea persists, an antiemetic (medication used to prevent or relieve nausea and vomiting), e.g., Prochlorperazine (Compazine)

D. Headache

1. Causes
   a) Common symptom during dialysis, the cause is largely unknown.

2. Management of Headache with medications
   a) Acetaminophen (Tylenol)

E. Fever/Chills

1. Causes
   a) Low grade fever during hemodialysis may be related to pyrogens present in the dialysate
   b) A pyrogen reaction should be suspected whenever shaking chills, usually accompanied by hypotension, occur anytime during the course of hemodialysis.
   c) A subsequent rise in body temperature (1-2 hours later) is a confirmatory sign that a pyrogen reaction has occurred.
   d) Other symptoms may accompany a pyrogen reaction such as nausea, vomiting, thirst, and tenderness or pain in the muscles.

2. Management and treatment of fever and chills
   a) Administer antipyretics such as acetaminophen
   b) Need to distinguish between endotoxemia alone and bacteremia/endotoxemia, the later which usually requires hospitalization and intravenous antibiotic therapy.

F. Angina (chest pain) during Dialysis

1. Causes
   a) Associated with cardiovascular disease

2. Management of angina with medications
   a) If anginal episode is associated with hypotension, the initial treatment should be to raise the blood pressure.
   b) Sublingual nitroglycerin can be given as soon as the blood pressure has increased to an acceptable level.
   c) If the blood pressure is not low when angina first manifests, then sublingual nitroglycerin should be administered as initial therapy (a drop in blood pressure should however, be anticipated after administration of nitroglycerin).
   d) Predialysis administration of 2% nitroglycerin ointment may be beneficial when applied one hour prior to dialysis.
   e) Predialysis administration of beta blockers, oral nitrates, or calcium-channel blocker medications may be of benefit. These should be used cautiously due to the risk of hypotension during dialysis.

G. Pruritis (itching)

1. Causes
   a) Common problem among ESRD patients.
   b) Usually reversible by adequate dialysis.
   c) In some well-dialyzed individuals, itching persists and may increase in severity while on dialysis.

2. Management of Pruritis with medication
   a) Administration of sedatives and antihistaminic agents such as Temaril, and diphenhydramine.
   b) Administration of intravenous lidocaine during dialysis.

III. Dialysis and Its Effect on Drug Therapy

1. The individual with ESRD is predisposed to drug toxicity.

2. Careful management including drug dosage medication and plasma drug level surveillance is sometimes necessary to ensure effective but safe concentrations which may be altered by intermittent dialysis therapy.

3. The kidneys are the major route of excretion for drugs and drug metabolites.

4. Loss of renal function that necessitates dialysis also reduces elimination of many medications with potential for accumulation to toxic levels.

5. Metabolic effects of uremia alter drug disposition.

6. Increased magnitude and duration of drug effect may necessitate adjustment in dosage or frequency of administration.

7. Dialysis may affect drug disposition, requiring supplemental doses of drugs removed during dialysis.

8. If a drug is primarily excreted by the kidney, then it is usually also dialyzable through hemodialysis.

9. A drug is considered dialyzable if its serum concentration levels can be depleted through the interaction with a dialysis process.

Figure 8.2

Medication Quick-Reference Guide

Frequently Prescribed Medications

Medication Classification	Example (generic/brand name)	Function	Possible Side Effects
Analgesics	Acetaminophen/Tylenol Ibuprofen/Motrin, Nuprin, Advil	Relieve pain, some may reduce fever.	High dosages can cause liver toxicity; gastric discomfort.
Antacids & Phosphate Binders	Calcium carbonate/Oscal, Tums Calcium acetate/Phos Lo Aluminum hydroxide/Amphogel Aluminum carbonate/Basaljel Sevelamer hydrocloride/Renagel	Control phosphate level by binding with phosphates in food to prevent bone disease and calcium deposits.	Constipation, nausea; loss of appetite. hypercalcemia
Antianemics Iron Supplements	Ferrous Sulfate/Feosol, Slo-Fe Ferrous Gluconate/Fergon	Prophylaxis and treatment of iron deficiency anemia.	Stomach upset, nausea, vomiting, diarrhea, constipation, dark stools.
Anticoagulant	Warfarin/Coumadin	To prevent blood from clotting in the vascular access	Minor bleeding; Hemorrhage
Antihypertensives	Clonidine/Catapress; Propanolol/Inderal; Prezosin/Minipress, Labetalol/Normadyne; Hydralazine/Apresoline; Diltiazem/Cardizem; Nifedipine/Procardia; Captopril/Capoten; Enalapril/Vasotec Amiodipine/Norvasc; Nadolol/Corgard; Timolol/Blocadren; Terezosin/Hytrin; Candesartan/Atacand; Losarten/Cozaar	To manage high blood pressure when control of sodium and fluid does not maintain blood pressure in acceptable range.	Tiredness, lightheadedness, weakness, dizziness.
Antipruretics	Diphenhydramine/Benadryl; Trimeprazine/Temaril; Hydroxyzine/Atarax	Relieve itching	Drowsiness, dizziness, fatigue, dry mouth
Cardiovascular Drugs Cardiac Glycosides	Digitalis/Digoxin Digitoxin	Increases heart muscle contraction; decreases heart rate; decreases conduction of the heart cells.	Anorexia, diarrhea, nausea, vomiting, headaches, blurred vision

Figure 8.2 continued

Medication Quick-Reference Guide

Frequently Prescribed Medications

Medication Classification	Example (generic/brand name)	Function	Possible Side Effects
Antianginal	Nitroglycerin/Nitrostat Propranolol/Inderal Atenolol/Tenormin Verapamil/Calan Nifedipine/Procardia Diltiazem/Cardizem	Increases blood flow to the heart muscle by either increasing oxygen supply of by decreasing oxygen demand by the heart.	Headache, dizziness, faintness, nausea
Laxatives & Cathartics	Lactulose, Bisacodyl/Dulcolax; Senna/Senokot; Psyllium colloid/Metamucil; Dioctyl sodium sulfosuccinate/Colace	Prevent constipation	Diarrhea, nausea, vomiting, abdominal cramping
Vitamins	Multivitamins Nephrocaps Nephrovite Diatx Folic Acid	Vitamins are necessary for normal metabolic functions & for tissue growth and healing. Replace any vitamins lost during dialysis	Occasional nausea
	Vitamin D 　　1,25 dihydrochole-calciferol/Rocaltrol 　　Doxercalciferol/Hectorol	Enhances the absorption of calcium from the gastrointestinal tract; helpful in maintaining bone formation.	Nausea, vomiting, loss of appetite, constipation, headache, hypercalcamia

10. The effect of hemodialysis on the concentration (or half-life) of a drug, is dependent on the following factors:

　a) The blood flow and dialysate flow rates

　b) The dialysis membrane permeability and surface area

　c) The molecular weight of the drug

　d) The water solubility of the drug

　e) The percent of protein binding of the drug

　f) The lipid affinity of the drug

　g) The drug distribution volume

11. Drugs that are dialyzable are frequently withheld and given at the end of dialysis.

12. Drugs are sometimes given for their immediate effects during treatment.

13. With the exception of heparin, single dose intravenous medications are injected post dialyzer via the venous blood tubing, and modifications in dose may be indicated.

14. It may be necessary to administer supplemental doses of certain drugs at the conclusion of dialysis. This especially applies to dialyzable drugs that require maintenance of specific plasma levels for therapeutic effect, e.g., an antibiotic.

Figure 8.3

Medications Commonly Given During Dialysis

Medication Classification	Generic and/or Brand Name)	Route of Administration	Purpose
Analgesic	Acetaminophen/Tylenol	Oral	Medication used for mild to moderate pain and to reduce fever
Antianemic	Erythropoietin/Epogen Darbepoetin alfa/Aransep	IV or subcutaneously (beneath the skin)	This is a recombinant form of erythropoietin, which stimulates bone marrow to produce red blood cells. It is used to elevate and maintain the red blood cell level and to decrease the need for transfusions.
	Iron dextran/Infed Ferricgluconule/Ferrlecit Iron Sucrose/Venofer	IV	Used in the treatment of iron deficiency anemia. Infed is used when patients have an intolerance or are resistant to oral iron.
Antibiotics	Gentamicin sulfate/Gentamicin Tobramycin/Nebcin	IV (post dialysis)	An antibiotic used primarily for serious gram negative infections.
	Cefazolin/Ancef	IV (post dialysis)	An antibiotic used for infections caused by gram positive cocci, gram negative bacteria.
	Vancomycin	IV (as prescribed)	An antibiotic used in the treatment of penicillin-resistant Staphylococcal infections.
Anticoagulant	Heparin	IV	Used to prevent blood from clotting in the extracorporeal circuit during dialysis.
Antiemetic	Prochlorperazine/ Compazine	Oral, IV, or intramuscular (IM)	Used for relief of nausea and vomiting
	Trimethobenzamide/ Tigan	Rectal or IM	Used for relief of nausea and vomiting
Antihistamine	Diphenhydramine Hydrochloride/Benadryl	Oral or intravenous (IV)	Used for minor allergic reactions or pruritis (itching)

Figure 8.3 continued

Medications Commonly Given During Dialysis

Medication Classification	Generic and/or Brand Name)	Route of Administration	Purpose
Chelating Agents	Deferoxamine/Desferal, DFO	IV	Treatment of iron overload and aluminum toxicity
Colloids	Albumin; "salt poor" albumin	IV	Highly effective means of restoring blood volume and blood pressure.
Heparin antagonist	Protamine sulfate	IV	In dialysis, used as a heparin antagonist in the event of heparin overdose.
Hypertonic Solutions	10% sodium chloride or 23.5% sodium chloride/hypertonic sodium chloride 50% dextrose (D50W)/hypertonic glucose	IV	Transfers water osmotically into the blood compartment from surrounding tissues helping to maintain blood volume. Used to treat severe muscle cramps.
Local Anesthetic	Lidocaine/Xylocaine	Intradermal (into the skin)	A drug used to produce a localized insensitivity (anesthesia) to pain when injected intradermally.
	Ethylchloride	Topical	A vapocoolant intended for topical application to control pain associated with venipuncture.
	Lidocaine 2.5% & Prilocaine 2.5%/Emla cream	Topical	A topical anesthetic applied for under an occlusive dressing for at least 1 hr., to provide analgesia for venipuncture.
Osmotic Solution	Mannitol (25%)	IV	Used to help maintain blood pressure and reduce dialysis symptoms by expanding the blood volume.

Figure 8.3 continued

Medications Commonly Given During Dialysis

Medication Classification	Generic and/or Brand Name)	Route of Administration	Purpose
Thrombolytic Agent	Streptokinase **Activase-TPA/Alteplase** Alteplase/Cathflo Activase	IV	Restore patency to intravenous catheters obstructed by clotted blood or fibrin
Vitamin D	Calcitriol/Calcijex **Paricalcitol/Zemplar** Doxercalciferol/Hectorol	IV	Enhance the absorption of calcium from the gastrointestinal tract. Helpful in maintaining bone formation.

Suggested Readings

Daugirdas, JT, Blake, PG and Ing, TS, editors (2001), *Handbook of Dialysis*, Third Edition, Boston: Little, Brown and Co.

Gutch, C.F., Stoner, M.H., Corea, A.L.(1999), *Review of Hemodialysis for Nurses and Dialysis Personnel*, Sixth Edition, Mosby.

Kee, J.L. and Hayes, E.R. (1993), *Pharmacology: A Nursing Approach*, Philadelphia: W.B. Saunders.

Lancaster, L., Editor (2001), *ANNA Core Curriculum for Nephrology Nursing*, Fourth Edition, Pitman, New Jersey: Anthony J. Jannetti, Inc.

Newberry, M.A.(1989), *Textbook of Hemdialysis for Patient Care Personnel*, Springfield, Ill.: Charles C. Thomas.

Nissenson, AR and fine, RN Editors (2002), *Dialysis Therapy*, Third Edition, Philadelphia; Henley and Belfus, Inc.

Chapter 9
Dialyzer Reuse

Contributing Author:
Philip M. Varughese, BS, CHT
Philip Andrysiak, BS, MBA, CHT

Chapter Outline

I. Purpose of Dialyzer Reprocessing

A. The multiple use of hemodialyzers was originally performed to conserve precious resources. The labor-intensive practice of cleaning and reassembling Kiil dialyzers led to the practice of flushing them and storing them in formaldehyde.

B. The relatively expensive high efficiency and high flux dialyzers led to a resurgence of reuse in the mid to late 1980s. Dialyzer reuse is the practice whereby the same dialyzer is used for multiple dialysis treatments to the same patients. High flux and high efficiency dialyzers aided in reducing treatment time. This treatment was welcomed by patients who spent more than 4 hours three times a week in dialysis. High flux dialyzers are a major cost consideration in dialysis; dialyzer reuse became more popular because it reduced the cost of dialysis.

C. Presently, dialyzer manufacturers produce dialyzers that are suitable for reprocessing. These multiple use dialyzers are the only ones approved by the FDA for reprocessing. It is recommended that units strictly follow procedures recommended by the manufacturer when reprocessing these dialyzers.

II. Types of Reuse Systems

A. Automated:

  1. Machines are available on the market for dialyzer reprocessing. These machines use microprocessors, electronic, and hydraulic components to perform the necessary steps. They automatically reprocess the dialyzer. The operator only has to put it on the machine and take it off. They also provide complete documentation for the entire process. Failure rate for an automated process is quite low.

B. Manual:

  1. Manual systems utilize valves and treated water to perform the reprocessing. They require an operator to open and close the valves at specified times to accomplish the procedure. They also require the operator to test the dialyzer. The failure rate for this process is quite high.

III. Reprocessing Procedures

A. Label: The reuse dialyzer is labeled with the name of the patient, number of previous uses, and date of the last reprocessing. Additional labeling may also be applied in the event that patients have the same or similar last names in order to prevent any mishaps. The dialyzer may also be labeled with test results and identification of the person performing the various steps of the reprocessing procedure.

B. Collection from unit

  1. Dialyzers should be collected from the patient care area in a container to prevent the splashing or dripping of blood throughout the facility.

  2. Generally, policies require that refrigeration of dialyzers should take place if reprocessing will not take place for at least 2 hours.

  3. Universal Precautions: protecting staff from contact with possibly contaminated blood and products, and preventing the spread of bacteria and viruses to other areas where they may cause infections in other staff or patients. Durable gloves and protective clothing should be worn during the reprocessing procedure. Gloves impervious to the disinfectant used are also required. These are usually not latex gloves. Universal precautions, including protective glasses, gloves, and fluid resistant gowns, should be observed throughout all processing procedures.

C. Cleaning blood from the dialyzer

  1. Diluted solutions of hydrogen peroxide, sodium hypo-chlorite, peracetic acid or other chemicals may be used as cleaning agents for the blood compartment. The cleaning agents must remove contaminants from the dialyzer without compromising the performance or the structural integrity of the dialyzer.

      a) Bleach
        (1) Effective agent for removing blood from a dialyzer; will also remove secondary membrane and can increase KUF of some dialyzers.

      b) Renalin
        (1) effective agent for removing blood from a dialyzer; does little to strip secondary membrane from fibers.

  2. Flushing removes blood from the blood compartment of the dialyzer; accomplished by running treated water through the dialyzer.

      a) The dialyzer must be flushed until its effluent is clear and the brown or pink tint disappears. Use <1ng/ml of endotoxin contained treated water during reprocessing. This is important because the blood side of the dialyzer might take up endotoxin that could be released into the circulation during the subsequent dialysis. Visual checks of the dialyzer should be done to ensure that only a minimal amount of fiber clots is present.

3. Head caps: Remove caps and remove clot from the pockets and check the 'o' rings. Residual clots located at the dialyzer may be released during subsequent reuse and cause patient embolism or other symptoms.

D. Reverse Ultra filtration

1. Moving fluid through the dialyzer membrane from the dialysate compartment into the blood compartment to remove the protein layer that occurs during treatment. This process can sometimes open clotted fibers.

E. Testing of the dialyzer to assure its efficacy in subsequent uses:

1. Clearance measurements

a) These are expressed in terms of the volume of blood from which the solute is completely removed or cleared per unit time, the unit of measure being milliliters per minute. Clearance of a reuse dialyzer should be maintained within a range of performance recommended by the manufacturer. The urea clearance should be the recommended criterion for rejecting a dialyzer. Acceptable clearance tolerance is +/- 10 percent of the originally suggested performance.

2. TCV

a) Facilities should use the total cell volume (TCV) measurement, the most widely accepted rejection parameter, as an indirect indicator of clearance performance. TCV is not a fiber Bundle Volume (FBV) test. The FBV is only the volume of the fibers. The TCV is the volume of the FBV and the header cap volume. Dialyzers must be discarded when this value changes by more than 20% of the original value. The effect of germicide can increase or decrease the clearance and these changes in clearance cannot be detected by TCV measurement.

b) Changes in TCV directly correlate with changes in diffusive capabilities of the dialyzer. When individual fibers become plugged, fibers are lost to solute transport and there is a decrease in overall clearance. This loss in transport is non-linear because the higher velocity in the remaining fibers causes an increase in the diffusion rate inside the fiber. This explains why a 20 percent loss in surface area only yields about a 10 percent loss in urea clearance.

c) 80% of initial volume is the cutoff point at which the dialyzer must be discarded.

(1) Example: Dialyzer has an initial volume of 150 ml. This dialyzer must be discarded if the volume falls below 120 ml.

F. Leak Test

1. Leak tests are performed to test for broken fibers or cracked potting compound. The pressure should be created 20% higher than the maximum operating TMP. The rate of pressure decrease must be equal to or less than that of a new dialyzer. All modern automated reprocessing units do this test automatically.

2. Also called pressure test. Pressure is applied to blood compartment of dialyzer and held. Rapid change in pressure would indicate a broken fiber, which would cause a blood leak during dialysis.

a) Failure of this test requires that dialyzer be discarded.

G. KUF Test

1. Measurement of dialyzer ultra filtration rate, and the changes with use and reprocessing

2. This is not an adequate indicator of diffusive clearance changes.

3. Evidence suggests that in-vivo KUF testing could be an indicator of convective and large molecule clearances.

H. Visual Inspection

1. There should be minimal signs of clotting in the fibers or the header of the dialyzer.

2. The dialyzer should be inspected for cracks and breakage.

3. The dialyzer should be filled with an adequate amount of disinfectant.

4. The dialyzer must be properly labeled with patient and dialyzer information.

I. Disinfection of the dialyzer to assure that all-microbial contamination is eliminated.

1. AAMI recommends that dialyzers be filled with germicide repeatedly until the effluent germicide concentration is within 10% of the original concentration and that the dialyzer ports then be disinfected and sealed with new or disinfected caps.

2. Monthly tests for total bacteria/ and or endotoxin levels in the water used to make up the germicide should be conducted. Testing of the germicides final use concentration should be part of the center's Quality Control program as well as verifying that each dialyzer was filled with germicide.

   a) The duration of storage should be appropriate for the agent used to disinfect the dialyzer.

3. The presence of the germicide should also be checked before the dialyzer is stored for the next treatment.

4. Renalin

   a) Contains peracetic acid which is acetic acid, and hydrogen peroxide

   b) Effective with all microorganisms, such as bactericidal, sporicidal, fungicidal, virucidal.

   c) Required dwell time
      (1) Minimum 11 hours

   d) Appropriate concentration is 3% when instilled into the dialyzer

   e) Renalin solution used by Renatron and has a shelf life of one week after dilution.

   f) Renalin containers and reprocessed dialyzers must be stored out of direct sunlight and in a temperature range of 32°F to 75°F.

5. Formaldehyde

   a) The oldest agent used for disinfection of reused dialyzers; does not degrade or change membrane properties.

   b) Formalin, is a saturated solution of formaldehyde in water. 100% of formalin solution contains 37 - 40 % formaldehyde.

   c) Formaldehyde allows the use of low concentrations if constant incubation at 40°C accompanies the reuse process.

   d) Low cost, stable solution, good high level disinfectant

   e) Carcinogenic, patient and staff acceptance low, offensive odor and irritation to skin and eyes

   f) Required dwell time is 24 hours contact time recommended.

   g) Appropriate concentration:

      (1) 4% when stored at room temperature
      (2) 1% when incubated at 100°F

6. Citric acid is used with heat to disinfect the dialyzer. This is also known as non-chemical dialyzer reprocessing. The dialyzers are filled with 1.5% of citric acid and heated at 95°C for 20 hours.

   a) Due to the increase in blood leaks for this process, the number of reuses per patient is low.

   b) Only certain dialyzers can be used in this process.

J. Exterior Disinfection:

1. Dialyzer exteriors must be cleaned and disinfected with low-level germicides, such as bleach diluted to a concentration of 1:100 of sodium hypochlorite.

K. Initiation of Dialysis Therapy:

1. Before initiating dialysis therapy, patient identification must be matched with the name shown on the dialyzer label. Two people verify identification and this step must be properly recorded. If possible, one of the persons checking identification should be the patient. Appropriate labeling of the dialyzer and successful completion of all necessary tests must be evident before initiation of treatment.

2. The absence of chemicals used in dialyzer disinfection must be confirmed before patient connection.

IV. Benefits of Dialyzer Reuse

A. Cost containment:

1. The dialyzer is the most expensive disposable used in the dialysis treatment, costing up to $30 or more. Reprocessing dialyzers saves considerable money for the facility.

2. Use of expensive high flux dialyzers is much more practical if the dialyzers are reprocessed.

B. Clinical Benefits:

1. Enhanced bio-compatibility

   a) The primary means of attenuating complement activation is the formation in the dialyzer of a secondary membrane that isolates the fiber from the patients' blood stream. If the reuse process does not remove this layer, the patients may have fewer reactions to the dialyzer during subsequent uses.

   b) Reduction or minimization of first use syndrome

   c) Decreased immune system activation

2. Decreased exposure to residual ethylene oxide

C. Dialysis patients should be carefully monitored for adverse reactions that may be related to reuse practices.

D. Priming the dialyzer and Rinsing of the germicides.

1. Prior to patient use, any disinfectant must be rinsed out of the dialyzer, and a test for the absence of the chemical must be performed.

2. Air bubbles in the fibers can cause individual fibers to become blocked. Be sure that the arterial line is fully primed before connection to the hemodialyzer. If peracetic acid-type germicide is used, be sure the blood side is flushed before beginning dialysate flow. The heat from the dialysate will cause air to be released from the peracetic acid thus air locking the fibers.

3. Germicide may back up into the heparin or monitor lines. Ensure that the heparin line is clamped and fluid is not forced into the monitor lines.

4. Discard the prime solution when beginning blood flow to the dialyzer. Do not connect the venous line to the venous needle until blood has reached the venous end of bloodline.

5. There is a possibility that germicide levels could increase if fluid circulating through the dialyzer is stopped before treatment is initiated. The rebound effect could expose the patient to germicide.

6. If the patient is exposed to the germicide they will feel a burning sensation at the access site at the very beginning of the initiation of treatment. Usually within five minutes.

E. Patient Monitoring:

1. Patient monitoring should include temperature measurement pre- and post-dialysis treatment. If fever (a temperature higher than 100°F) or chills are present during treatment or post-dialysis, a pyrogen reaction may be suspected, and should be promptly reported and investigated. This usually occurs at approximately thirty minutes after the initiation of treatment.

2. Patients should be monitored for other unexplained symptoms as well as allergic reactions or pain in the blood access arm at the beginning of the dialysis process. If these occur, it should be properly reported and the cause must be investigated and remedied appropriately. It is recommended that the operator stop the dialysis treatment when any reaction or unexplained symptoms occur that are thought to be related to the reprocessing.

F. Proper heparinization and priming procedures are critical in maintaining the efficacy of the dialyzers. This is especially true in the case of larger surface area and high flux dialyzers. It is recognized that larger molecule clearances are largely membrane limited as opposed to small molecule clearances which are largely flow rate limited. Inadequate anticoagulation can cause problems with residual blood clotting within the dialyzers. As a result, reduced dialysis efficacy through loss of dialyzer surface area can result. The number of reuses will also diminish due to lack of proper anticoagulation that causes a decrease in the TCV.

V. Risks and Hazards of Dialyzer Reuse

A. There is a potential for bacterial contamination if the dialyzer is not cleaned and disinfected properly.

B. Exposure of the patient to chemicals may also occur if the dialyzer is not properly prepared for use.

C. Reduced dialyzer efficiency can lead to under dialysis and increased mortality if dialyzers are not cleaned and tested properly.

D. With ever increasing dialyzer reuse numbers, the risk of blood leaks significantly increases. During a blood leak the dialysate can mix with blood which may expose the patient to pathogens.

E. Dialyzer used on wrong patient.

1. As long as the dialyzer is disinfected properly this risk is minimal.

F. Water Requirements:

1. AAMI Standards for chemical and microbiological contamination must be met at all times for reprocessing of dialyzers and for dilution of chemical disinfectants

a) Testing Water Quality: Both the blood and dialysate compartments of the dialyzer should be rinsed and cleaned with water that enables it to meet the AAMI standards. The water should have a bacterial colony count of less than 200 CFU per ml or a bacterial lipopolysaccharide (LPS) concentration of less than 1 ng/ml (5EU) as measured by the Limulus amebocyte assay.

VI. Documentation

A) All reuse records should meet the requirements for medical records. The following is the minimum recording requirements:

1. The dialyzer reprocessing Master Manual, with policies, procedures and training.

2. The patient reprocessing record should have information of each dialyzer process including:

   a) Rinsing and cleaning, Disinfection, Testing, Storage and Setup for reuse.

   b) Equipment Maintenance Record; repair, preventive maintenance and validation results

   c) Personnel Training and health monitoring records; reuse training, validation, periodical in service, auditing and physical health.

   d) Complaint/Failure investigation record. A record of complaints by patients and staff about failures of reprocessed dialyzers or possible adverse reactions to reprocessed dialyzer, the investigation results and corrective plan.

   e) Daily logs
   (1) Machine self-test, if applicable
   (2) TCV verification, if applicable

3. Disinfectant presence verification.

4. Maintenance logs:

   a) Maintenance and repairs must be maintained according to manufacturer's recommendations. Each piece of equipment used for reprocessing must be appropriately maintained and tested to perform its intended task. Along with complete documentation of system function, operation procedures, potential system failures and dialyzer reuse criteria must be in the dialyzer-reprocessing manual.

   b) Operational logs indicate when repairs were performed and who performed them.

5. Training and testing of staff.

   a) All staff performing dialyzer reprocessing must be trained according to unit policy and procedures. Competency testing must be done and documented.

6. Policy and procedures

   a) All policies and procedures used in the reprocessing of dialyzers must be documented and reviewed periodically.

VII. Quality Assurance

A. Reprocessing is the "re-manufacturing" of a medical device, which has direct contact with patient's blood. Therefore, the area should be clean and sanitary at all times. Storage areas for new dialyzers and reprocessing materials should be designed to facilitate rotation of stock. Vapors from reprocessing materials should be maintained below potentially toxic limits as per EPA standards.

B. Water cultures and LAL's:

1. Must be tested at least monthly, and must meet or exceed AAMI standards.

   a) Cultures: 200 CFU's per ml maximum

   b) LAL: 5 EU's per ml maximum

C. Air quality testing

1. Performed quarterly in reuse area

D. Maximum formaldehyde vapor levels

1. TWA (Time Weighted Average) 0.75 ppm

2. STEL (Short Term Exposure Limit) 3 ppm

E. Maximum Renalin vapor levels

1. Acetic acid- 10 ppm

2. H_2O_2- 1 ppm

F. Peracetic acid

1. None developed

G. Maximum Gluteraldehyde vapor levels

1. 0.2 ppm.

H. Trend analysis

1. Dialyzer failures and unusual occurrences must be reviewed for trends that could lead to adverse patient outcomes.

I. Reasons for dialyzer failures

1. Blood leaks

2. Pyrogenic reactions (elevated temperatures)

3. Patient reactions to chemicals

4. Patient complaints

J. Dialyzer performance validation

1. In-vivo testing of dialyzer clearances

2. Changes in dialyzer clearance should correlate with changes in TCV

3. A 20% drop in TCV should equal an approximate drop in clearance of 10%

4. Monitoring delivered dose of dialysis (URR or Kt/V)

5. A decrease in the delivered dose of dialysis should result in an investigation into the reasons, which would include the reprocessed dialyzer as well as access problems, time on dialysis, and heparinization.

Suggested Readings

AMGEN, Inc. (1992), *Core Curriculum for Dialysis Technicians,* Wisconsin: Medical Media Publishing, Inc.

Daugirdas, John T. and Ing, Todd S., Editors (1993), *Handbook of Dialysis, Second Edition.* Little, Brown and Co.

HCFA Pub. 7 - Rev.286. 01-98, State Operations Manual Provider Certification

Renal Systems, Dialyzer Reprocessing, 1990.

AAMI (1998), *AAMI Standards and Recommended,* Volume 3, 1998 Edition

Chapter 10
Infectious Disease and Infection Control

Contributing Authors:
Matthew J. Arduino, Dr.P.H

Chapter Outline

I. Introduction

Patients with end stage renal disease (ESRD) are often at an increased risk of developing infections because they suffer from abnormal immune responses. These patients can develop serious infections when exposed to various infectious agents. In this chapter a number of potential problem areas for hemodialysis patients and staff will be discussed. The main infections and adverse events caused by microbial byproducts discussed here will be those of importance in maintenance hemodialysis centers. These include the three major bloodborne pathogens (hepatitis B and C, and the human immunodeficiency virus [HIV]), and, in particular, antimicrobial-resistant bacteria. However, there are a number of microbial products, which can also produce disease in hemodialysis patients. These products include a number of microbial toxins, which can enter the patient's bloodstream via contaminated water and dialysate or contaminated hemodialyzers.

II. Non-infectious Agents in Hemodialysis Patients

A. Endotoxin.

Endotoxin is a component of the cell wall of gram-negative bacteria. Endotoxin is responsible for causing pyrogenic reactions during hemodialysis and may also play a role in what is now referred to as the chronic inflammatory response syndrome.

Pyrogenic reactions are usually defined as fever ≥38°C in a patient who was afebrile at the start of the treatment, with no obvious signs of infection. In addition to fever, these signs and symptoms usually include rigors (shaking chills) and hypotension, and may also include nausea, vomiting, and backache. Pyrogenic reactions usually occur within 1.5 hrs of initiation of hemodialysis.

These reactions are usually caused by hemodialyzers that were reprocessed with water containing >5 endotoxin units (EU)/ml. Dialysate containing >2,000 colony forming units (CFU)/ml of bacteria has also been shown to produce pyrogenic reactions. Commercial test-kits (*Limulus* amebocyte lysate tests) are available to test water and dialysate for bacterial endotoxin.

B. Exotoxin A

Exotoxin A is produced by a common water organism, *Pseudomonas aeruginosa*. This toxin may also be involved in producing chronic inflammatory responses in dialysis patients. There are no commercially available test kits for this toxin.

C. Other Biological Toxins

Other toxins include those produced by toxigenic cyanobacteria. In an outbreak in Brazil in a facility that received untreated raw water from a tanker truck, approximately half of the patients died from liver failure after being treated with dialysate made from the contaminated water. The water was found to contain both a neurotoxin (anatoxin-A) and hepatotoxin (microcystin-LR). The outbreak could have been prevented by using appropriate water treatment methods such as reverse osmosis [1].

III. Bloodborne Pathogens

Three major bloodborne pathogens are important to both patients and staff of the hemodialysis community. All of these agents are viruses and include the hepatitis B virus (HBV), hepatitis C virus (HCV), and the HIV. HBV is the most efficiently transmitted bloodborne virus within the hemodialysis unit.

A. Hepatitis B Virus

HBV has historically been a major health hazard for both patients and staff in dialysis centers. It is by far the most efficiently transmitted bloodborne pathogen in this setting. Most HBV infections in dialysis patients are subclinical, and a large percentage of these patients are persistently hepatitis B surface antigen (HBsAg) positive. Clinical features may include jaundice, fatigue, abdominal pain, loss of appetite, intermittent nausea, and vomiting.

HBV tends to become endemic because dialysis patients are likely to become chronic asymptomatic HBsAg carriers, and also because these carriers become a source of contamination for many environmental surfaces. HBV can enter the body through:

(1) direct percutaneous inoculation by needle of contaminated serum or plasma or transfusion of infected blood or blood products; (2) percutaneous transfer of infected serum or plasma into cuts, scratches, abrasions, or other overt or inapparent breaks in the skin; (3) introduction of infective serum or plasma into the mouth or eyes; (4) introduction of other known infective secretions such as saliva and peritoneal fluid into mucosal surfaces or indirect transfer of serum or plasma via vectors or inanimate environmental surfaces.

Dialysis staff members may become infected with HBV through accidental needle puncture, breaks in their skin, or mucous membranes from their frequent and continuous contact with blood and blood-contaminated surfaces in the unit. Dialysis patients may become infected in the unit by several mechanisms: (1) through internally contaminated dialysis equipment such as venous pressure gauges or venous pressure isolators or filters (used to prevent reflux of blood into gauges) that are not routinely changed after each use; (2) through injections if the site of injection is contaminated with HBV; (3) through breaks in skin or mucous membranes when in contact with contaminated objects. There has been no documented evidence of disease transmission from infected dialysis staff to dialysis patients. However, dialysis staff may physically carry HBV from infected to susceptible patients via contaminated hands, gloves, and other objects.

Environmental surfaces in the dialysis area may constitute a major mechanism of disease transmission. HBsAg has been detected on clamps, scissors, dialysis machine control knobs or panels, intravenous (IV) poles mounted on dialysis machines, interior of the connecting tube on arterial or venous-pressure monitors, tops of centrifuge cups, wintrobe tube racks, telephones, marking pens, walls, and surfaces of dialysis machines in hemodialysis units.

Since HBV is most efficiently transmitted in the dialysis setting, the infection control precautions recommended for dialysis units were developed to prevent transmission of this agent. The primary rationale is that infection control practices that effectively control the transmission of HBV would also be effective in preventing the transmission of other microorganisms (bacteria and viruses).

Testing and Diagnosis. In newly infected individuals, HBsAg becomes detectable about 8 weeks after exposure. Conversion from HBsAg negative to positive is essentially synonymous with newly acquired HBV infection, and the presence of HBsAg is indicative of ongoing HBV infection and potential infectiousness.

Antibody to hepatitis B core antigen (anti-HBc) appears at the onset of symptoms or liver test abnormalities in acute HBV infection, rapidly rises to high levels, and persists for life. The presence of anti-HBc indicates previous or ongoing infection with HBV. Recently acquired infection can be distinguished by the presence of IgM anti-HBc, which is detected at the onset of acute hepatitis B and remains detectable for about 6 months.

In persons who recover from HBV infection, HBsAg is usually cleared from the blood in 2-3 months, and antibody to HBsAg (anti-HBs) develops during convalescence. The presence of anti-HBs is generally interpreted as indicating recovery and immunity from HBV infection. After recovery from natural infection, most persons will be positive for both anti-HBs and anti-HBc, whereas only anti-HBs develops in persons who are successfully vaccinated against hepatitis B.

In persons who do not recover from HBV infection and become chronically infected with HBV, HBsAg (and anti-HBc) remain detectable. HBV infection is likely to become chronic in dialysis patients. For testing recommendations see Section V.

B. Hepatitis C Virus

HCV is the etiologic agent of most parenterally transmitted non-A, non-B (NANB) hepatitis worldwide. HCV is an RNA virus classified in the Flavivirus family and, since its discovery in 1988, has been shown to be a major cause of acute and chronic hepatitis. There are multiple HCV genotypes and within genotypes there are closely related genotypes or quasi-species. Antibody elicited by infection with one genotype fails to cross-neutralize virus of another genotype and prior infection does not produce immunity. It is estimated that there are some 35,000-180,000 HCV infections per year and approximately 3.5 million chronic cases in the United States.

Interpretation of enzyme immunoassays is limited by several factors. These assays do not detect anti-HCV in all infected persons, and about 5% of HCV-infected persons may be anti-HCV negative (this proportion may be higher in immuno- compromised, including chronic hemodialysis, patients). These assays do not distinguish between acute, chronic, or resolved infections. They also may yield falsely positive results, which can be as high as 50% in populations with a low prevalence of HCV infection.

HCV is primarily transmitted by direct percutaneous exposure to blood. In the dialysis environment, staff members may become infected with HCV through percutaneous or permucosal exposures to anti-HCV-positive blood. Dialysis patients presumably may acquire HCV infection through similar exposures, but the risk factors for transmission of HCV infection among dialysis patients have not been well studied. Other than receipt of blood and blood products prior to donor screening for anti-HCV, the only risk factor identified has been increasing years on long-term dialysis. The association between HCV infection and length of time on dialysis suggests that cumulative exposures in the dialysis setting may be important. In contrast to HBV, HCV circulates at lower titers in infected blood, and its ability to survive in the environment is questionable. In the hemodialysis environment, where the potential for contamination with blood is high, short-term survival may be sufficient to facilitate transmission if there is contamination of supplies and articles that are shared among patients. In addition, most patients infected with HCV remain persistently infected and provide a large reservoir that serves as a potential source of transmission to others.

C. *Human Immunodeficiency Virus /Acquired Immunodeficiency Syndrome (AIDS)*

During 1985 - 1997, the percentage of U.S. centers that reported providing hemodialysis for patients with HIV infection increased from 11% to 39% and the number of hemodialysis patients with known HIV infection increased from 0.3% to 1.3% [2]. There has been a report of one confirmed and two possible cases of HIV transmission in U.S. dialysis centers from an infected dialysis patient to a dialysis staff member. In the confirmed case the dialysis worker sustained a needlestick with a large bore acccess needle while performing dialysis on a patient who was known to be HIV positive and was undergoing dialysis in a private room. The dialysis worker had no known HIV risk factors, was HIV negative at the time of the exposure, and subsequently became HIV positive (CDC, unpublished data). Outside of the United States there have been reports of transmission of HIV from patient to patient in developing countries. Breaks in infection control measures, especially sharing of syringes or needles, appear to be the most likely modes of transmission in these outbreaks. Other than the needlestick incidents reported above, transmission of HIV has not been reported in U.S. hemodialysis centers.

HIV is transmitted much less efficiently than HBV, presumably because of the significantly lower levels of HIV in the blood of infected individuals. Therefore, the dialysis unit precautions presented below, in our opinion, are adequate to prevent transmission of HIV from patients to staff members and from patient to patient. Patients with HIV infection can be treated with either hemodialysis or peritoneal dialysis; the type of dialysis treatment should be based on the needs of the patient. They need not be isolated from other patients, either in separate rooms or by using dedicated

machines, and HIV-positive patients can participate in dialyzer reuse programs. Disinfection and sterilization strategies routinely practiced in dialysis centers, and discussed elsewhere in this chapter, are adequate to prevent the transmission of HIV.

Routine testing of dialysis patients or staff members for HIV antibody is not necessary for infection control purposes. HIV testing for patient management, antimicrobial prophylaxis, and other reasons, however, may be desirable.

IV. Bacterial Infections

Bacterial infections are thought to be common in hemodialysis patients, but there have been few formal studies of this topic. From the data published in the literature, the rate of bacteremia was 0.7 per 100 patient-months (8.4 per 100 patient-years), and, contrary to expectation, nonbacteremic infections and infections not involving the vascular-access site predominated in these studies. Independent risk factors for infection in hemodialysis patients include type of vascular access, serum albumin level, and race. Use of bio-incompatible membranes also is a reported risk factor for infection.

Staphylococcus aureus is the most common cause of vascular-access infection and bacteremia in hemodialysis patients. In patients receiving dialysis through a central catheter, *S. epidermidis* is an important pathogen. Gram-negative bacteria may have a larger role when the patient's access site is in the lower extremities. Other causes of bacteremia (*Mycobacterium abscessus*, enterococci, and a variety of gram-negative bacteria) have also been associated with contaminated dialysis machines and improperly reprocessed hemodialyzers.

A. *Vascular-Access Infections*

As noted above, bacterial infections in hemodialysis patients most commonly arise from the vascular-access site. Vascular- access site infections may metastasize to the lung, skin, heart, central nervous system, bone or joint, or kidney.

Local signs of vascular-access infection include erythema, warmth, induration, swelling, tenderness, breakdown of skin, loculated fluid, or purulent exudate. Some of the risk factors for vascular-access infection include: (1) type of vascular access (fistula, graft, or catheter); (2) location of access in the lower rather than upper extremity; (3) recent thrombectomy, graft revision, or reconstructive procedure; (4) local access trauma or hematoma; (5) dermatitis overlying the site; (6) scratching of insertion sites; (7) poor patient hygiene; (8) poor needle insertion technique; (9) older age; and (10) diabetes.

Native arteriovenous fistulas are associated with lower rates of thrombosis and infection than are synthetic grafts. Despite their lower complication rate, the use of fistulas appears to be decreasing. At the end of 1997, 59.7% of hemodialysis patients were receiving dialysis through grafts, 22.8% through fistulas, and 17.5% through temporary or permanent central catheters [2].

Central catheters are associated with higher rates of bacteremia than are either fistulas or grafts. Cuffed, dual-lumen, silicone catheters have lower rates of bacteremia (25-29 per 100 patient-years) than do other catheters, but these rates still exceed those reported in patients with permanent accesses (8.4 per 100 patient-years). In 1991, CDC investigated 35 bloodstream infections among 68 patients receiving hemodialysis through central catheters of which, many that were being used for permanent access; one patient died and one developed endocarditis and required aortic valve replacement. To minimize infectious complications, patients should be referred early for creation of an implanted access, thereby decreasing the time receiving dialysis through a temporary catheter. Additionally, permanent catheters should be used only in patients for whom implanted access is impossible.

CDC has published guidelines for prevention of central catheter-associated infections [3]. The following recommendations are intended for all types of central catheters (i.e., not specifically hemodialysis catheters): use sterile technique during catheter insertion; do not use antimicrobial prophylaxis before insertion or during the use of the catheter to prevent infections; and do not routinely replace the catheter to prevent infections.

Recommendations specific for hemodialysis catheters:

(1) use a cuffed catheter if the period of access is anticipated to be ≥1 month

(2) use the catheter solely for hemodialysis unless there is no alternative access

(3) restrict manipulation of the catheter to trained dialysis personnel

(4) replace the catheter site dressing at each hemodialysis or when the dressing becomes damp, loosened, or soiled

(5) apply povidone-iodine ointment to the catheter insertion site at each dressing change

Patients who are nasal carriers of *S. aureus* have an increased risk of *S. aureus* vascular-access infection. Treatment of these colonized patients with oral rifampin or intranasal mupiricin has been shown to decrease the

S. aureus bacteremia rate, but in one of these studies this reduction may have been accompanied by an increase in bacteremias caused by other organisms. Resistance to mupiricin is common with frequent or continuous application, and uncommon when the agent is used in periodic short courses.

B. Infections Through Contaminated Hemodialysis Equipment or Dialysate, or Errors in Reprocessing

In the early days of hemodialysis, bacteremias were often associated with dialysate containing > 2,000 CFU/ml of microorganisms. In addition the increased use of bicarbonate-based dialysate, which can support prolific growth of gram- negative bacteria and dialyzer reuse have been linked to episodes of bacteremia. Many of the CDC outbreaks over the last 11 years have been associated with errors in hemodialyzer reprocessing, *i.e.*, failure to ensure proper concentration of germicide in the hemodialyzer or improperly making up germicide from concentrates for use in a manual system; disassembly of hemodialyzers without proper disinfection of O-rings, caps, and headers (header sepsis); and failure to mix germicide when diluting concentrate with water.

Recent outbreaks of bacteremia have been associated with the waste-handling option of the Cobe CentryIII machines. In each of these cases, there were breaks in disinfection practices, insufficient maintenance schedules for replacement of check valves, or lapses in daily quality control protocols [4,5]. Outbreaks of bacteremia in each of these cases resolved with discontinuation of use of the waste handling option. The manufacturer has now developed a training program, which addresses the appropriate use of this option for owners of these machines.

C. Vancomycin-Resistant Enterococci and Other Antimicrobial-Resistant Bacteria

Dialysis patients are an important part of the epidemic of vancomycin resistance. A study at 49 hospitals showed that dialysis was an independent risk factor for bacteremia due to vancomycin-resistant enterococci (VRE). In outbreaks in hospitals, patients on dialysis or with renal insufficiency have constituted a significant portion of VRE case-patients The percentage of hemodialysis centers reporting ≥1 patients with VRE colonization or infection increased from 11.5% in 1995 to 29.8% in 1997 [2]. In addition, of four reported patients having cultures positive for vancomycin intermediate *S. aureus* (VISA), two were on chronic peritoneal dialysis and one was on temporary peritoneal dialysis.

V. Infection Control Precautions for Dialysis Units

A. Dialysis Unit Precautions

In 1977, CDC published precautions to prevent transmission of HBV in dialysis centers [6]. In 1987, universal precautions were developed to prevent transmission of all bloodborne pathogens, including HBV and HIV, in health care and other settings [7]. In 1996, an updated system of precautions, termed standard precautions, was published to replace universal precautions for the hospital and most healthcare settings [8]. The infection control measures currently recommended for dialysis units incorporate features of each of these guidelines. These measures are effective against HBV, the most highly transmissible organism in hemodialysis units; therefore, they should also be effective against other viruses (e.g., HCV) and bacteria (e.g.,VRE).

Note that dialysis unit precautions are more stringent than universal or standard precautions. For example, standard precautions require the use of gloves only when touching blood, body fluids, secretions, excretions, or contaminated items. In contrast, dialysis unit precautions require glove use whenever patients or hemodialysis equipment is touched. Standard precautions do not restrict the use of supplies, instruments, and medications to a single patient however, dialysis unit precautions specify that no supplies, instruments or medications be shared between any patients.

Since dialysis patients may be infected or colonized with a variety of bacteria and viruses, the following precautions should be used during care of **all dialysis patients at all times**.

- Assign each patient a dialysis chair or bed and machine and supply tray (tourniquet, antiseptics, if possible blood pressure cuff). Avoid sharing these items. Do not share clamps, scissors, other nondisposable items unless sterilized or disinfected between patients.

- Prepare and distribute medications from a centralized area. Medication carts should not be used. Separate clean and contaminated areas; for example, handling and storage of medications

and hand washing should not be done in the same or adjacent area to that where blood samples or used equipment are handled.

- Disposable gloves should be worn by staff members for their own protection when handling patients or dialysis equipment and accessories. Gloves should be worn when taking blood pressure, injecting saline or heparin, or touching dialysis machine knobs to adjust flow rates. For the patient's protection, the staff member should use a fresh pair of gloves with each patient to prevent cross-contamination. Gloves also should be used when handling blood specimens. Staff members should wash their hands after each patient contact.

- Avoid touching surfaces with gloved hands that will subsequently be touched with ungloved hands before being disinfected.

- Staff members may wish to wear protective eyeglasses and masks for procedures in which spurting or spattering of blood may occur, such as cleaning of dialyzers and centrifugation of blood.

- Staff members should wear gowns, scrub suits, or the equivalent while working in the unit and should change out of this clothing at the end of each day.

- After each dialysis, (1) change linen and (2) clean and disinfect the dialysis bed/chair and nondisposable equipment (especially control knobs and other surfaces touched by gloved hands).

- Crowding patients or overtaxing staff may facilitate cross-transmission. Avoid clutter and allocate adequate space to facilitate cleaning and housekeeping.

- Staff members should not smoke, eat, or drink in the dialysis treatment area or in the laboratory. There should be a separate lounge for this purpose. However, all patients may be served meals. The glasses, dishes, and other utensils may be cleaned in the usual manner by the hospital staff. No special care of these items is needed.

B. Control Measures for Hepatitis B Virus

Because HBV is so highly transmissible in hemodialysis centers, several precautions in addition to those outlined above have been recommended specifically to deal with this pathogen.

- Patients and staff should be vaccinated and screened as per recommended schedules (see below).

- HBsAg-positive patients should undergo dialysis in a separate room designated only for HBsAg-positive patients. They should use separate machines, equipment, and supplies, and most importantly, staff members should not care for both HBsAg-positive and susceptible patients on the same shift or at the same time. If a separate room is not possible, HBsAg-positive patients should be separated from HBV- susceptible patients in an area removed from the mainstream of activity and should undergo dialysis on dedicated machines. Anti-HBs-positive patients may undergo dialysis in the same area as HBsAg-positive patients, or they may serve as a geographic buffer between HBsAg-positive and HBV-susceptible patients; in either instance they may be cared for by the same staff member. When the use of separate machines is not possible, the machines can be disinfected by using conventional protocols, and the external surfaces can be cleaned with soap and water or a detergent germicide and disinfected.

Although there is no evidence that patients or staff members in centers that reuse dialyzers are at greater risk of acquiring HBV infection, it might be prudent that HBsAg-positive patients not participate in dialyzer reuse programs. HBV can occur in high concentration in blood, and handling dialyzers used on HBsAg-positive patients during the reprocessing procedures might place staff members at risk for HBV infection.

The Centers for Disease Control and Prevention (CDC) and the Advisory Committee on Immunization Practices (ACIP) have published guidelines for protection against infection with HBV [9]. This section is meant to collate, summarize, and update, but not replace, sections of these guidelines that deal specifically with hemodialysis patients and staff. If a patient or staff member is exposed to HBV, the recommendations of the ACIP [10] should be followed.

Initial Testing for Hepatitis B Virus Markers

Hemodialysis patients and staff should be tested for HBsAg and anti-HBs when they begin dialysis or employment in the center. They should be classified as infected if HBsAg positive; immune if anti-HBs positive (≥10 milli-international units per milliliter [mIU/ml]) on at least two consecutive occasions; or susceptible if HBsAg negative and anti-HBs negative (<10 mIU/ml).

For infection control purposes, testing anti-HBc is not necessary. However, if testing is done, individuals who are HBsAg negative and anti-HBc positive have had past HBV infection and are immune.

Hepatitis B Vaccination

All susceptible patients and staff should receive hepatitis B vaccine (dosage schedules in Table 1), be tested for anti-HBs 1-2 months after the final dose of vaccine, and be followed up as outlined below. Vaccination of immune (anti-HBs ≥10 mIU/ml on two consecutive occasions) persons is not necessary, but also is not harmful.

Screening and Follow-up

Screening and follow-up depends on the result of anti-HBs testing 1-2 months after the final dose of vaccine (Fig. 10.2). Unvaccinated immune individuals can be screened and followed up as if they were vaccine responders.

Patients who are anti-HBs positive (≥10 mIU/ml) after vaccination are responders. They should be tested for anti-HBs each year (Fig. 10.2). If the level of anti-HBs falls below 10 mIU/ml, they should receive a booster dose of hepatitis B vaccine and continue to be tested for anti-HBs each year.

Patients who are anti-HBs negative (<10 mIU/ml) after vaccination are non-responders. They should be revaccinated with second three dose vaccine series and retested for anti-HBs 1-2 months later. If they are then anti-HBs positive (≥10 mIU/ml), they can be reclassified and treated as responders (see above). If they continue to be non-responders (anti-HBs <10 mIU/ml), they should be considered susceptible to HBV infection and tested for HBsAg every month and anti-HBs every 6 months (Table 2).

Staff who are anti-HBs positive (≥10 mIU/ml) after vaccination are responders. They do not need any further routine anti-HBs testing (Table 2). If exposed to blood from a patient known to be HBsAg-positive no further action is required [9].

Staff who are anti-HBs negative (<10 mIU/ml) after vaccination are non-responders. They should be revaccinated with a second three-dose vaccine series, and retested for anti-HBs 1-2 months later. If they then become anti-HBs positive (≥10 mIU/ml), they should be reclassified and treated as responders (see above). If they are not revaccinated, or are still anti-HBs negative (<10 mIU/ml) after re-vaccination, they continue to be non-responders. Non-responders should be considered susceptible to HBV infection and tested for HBsAg and anti-HBs every 6 months (Table 2). If they are exposed to the blood of a person known to be HBsAg-positive, they should either receive 2 doses of hepatitis B immune globulin (HBIG), or if not previously re-vaccinated receive 1 dose of HBIG and initiate re-vaccination.

C. *Drug Resistant Microorganisms (Vancomycin Resistant Enterococci, Methicillin Resistant Staphylococcus aureus, Staphylococci with reduced susceptibility to glycopeptide antimicrobial agents)*

CDC recommends contact precautions for care of hospitalized patients infected or colonized with MRSA, VRE, or certain other antimicrobial-resistant bacteria [8,11]. Dialysis unit precautions as outlined above include many of the measures recommended under contact precautions. However, under contact precautions (but not dialysis unit precautions) a private isolation room and (in certain instances) a separate gown are recommended. These measures were recommended to prevent possible transmission via contaminated environmental surfaces such as counter tops and bed rails. Hospitalized patients spend nearly 24 hours a day in their hospital bed, whereas dialysis patients spend only 3-5 hours three times a week in the dialysis unit. Note that feces are the main reservoir for VRE. The potential for bacterial contamination of environmental surfaces would appear to be much greater in hospitalized patients than in most dialysis outpatients.

Dialysis unit precautions should be used for care of all patients; at present we do not advise additional precautions for most patients with MRSA or VRE. However, additional precautions would be prudent for patients with infective material that can not be contained (e.g., wound drainage that can not be contained by dressings and is culture-positive for MRSA or VRE, or a positive stool culture for VRE and fecal incontinence, a colostomy, diarrhea, or poor hygiene). For these patients, if an isolation room is not available, enhanced attention to patient separation and environmental cleaning might be sufficient. Staff should wear a separate gown when caring for such patients.

Dialysis units should reevaluate their compliance with dialysis center precautions and improve precautions for care of all patients where necessary. Another approach would be cohorting—assign patients with known MRSA or VRE to certain dialysis stations at one end of the unit, use dedicated staff to care for them, and ensure that strict precautions are used at these stations.

Figure 10.1

Hepatitis B Vaccine Dosage Schedules

Product/Group		Dose	Schedule
Recombivax HB			
	Patients	40 µg (1 ml)*	3 doses at 0, 1, and 6 months
	Staff	10 µg (1 ml)	3 doses at 0, 1, and 6 months
Engerix-B			
	Patients	40 µg (2 ml)**	4 doses at 0, 1, 2, and 6 months
	Staff	20 µ(1ml)	3 doses at 0, 1, and 6 months or 4 doses at 0, 1, 2, and 6 months

*Special formulation
** Two 1.0-ml doses administered at one site

Prudent Vancomycin Use

Prudent vancomycin use is another important issue discussed in the CDC guideline "Recommendations for Preventing the Spread of Vancomycin Resistance" [11]. Antibiotic use can be considered in three categories: prophylaxis given to uninfected patients in an attempt to prevent infection; empiric therapy, given to patients with signs and symptoms of infection, pending culture results; and continuing therapy, given after culture results are known.

Prophylaxis with vancomycin should not be given, other than for certain surgical procedures [11].

Empiric treatment with vancomycin is appropriate, pending culture results, in patients with beta-lactam allergy, or in instances where serious infection with beta-lactam-resistant gram-positive bacteria (i.e., MRSA or *Staphylococcus epidermidis*, which are generally beta-lactam resistant) is likely. Knowing the percent of *S. aureus* that are methicillin-resistant in your area, and the percent of serious infections due *to S. epidermidis*, is important in determining empiric antimicrobial-coverage.

Continuing treatment depends on culture results. If the patient has allergy to beta-lactam antimicrobials, or if beta-lactam resistant bacteria are isolated (with the exception of single blood cultures positive for S. epidermidis), vancomycin is appropriate. Depending on susceptibility results, alternative antimicrobial agents

(*e.g.,* cephalosporins) with dosing intervals ≥ 48 hours, which would allow post-dialytic dosing, could be used. Recent studies suggest that cefazolin given 3 times a week provides adequate blood levels [12,13].

D. Recommendations for Screening for Hepatitis C

The only assays approved by the U.S. Food and Drug Administration for diagnosis of HCV are those that measure anti-HCV. These tests can detect anti HCV in ≥ 97% of infected patients. Supplemental testing with a more specific assay (*i.e.,* recommbinant immunoblot assay or RIBA™) prevents the reporting of false positive results, particularly in settings where asymptomatic persons are being tested. For patients with acute HCV, however, there may be a prolonged interval between exposure or onset of hepatitis and antibody seroconversion. Persons negative for anti-HCV during their acute illness should be retested at least six months later to make a final diagnosis. Anti-HCV can be detected in 80% within 15 weeks, in 90% within 5 months, and in more than 97% within 6 months after exposure [14].

Patients with a diagnosis of non-A, non-B hepatitis who remain negative for anti-HCV may have hepatitis C but fail to elicit an immune response detectable by the current assay, they may be infected with a second agent of non-A, non-B hepatitis, or their hepatitis may have another cause (viral or

Figure 10.2

Recommendations for Serologic Surveillance for Hepatitis B Virus (HBV) among Patients and Staff of Chronic Hemodialysis Centers

Vaccination/Serologic Status and Frequency of Screening			
Group/Screening Test	Vaccine Non-Responder or Susceptible*	Vaccine Responder or Natural Immunity**	Chronic HBV Infection***
Patients			
HBsAg	Every Month	None	Every Year
Anti-HBs	Every 6 Months	Every Year	If HBsAg becomes negative
Staff			
HBsAg	Every 6 Months	None	Every Year
Anti-HBs	Every 6 Months	None	If HBsAg becomes negative

*Anti-HBs < 10 mIU/ml
**Anti-HBs ≥ 10mIU/ml
***HBsAg positive for at least 6 months; or HBsAg positive, anti-HBc positive, IgM anti-HBc negative

nonviral). Thus, the diagnosis of acute non-A, non-B hepatitis must continue to rely on the exclusion of other etiologies of liver disease even with the availability of a licensed test for anti-HCV.

The recommendations are as follows:

- Dialysis unit precautions as outlined above should be used for all patients.

- Patients who are positive for anti-HCV or have a diagnosis of non-A, non-B hepatitis do not have to be isolated from other patients or receive dialysis separately on dedicated machines. In addition, they can participate in dialyzer reuse programs.

- Patients should be monitored for elevations in ALT and AST monthly. Elevations in liver enzymes may be detected earlier than anti-HCV in patients with acute hepatitis.

- Routine screening of patients or staff for anti-HCV is not currently recommended for purposes of infection control. Dialysis centers may wish to conduct serologic surveys of their patient populations to determine the prevalence of the virus in their center, and in the case of patients or staff with a diagnosis of non-A, non-B hepatitis, to determine medical management. In addition, if liver enzyme screening indicates the occurrence of an epidemic of non-A, non-B hepatitis in the dialysis setting, anti-HCV screening on serum samples collected during and subsequent to outbreaks may be of value. However, since anti-HCV in an individual cannot measure infectivity, its usefulness for infection control in the dialysis center setting is limited. (The recommendation in this last bullet is currently undergoing review and revision and may change).

References

Cited References

1. Jochimsen EM, Carmichael WW, An JS, Cardo DM, Cookson ST, Holmes CE, Antunes MB, de Melo Filho DA, Lyra TM, Barreto VS, Azevedo SM, Jarvis WR. "Liver failure and death after exposure to microcystins at a hemodialysis center in." *N Engl J Med* 1998;338(13): 873-878

2. Tokars JI, Miller ER, Alter MJ, Arduino MJ. National Surveillance of Dialysis Associated Diseases in the United States, 1997. National Center for Infectious Diseases, Centers for Disease Control and Prevention, Public Health Service, Department of Health and Human Services, Atlanta, GA 30333, 1998. (http://www.cdc.gov/ncidod/hip/Dialysis.htm)

3. Pearson ML, HICPAC. "Guideline for prevention of intravascular device related infections." *Am J Infect Control* 1996;24:262-293 (http://www.cdc.gov/ncidod/hip/iv/iv.htm)

4. Centers for Disease Control and Prevention. "Outbreaks of gram-negative bacterial bloodstream infections traced to probable contamination of hemodialysis machines" —Canada, 1995; United States, 1997; and Israel, 1997. *MMWR* 1998;47:55-59

5. Jochimsen EM, Frenette C, Delorme M, Arduino M, Aguero S, Carson L, Ismail J, Lapierre S, Czyziw E, Tokars JI, Jarvis WR. "A cluster of bloodstream infections and pyrogenic reactions among hemodialysis patients traced to dialysis machine waste-handling option units." *Am J Nephrol* 1998;18(6):485-489

6. Centers for Disease Control and Prevention. "Control measures for hepatitis in dialysis centers." Viral Hepatitis Investigations and Control Series. November 1977.

7. Centers for Disease Control and Prevention. "Recommendations for prevention of HIV transmission in health-care settings." *MMWR* 1987;36 (No. 2S):3S-18S

8. Garner JS, the Hospital Infection Control Practices Advisory Committee. "Guideline for isolation precautions in hospitals." *Infect Control Hosp Epidemiol* 1996;17:53-80

9. Advisory Committee on Immunization Practices and Hospital Infection Control Practices Advisory Committee. "Immunization of Health-Care Workers: Recommendations of the Advisory Committee on Immunization Practices and the Hospital Infection Control Practices Advisory Committee." *MMWR* 1997; 46 (RR-18).

10. Centers for Disease Control. "Hepatitis B virus: a comprehensive strategy for eliminating transmission in the United States through universal childhood vaccination." *MMWR* 1991;40 (no. RR-13): 1-42

11. Centers for Disease Control and Prevention. "Recommendations for preventing the spread of vancomycin resistance." *MMWR* 1995;44 (No. RR-12):1-13.

12. Marx MA, Frye RF, Matzke GR, Golper TA. "Cefazolin as empiric therapy in hemodialysis-related infections: efficacy and blood concentrations." *Am J Kidney Dis.* 1998;32:410-414

13. Fogel MA, Nussbaum PB, Feintzeig ID, Hunt WA, Gavin JP, Kim RC. "Use of cefazolin in chronic hemodialysis patients: a safe and effective alternative to vancomycin." *Am J Kidney Dis* 1998;32:401-409

14. CDC. "Recommendations for prevention and control of hepatitis C virus (HCV) infection and HCV-related chronic disease." *MMWR* 1998;47 (RR-19):1-38

Additional References

Favero MS, Alter MJ, Tokars JI, Arduino MJ. Dialysis-associated infections and their control, pp 357-380. In JV Bennet and P Brachman (eds), *Hospital Infections*, Fourth Edition, Lippencott-Raven Publishers, Philadelphia, 1998

Kessler M, Hoen B, Mayeux D, Hestin D, Fontenaille C. "Bacteremia in patients on chronic hemodialysis." *Nephron* 1993;64:95-100

Kaplowitz LG, Comstock JA, Landwehr DM, Dalton HP, Mayhall CG. "A prospective study of infections in hemodialysis patients: patient hygiene and other risk factors for infection." *Infect Control Hosp Epidemiol* 1988;9:534-541

Churchill DN, Taylor DW, Cook RJ, et al. "Canadian hemodialysis morbidity study." *Am J Kidney Dis* 1992;19:214-234.

Churchill DN. "Clinical impact of biocompatible dialysis membranes on patient morbidity and mortality: an appraisal of the evidence." *Nephrol Dial Transplant* 1995;10:52-56.

Theresa L. Smith, Michele L. Pearson, Kenneth R. Wilcox, Cosme Cruz, Michael V. Lancaster, Barbara Robinson-Dunn, Fred C. Tenover, Marcus J. Zervos, Jeffrey D. Band, Elizabeth White, William R. Jarvis, for the Glycopeptide-Intermediate Staphylococcus aureus Working Group. "Emergence of Vancomycin Resistance in Staphylococcus aureus." *New Engl J Med* 1999;340:493-501

Chapter 11
Safety in Dialysis

Contributing Author:

Lawrence K. Park, MSPH, CHM

In this chapter we will be discussing safety in a dialysis clinic. An effective approach would be to look at the Occupational Safety and Health Administration (OSHA) and their requirements where their primary focus is safety.

According to Title 29 Part 1903, Section 1 of the Code of Federal Regulations:

The Williams-Steiger Occupational Safety and Health Act of 1970 (84 Stat. 1590 *et seq.*, 29 U.S.C. 651 *et seq.*) requires, in part, that every employer covered under the Act furnish to his employees employment and a place of employment which are free from recognized hazards that are causing or are likely to cause death or serious physical harm to his employees. The Act also requires that employers comply with occupational safety and health standards promulgated under the Act, and that employees comply with occupational safety and health standards promulgated under the Act, and that employees comply with standards, rules, regulations and orders issued under the Act which are applicable to their own actions and conduct. The Act authorizes the Department of Labor to conduct inspections, and to issue citations and proposed penalties for alleged violations.

In reviewing the above paragraph, let us address the first issue of the employer providing a place of employment free from recognized hazards that are likely to cause death or serious physical harm to his employees.

An example of this type of hazard in a dialysis facility would be tuberculosis. According to the OSHA Fact Sheet 93-43 entitled "Enforcement Policy on Tuberculosis (TB)," (which is based on the October 8, 1993 agency wide enforcement policy):

Inspection for occupational exposure to TB shall be conducted in response to employee complaints and as part of all industrial hygiene compliance inspections in workplaces where the Centers for Disease Control (CDC) has identified workers as having a greater incidence of TB infection. These workplaces are health care settings, correctional institutions, homeless shelters, long-term care facilities for the elderly and drug treatment centers.

Citations based on the general duty clause will be issued only to employers whose employees work on a regular basis in one of the five types of facilities listed above by the CDC as having a higher incidence of TB than the general population, and whose employees 1) have potential exposure to the exhaled air of an individual with suspected or confirmed tuberculosis, or 2) were exposed to a high

hazard procedure performed on an individual who may have tuberculosis and which has the potential to generate potentially infectious airborne respiratory secretions.

To prove a violation of the general duty clause, it must be shown that the employer *failed* to keep the workplace free of a *hazard* to which his or her employees were exposed, that the hazard was recognized, that the hazard was causing or likely to cause death or serious physical harm, and that a feasible and useful method to correct the hazard existed.

Second, the employer must comply with occupational safety and health standards promulgated with the Act designed to promote health and safety. Please find below a listing of OSHA programs which may be relevant to your dialysis facility (as cited in Title 29 Code of Federal Regulations):

- 1903.2 (Posting of job safety and health notice)
- 1904.1 (Purpose and Scope - Recording and Reporting Occupational Injuries and Illnesses)
- 1904.2 (Log and Summary of Occupational Injuries and Illnesses)
- 1910.35 (Definitions – Means of Egress)
- 1910.36 (General Requirements – Means of Egress)
- 1910.37 (General Means of Egress)
- 1910.38 (Employee Emergency Plans and Fire Prevention Plans)
- 1910.95 (Occupational Noise Exposure)
- 1910.101 (Compressed Gases – General Requirements)
- 1910.132 (General Requirements – Personal Protective Equipment)
- 1910.133 (Eye and Face Protection)
- 1910.134 (Respiratory Protection)
- 1910.145 (Specification for Accident Prevention Signs and Tags)
- 1910.146 (Permit Required Confined Spaces)
- 1910.147 (The Control of Hazardous Energy - Lockout/ Tagout)
- 1910.151 (Medical Service and First Aid)
- 1910.157 (Portable Fire Extinguishers)
- 1910.158 (Standpipe and Hose Systems)
- 1910.159 (Automatic Sprinkler System)
- 1910.1000 (Air Contaminants)

- 1910.1001 (Asbestos)
- 1910.1020 (Access to Employee Exposure and Medical Records)
- 1910.1030 (Bloodborne Pathogens)
- 1910.1048 (Formaldehyde)
- 1910.1200 (Hazard Communication)

In reference to the above topics, there are numerous questions which could be asked to ensure safety. Examples include:

- Are compressed oxygen cylinders secured?
- Is there 3 foot access to the electrical panels?
- Are the electrical panels labeled as to function?
- Are there portable fire extinguishers on site?
- Are the extinguishers appropriate for the class of commodity stored?
- Are fire extinguishers checked monthly and certified annually?
- Is the emergency evacuation plan in place?
- Are the emergency evacuation routes posted?
- Does the site plan denote you are here, exits, pull stations, fire extinguishers, smoke detectors, arrows showing the shortest route of egress, etc.?
- Are the exit lights all lit?
- Are the exits kept clear and unobstructed?
- Is the fire alarm system tested?
- Is the sprinkler system tested?
- Is each electrical circuit marked to indicate its purpose?
- Is there a chemical inventory list?
- Are there Material Safety Data Sheets for all items on the chemical inventory list?
- Are all hazardous chemicals labeled?
- Are chemicals properly stored and handled?
- Is there a drench shower/eyewash, when required?
- Are appropriate personal protective equipment being selected and worn by personnel?
- Is air sampling conducted for chemical contaminates, when required?
- Are appropriate respirators utilized, when required?

- Is fit testing, medical surveillance and training conducted for respirator wearers?
- Is personal protective equipment available for employees based on potential hazards?

As with any program, training is essential to safety. Examples of training in dialysis may include the following:

- Bloodborne Pathogen
- Formaldehyde
- Hazard Communication
- Electrical Safety
- Back Injury Prevention
- Needlestick Prevention
- Respiratory Protection
- Portable Fire Extinguisher
- The Control of Hazardous Energy
- Asbestos
- Airborne Pathogen
- Personal Protective Equipment
- Workplace Violence
- Accident Investigation
- Defensive Driving

In addition, there are resources available from OSHA which can be used as a reference to assist in the health and safety effort in the *dialysis clinic* and some of them are listed below:

1. US Department of Labor Program Highlights Fact Sheets

   - No. OSHA 93-02 "Inspecting for Job Safety and Health Hazards"
   - No. OSHA 93-05 "Record Keeping Requirements"
   - No. OSHA 93-09 "Back Injuries – Nation's Number One Workplace Safety Problem"
   - No. OSHA 95-24 "Safety with Video Display Terminals"
   - No. OSHA 93-32 "Control of Hazardous Energy Sources"
   - No. OSHA 93-43 "Enforcement Policy for Tuberculosis"
   - Bloodborne Facts – 1992

- No. OSHA 92-27 "Occupational Exposure to Formaldehyde"

- No. OSHA 93-41 "Workplace Fire Safety"

- No. OSHA 93-44 "OSHA Emergency Hotline"

- No. OSHA 92-19 "Responding to Workplace Emergencies"

- No. OSHA 93-03 "Eye Protection In the Workplace"

- No. OSHA 93-26 "Hazard Communication Standard"

- No. OSHA 92-01 "Job Safety and Health"

- No. OSHA 93-07 "Improving Workplace Protection For New Workers"

- No. OSHA 92-46 "Bloodborne Pathogens Fact Sheet – Summary of Key Provisions."

- No. OSHA 92-08 "Protecting Yourself with Personal Protective Equipment."

2. US Dept. of Labor Booklets

- Access to Medical and Exposure Records – OSHA 3110 (1993)

- All About OSHA – OSHA 2056 (1995)

- Asbestos Standard for General Industry – OSHA 3095 (1995)

- Employee Workplace Rights – OSHA 3021 (1994)

- Chemical Hazard Communication – OSHA 3084 (1995)

- Consultation Services for the Employer – OSHA 3047 (1997)

- How to Prepare for Workplace Emergencies – OSHA 3088 (1995)

- Occupational Exposure to Bloodborne Pathogens – OSHA 3127 (1996)

- Bloodborne Pathogens and Acute Care Facilities – OSHA 3128 (1992)

- Personal Protective Equipment – OSHA 3077 (1998)

- Brief Guide to Recordkeeping Requirements for Occupational Injuries and Illnesses – OMB No. 1220-0029

- Log and Summary of Occupational Injuries and Illnesses (Form OSHA 200)

- Hospitals and Community Emergency Response – What You Need to Know – OSHA 3152 (1997)

- Recordkeeping Guidelines for Occupational Injuries and Illnesses – OMB No. 1220-0029

- Supplementary Record of Occupational Injuries and Illnesses (Form OSHA 101)

- Hearing Conservation – OSHA 3074 (1995)

- (Lockout/Tagout) Control of Hazardous Energy – OSHA 3120 (1994)

- Material Safety Data Sheet – OSHA 174

- OSHA Inspections – OSHA 2098 (1996)

- OSHA Publications and Audiovisual Programs – OSHA 2019 (1998)

- Respiratory Protection – OSHA 3079 (1993)

- Video Display Terminals – OSHA 3092 (1996)

3. US Department of Labor Field Inspection Reference Manual (FIRM)

4. US Department of Labor Directives – developed by OSHA to provide a standardized system of inspection procedures for compliance staff and contains information on the application of a particular standard, or providing guidance regarding OSHA's policies and procedures.

5. US Department of Labor Technical Manual

6. US Department of Labor Posters

- Attention Drivers OSHA 3113 (1994)

- Confined Spaces Can Kill – OSHA 3140 (1994)

- Job Safety and Health Protection – OSHA 2203 (1997)

7. Code of Federal Regulations

- Title 29 Code of Federal Regulations Parts 1901.1 to 1910.999 (General Industry)

- Title 29 Code of Federal Regulations Parts 1910.1000 to End (General Industry)

Finally, to enforce safety in the workplace, OSHA has established a system of inspection priorities and they are listed below as stated in OSHA's Publication No. 2056:

- Imminent Danger – First priority is imminent danger. Imminent danger is any condition where there is reasonable certainty that a danger exists that can be expected to cause death or serious physical harm immediately or before the danger can be eliminated through normal enforcement procedures.

- Catastrophes and Fatal Accidents – Second priority is given to investigation of fatalities and catastrophes resulting in hospitalization of three or more employees.

Such situations must be reported to OSHA by the employer within 8 hours. Investigations are made to determine if OSHA standards were violated and to avoid recurrence of similar accidents.

- Employee Complaints – Third priority is given to employee complaints of alleged violation of standards or of unsafe or unhealthful working conditions.

- Programmed High-Hazard Inspections – Fourth in priority are programs of inspection aimed at specific high-hazard industries, occupations or health substances. Industries are selected for inspection on the basis of such factors as the death, injury and illness incidence rates and employee exposure to toxic substances. Special emphasis may be regional or national in scope, depending on the distribution of the workplaces involved. Comprehensive safety inspections in manufacturing will be conducted only in those establishments with lost work-day injury rates at or above the most recently published BLS national rate for manufacturing. States with their own occupational safety and health programs may use somewhat different systems to identify high-hazard industries for inspection.

- Follow-up Inspections – Finally, a follow-up inspection is conducted to determine if the previously cited violations have been corrected. If an employer has failed to abate a violation, the compliance officer informs the employer that he/she is subject to "Notification of Failure to Abate" alleged violations and propose additional daily penalties while such failure or violation continues.

In conclusion, there are many resources to assist you in your efforts in safety and dialysis. But always remember that safety is everyone's responsibility and safety starts with each one of us.

Chapter 12
Machine Functions

Contributing Author:
Danilo Concepcion, CHT

Chapter Outline

Figure 12.1

Schematic Representation of Extracorporeal Blood Circuit and Dialysate Delivery System Supplying Dialysate to the Dialyzer

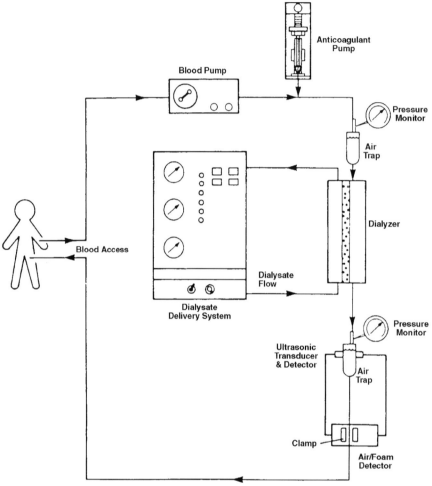

Source: Clinical Dialysis, p. 60, fig. 3-2.

I. Machine Functions

A. Dialysate Delivery

1. Concentrate proportioning is achieved by volumetric proportion or servo controlled proportioning.

   a) Different systems proportion at different ratios (e.g., 35X, 36.83X, 45X). Geometrical symbols on manufacturing package or container indicates the type of proportioning ratio the concentrate is to be calibrated to:

   (1) Square symbol denotes a 35X proportioning ratio

   (2) Circle symbol denotes a 36.83X proportioning ratio

   (3) Triangle symbol denotes a 45x proportioning ratio

   (4) Diamond symbol denotes a 36.1 bicarb concentrate generator

   b) In volumetric proportioning, all three streams (water, acid and bicarbonate) are calibrated to deliver a fixed volume.

   c) In a servo controlled proportioning, the operator enters a desired conductivity, and a servo. Feedback control system compares the conductivity measured by the acid/acetate or

Figure 12.2

Single Proportioning System

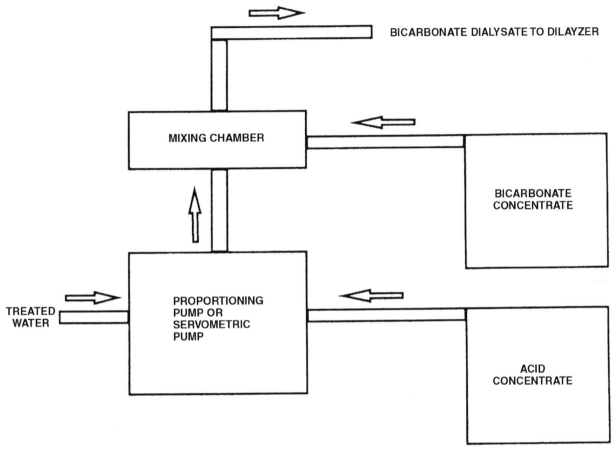

BICARBONATE DIALYSATE TO DILAYZER

MIXING CHAMBER

BICARBONATE CONCENTRATE

TREATED WATER

PROPORTIONING PUMP OR SERVOMETRIC PUMP

ACID CONCENTRATE

Reprinted with permission of the American Nephrology Nurses' Association, publisher, ANNA Core Curriculum for Nephrology Nursing, *Third Edition 1995.*

bicarbonate control conductivity cells with the value selected by the operator. If the values differ, the system sends an error-correction signal that adjusts the delivery rate of the appropriate pump.

d) Bicarbonate dialysis requires two concentrates since concentrated calcium (from the acid component) and bicarbonate will produce a precipitate.

e) Some systems use dry bicarbonate alone, while other systems use concentrates that are bicarbonate mixed with sodium chloride.

f) Mismatch of the different types of concentrates available can yield an alarm free

conductance value, but contain an improper electrolyte concentration.

g) Reliance solely on the conductivity to ensure safety is cautioned: all relevant factors should be considered (including pH).

h) AAMI standard A3.1.1 states "Recognition and application of appropriate concentrates to produce the desired dialysate is the responsibility of the operator."

i) Alarm set points shall be set at ± 5 percent from the nominal value of the particular dialysate in use and shall activate a visual and an audible alarm.

Figure 12.3

Air Removal System

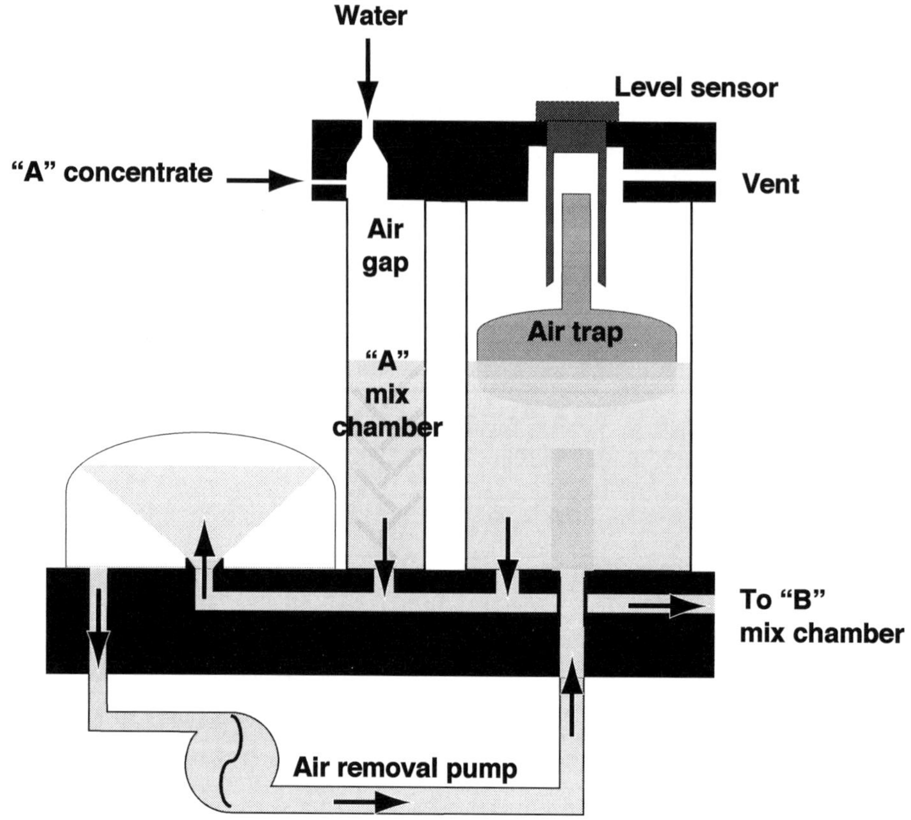

Reprinted with permission from Althin System 1000 Maintenance Manual, *p. 4. © Althin Medical, Inc.*

j) Dialysate flow will be diverted from the dialyzer during a conductivity alarm.

k) A volumetric proportioning system must have an on-line conductivity monitor downstream of the mixing point.

   (l) Systems for dual proportioning to produce bicarbonate dialysate using conductivity servo control shall have separate on-line conductivity cells to control and monitor each proportioning system.

2. Sodium/bicarbonate profiling allows for the modification of the sodium/bicarbonate concentration according to a predetermined profile. The profile provides an automated method of increasing and decreasing the sodium/bicarbonate concentration per physician prescription.

B. The deaeration device (as described by AAMI) "should remove all entrained air as well as any air which could potentially come out of the solution in the dialysate circuit at both maximum operational temperature and minimal operational pressures occurring within the circuit."

1. Dissolved air in the dialysate circuit may adversely affect the dialysis system monitors, hemodialyzer efficiency, ultrafiltration control, and patient safety.

2. Air in the dialysate compartment, or within the fiber of the dialyzer, can reduce dialyzer efficiency by displacing dialysate fluid. This effectively reduces dialyzer surface area.

3. Air may cross the membrane and create foam in the blood compartment.

C. *Temperature control and monitoring maintains the dialysate within the physiological range.*

1. A temperature greater than 42 degrees centigrade denatures protein and results in hemolysis.

2. A temperature less than 35 degrees centigrade may produce chilling and hypothermia, and clotting of the hemodialyzer can occur.

3. A visual and an audible response are required for a temperature alarm.

4. Dialysate flow will be diverted from the dialyzer during a temperature alarm.

D. *A blood leak detector is designed to monitor the occurrence of a rupture in the membrane of a dialyzer during a patient's treatment by detecting changes in optical density in dialysate downstream of the dialyzer. This is usually accomplished by emitting an infrared light beam across an optical path through the dialysate onto a receiver opposite the light source. Blood entering the optical path would decrease the intensity of the light and signal a change in optical density of the dialysate. The change in optical density activates the alarm sequence.*

1. The sensitivity of the blood leak alarm system is 0.35 ml of blood per liter of dialysate for a fixed alarm limit and less than 0.45 ml of blood per liter of dialysate for an adjustable limit at a hematocrit of 25%.

2. The blood pump should stop automatically for a blood leak alarm.

3. Blood-side pressure should never be less than dialysate-side pressure.

4. Ultrafiltration should be minimized automatically or manually to decrease the loss of blood.

E. *The bypass function is to interrupt the flow of dialysate to the dialyzer during an improper dialysate condition. Dialysate flow will be automatically diverted from the dialyzer to the drain during a dialysate alarm condition.*

1. An audible and visual alarm response will be evident during a bypass condition.

2. Temperature limits are usually set at 35 degrees centigrade for the low limit and 39 degrees centigrade for the high limit.

3. Dialysate conductivity varying more than ± 5 percent from the nominal value of the concentration in use shall cause a dialysate alarm.

F. *Ultrafiltration control determines the amount of fluid withdrawn from the extracorporeal circuit through the dialyzer membrane. Current hemodialysis systems design incorporates varying principles and techniques in performing fluid removal.*

1. Transmembrane pressure type machines are not dependent on dialysate volume control.

   a) Fluid removal is dependent upon the transmembrane pressures created by the differential between the blood-side and dialysate-side pressures.

   b) The blood side pressure is dependent on the blood pump rate, the gauge of the fistula needle in use, and the adequacy of the access flow.

   c) The dialysate-side pressure is regulated by an adjustable restrictive valve located in the dialysate flow path.

2. Transmembrane pressure (TMP) can be defined as:

   a) $TMP = (Pbi + Pbo)/2 - (Pdi + Pdo)/2$

   b) This can be approximated by the equation $(Pbo - Pdo)$. This is only correct when the blood and dialysate pressure drops are equal.

      (1) Pbi = Pressure of blood at dialyzer inlet

      (2) Pbo = Pressure of blood at dialyzer outlet

      (3) Pdi = pressure of dialysate at dialyzer inlet

      (4) Pdo = pressure of dialysate at dialyzer outlet

Figure 12.4

Flow Equalizer (Volumetric UF Control)

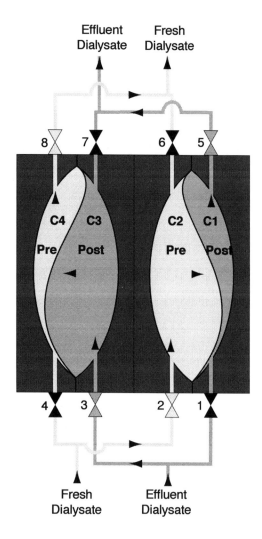

G. *A volumetric UF controlled machine is dependent on a balancing chamber system. The balance chamber ensures that equal amounts of fluid enter and exit the dialyzer.*

1. The chamber is divided into two equal chambers, with each chamber divided by an elastic membrane. The principle is based on displacing a volume of fluid on one side of the membrane by the introduction of fluid into the opposite side of the membrane. The two equal chamber halves operate alternatively to maintain a consistent flow of dialysate to the dialyzer. The dialysate circulates through a closed loop. With flow rate equal in and out of the dialyzer, the UF is zero.

2. To achieve ultrafiltration, a UF pump creates an imbalance by withdrawing fluid from the closed loop circuit at a rate determined by the machine operator. This pump is calibrated to remove a specific, known amount for each stroke.

3. The volume withdrawn from the loop is replaced by fluid crossing the dialyzer membrane from the blood side into the dialysate side. This fluid is therefore removed from the patient's blood stream.

H. *A flow metric control ultrafiltration system uses flow measuring devices that are in line before and after the dialyzer. The ultrafiltration is measured by the difference between the flow rate into the dialyzer and the flow rate out of the dialyzer. A microprocessor adjusts the TMP to achieve the desired ultrafiltration rate.*

I. *Ultrafiltration Profile in microprocessor controlled systems allows for the control and regulation of the ultrafiltration rate per hour according to a pre-programmed template.*

II. Extracorporeal Circuit

A. *The blood pump maintains a constant flow of blood through the dialyzer by means of a peristaltic action of the blood pump segment of the blood tubing.*

1. Blood pump segments are supplied in different diameters.

   Note: the proper blood pump I.D. setting must match the type of blood tubing used.

2. Self-occluding rollers applying pressure on the segment provides the peristaltic movement of blood through the extracorporeal system.

Figure 12.5

Ultrafiltration System

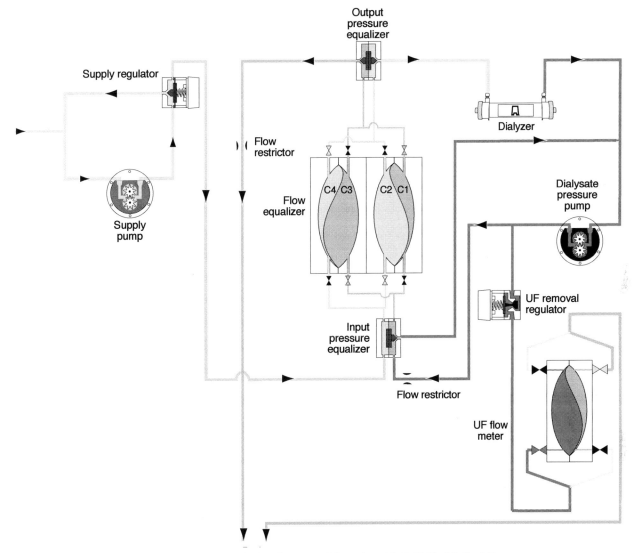

Reprinted with permission from Althin System 1000 Maintenance Manual, *p. 10.* © Althin Medical, Inc.

3. The volume of blood per minute is dependent on the revolutions per minute of the blood pump and the diameter of the pump segment.

4. Some systems maintain and display total blood volume processed, calculated by counting blood pump revolutions during a dialysis treatment.

B. Arterial and venous pressures are measured in mmHg (millimeters of mercury).

1. The arterial segment of the extracorporeal system is located pre dialyzer and contains the blood pump segment.

   a) According to the location of the arterial chamber in relation to the blood pump, arterial pressure may be monitored pre blood pump or post blood pump,

Figure 12.6

SPS 550 UF Control and Monitor System (Flow metric UF Control)

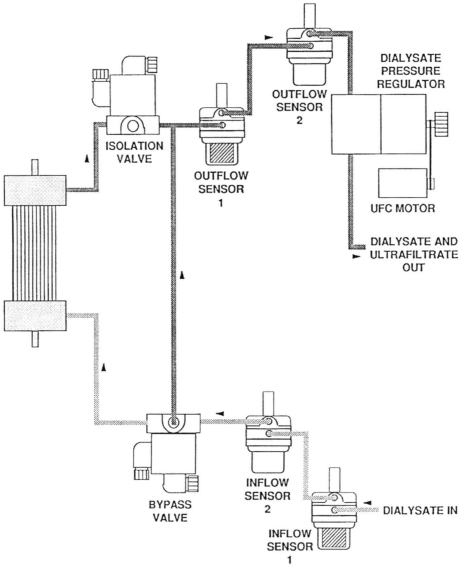

Reprinted with permission. © Baxter Healthcare Corporation

b) A pre blood pump arterial chamber position will result in an arterial negative pressure measurement.

    (1) A leak or line separation in the segment pre-blood pump would result in the introduction of air into the extracorporeal system.

    (2) An increase (more negative) in arterial negative pressure measurement would indicate an insufficient blood flow in relation to the pump rate speed. An increase in arterial negative pressure could be the cause of one of the following:

    kink in the arterial line, inappropriate fistula needle gauge, clotted access, inadequate needle placement, excessive blood flow rate, or a decrease in patient blood pressure.

Figure 12.7

Blood and Dialysate Circuits

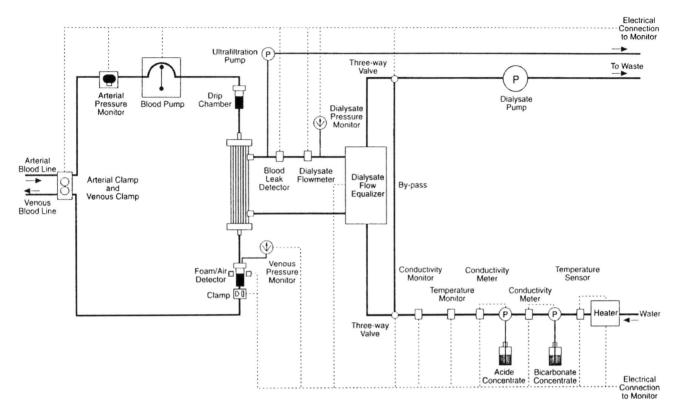

Source: Long-term Hemodialysis, *p. 34, fig. 4-2*

c) A post blood pump arterial chamber position will result in an arterial positive pressure measurement.

   (1) A leak or line separation in the extracorporeal system post blood pump would result in the loss of blood.

   (2) An increase in the arterial positive pressure measurement would indicate that there is a restriction to the blood flow through the dialyzer. This may be a result of a kinked line post chamber, clotting of the dialyzer, excessive blood flow rate, or a blockage of the venous segment of the extracorporeal circuit.

   (3) A decrease in the arterial positive pressure would indicate a disconnection of the extracorporeal circuit post-blood pump or a decrease in blood flow rate.

2. The venous segment of the extracorporeal system is located post dialyzer and contains the venous drip chamber.

   a) Venous pressure should always be maintained above zero (positive).

   b) A leak or line separation in the venous segment would result in the loss of blood.

   c) A high venous pressure would indicate a kink in the tubing distal to the venous chamber, a clotted access, a needle infiltration, low patient blood pressure, a clotted venous line, incorrect fistula needle gauge, or excessive blood flow rate, or recirculation.

   d) A low venous pressure would indicate a leak or line separation in the extracorporeal circuit post blood pump, a change in blood flow rate, or dialyzer clotting.

Figure 12.8

Venous and Arterial Tubing Sets

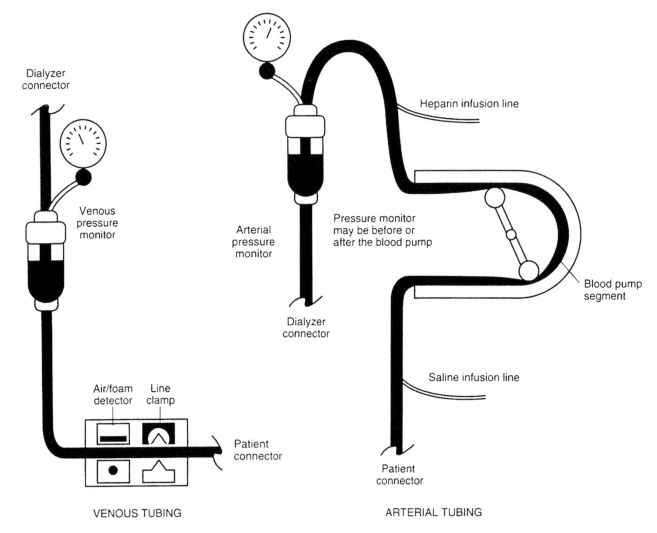

Dialyzer connector

Venous pressure monitor

Air/foam detector

Line clamp

Patient connector

VENOUS TUBING

Heparin infusion line

Arterial pressure monitor

Pressure monitor may be before or after the blood pump

Blood pump segment

Dialyzer connector

Saline infusion line

Patient connector

ARTERIAL TUBING

Reprinted with permission from AMGEN Core Curriculum, *p. 41, fig. 14*

3. In some machines, a venous level adjustment devices are incorporated into the internal component of the monitoring line. The device is a peristaltic pump parallel to the pressure transducer system.

   a) A switch operates the level adjustment. Switch up raises the level in the drip chamber; switch down lowers the level in the drip chamber.

C. Air-in-Blood Detector. This device monitors the fluid or blood level in the venous drip chamber for air in the extracorporeal system. Any air in this system that gets past the venous drip chamber could go directly into the patient's vascular system, causing an air embolus.

1. A.A.M.I. recommendation states, "The protective system shall include an air/foam detector and a venous-return-line occlusion clamp, which will prevent an air embolus to the patient.

Figure 12.9

Air/Foam Monitor

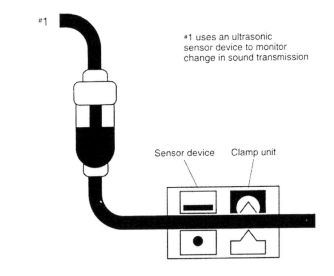

#1

#1 uses an ultrasonic sensor device to monitor change in sound transmission

Sensor device   Clamp unit

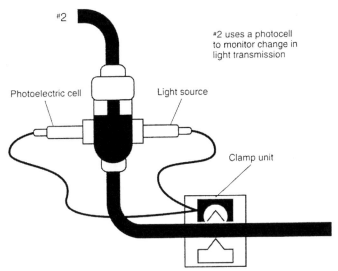

#2

#2 uses a photocell to monitor change in light transmission

Photoelectric cell   Light source

Clamp unit

Reprinted with permission from AMGEN *Core Curriculum, p. 41, fig. 14*

2. An air-in-blood detector alarm will cause the following safety logic response:
   a) An audible and visual alarm
   b) Disabling of an integral or external blood pump
   c) Occlusion of the venous return line by the venous occlusion clamp
   d) Reduction of the ultrafiltration rate (ultrafiltration controlled systems).

D. Heparin pumps are used to infuse anticoagulant into the extracorporeal system during a treatment.

1. Use a syringe type and size specific for the design of the heparin pump in use. Incorrect syringe size will cause inaccurate delivery of heparin.

2. All air should be removed from the syringe and the heparin infusion line.

III. Alarm Functions

A. *Alarm functions can be divided into two categories: extracorporeal alarms and dialysate alarms. All alarms will be evident by audio and visual indicators.*

1. Extracorporeal alarms are: the level (air in blood) detector, arterial pressure, venous pressure, blood leak detector, and transmembrane pressure alarm (TMP). An extracorporeal alarm will stop the blood pump and clamp the venous line clamp.

    a) The level/air detector is to detect air in the venous drip chamber, or venous blood line. The principle used is ultrasonic. Ultrasonic transducers are fitted on each side of the venous line or drip chamber, one being a transmitter and the other being a receiver. A signal is sent through the blood and received and measured on the receiving side. Any air in the blood will decrease the density of the fluid, creating a change in the signal that is then sensed at the receiver, causing a level detector alarm.

    b) The arterial pressure is monitored by means of a pressure transducer. A transducer is the electronic component that translates pressure into an electronic reading. Connection to the transducer is achieved via the arterial monitor port and the arterial monitor line, attached to the arterial drip chamber. A transducer protector must be placed in line to prevent contamination of the pressure transducer. Upper and lower alarm limits must be set by the operator to create an alarm if the arterial pressure changes.

    c) The venous pressure is measured in the same manner as the arterial pressure. In addition to its venous alarm function, the venous pressure is an integral part of the transmembrane pressure (TMP). The appropriate value of the venous pressure varies from patient to patient.

    d) The appropriate value for TMP is dependent on the KUF of the dialyzer and the rate of fluid removal. The monitor alarms are set to detect changes in TMP during a treatment. Increase in TMP during a treatment can result from a decrease in dialyzer total cell volume, increase in UFR rate, or recirculation.

IV. Equipment Disinfection

A. *Chemical disinfection procedures introduce unsafe chemicals into the dialysate system that may adversely affect the patient. As required by AAMI, "provisions should be made for restoring the dialysate system to physiological conditions after disinfection."*

1. Disinfection/rinse interlock switch protection must be incorporated into all systems during a chemical disinfection procedure to prevent the possibility of performing dialysis prior to elimination of residual chemicals from the system.

2. Residual chemicals shall be tested for and their absence verified according to the manufacturer's recommendation.

B. *Heat disinfection is performed by achieving temperatures of greater than 80 degrees centigrade in the dialysate system.*

1. The equipment must be designed so as not be able to dialyze a patient during the disinfection procedure.

2. The 80 degree temperature must be maintained for a period of time, generally 15 to 20 minutes, as recommended by the manufacturer.

3. Follow the manufacturer's recommended minimum frequency of disinfection.

4. Heat disinfection is effective for killing bacteria, but does not kill spores or viruses. Periodic disinfection with chemicals is still required.

V. Maintenance and Repairs

A. Maintenance and repair recommendations are outlined by the manufacturer.

1. Maintenance may be recommended on the following frequency:
   a) Per treatment
   b) Daily
   c) Weekly
   d) Monthly
   e) Quarterly
   f) Semiannually
   g) Annually
   h) Based on machine hours

B. Repairs should be performed by trained and qualified personnel only.

1. Equipment needing repairs must be isolated and labeled to prevent the use of equipment.

C. To assure proper machine function, records must include the date of preventative maintenance procedures and the date and results of scheduled testing or calibration of the equipment.

1. Maintenance procedures should be written and a schedule of preventative maintenance activities should be outlined and adhered to.

2. Documentation of all work performed on equipment must bear the signature of the person performing the work.

Suggested Readings

AAMI (1996), *AAMI Standards and Recommended Practices,* 1996 Edition, Arlington: Association for the Advancement of Medical Instrumentation.

AMGEN, Inc. (1992), *Core Curriculum for Dialysis Technicians,* Wisconsin: Medical Media Publishing, Inc.

Daugirdas, JT and Ing, TS, editors (1994), *Handbook of Dialysis,* Boston: Little, Brown and Co.

Repair and maintenance manuals from your dialysis machine manufacturer.

Chapter 13
Computers in Dialysis

Contributing Author:
Dr. Elizabeth J. Lindley, PhD

Chapter Outline

Computers in Dialysis

Renal units generate a vast quantity of data on each patient. This information often resides in a hand-written folder, but it is far more useful if it can be carefully organized in a computer. For individual patients, the computer can flag up problems, such as high potassium or a gradual increase in blood pressure. It can also be used to monitor the patient's response to changes in the dialysis prescription or medication, such as a new phosphate binder. Cumulative data can be used for clinical audits and to assess the outcome of actions taken to improve quality.

In some units the data is stored in a main-frame computer, usually running a UNIX operating system that supports multitasking and multiple users. The dialysis technician is usually not involved in the specification of these systems, so this chapter will focus on the 'microcomputer' or PC.

I. Purchasing Decisions

A. *Notebook PCs*

Now available with large, easily viewed displays, built-in CD-ROM and 3.5" disk drives and the usual communication ports. You need a good reason for purchasing a notebook as they are more expensive to buy and maintain, and more likely to be damaged or stolen, than a comparable desktop. The usual reason is that the PC will be used in several locations. Patient-related information on a portable PC must be adequately protected.

B. *Operating system*

The most popular are Microsoft Windows and the Macintosh operating system. Both have a graphical user interface (GUI) based on a desktop with icons and menus. The Mac system's fast, high quality graphics is popular with publishers and designers, and it can now emulate a PC to run more software, but it is only available on Apple computers.

C. *Central processing unit (CPU)*

The chip that carries out the arithmetic functions and logical tests and controls the movement of data between the other devices that make up the PC. Intel is the market leader and the chips are usually defined using Intel's nomenclature. The 386 and 486 are effectively obsolete. Pentiums come as standard or MMX (multi-media extension) with processing speeds up to 300MHz. The price of the PC may be much lower if it doesn't have an Intel processor.

D. *Cache*

Special memory that tries to minimize disk access time by storing chunks of the data that was close to the last location you accessed. A larger cache will enhance the performance of the PC.

E. *Random Access Memory (RAM)*

Memory that is lost when the computer is switched off. Static RAM (SRAM) consists of switches that stay in place when switched and works faster than dynamic RAM (DRAM) which has to be constantly refreshed. EDO (enhanced data out) is a form of DRAM. Inadequate RAM will dramatically reduce the performance of the PC. Most PC's can have extra RAM added.

F. *Hard disk*

Memory that is not lost when the computer is switched off. Usually defined by the size and the system controlling the way data is written to and read from the disk. IDE (or Integrated Drive Electronics) is a slower controller than SCSI (Small Computer Systems Interface). Hard disks can have a capacity of many Gigabytes, but modern software requires a lot of disk space. Buy a larger disk if you plan to install a lot of general software, or it you expect to store a lot of image files.

G. *Expansion slots*

Accommodate the cards that come with peripheral devices requiring hardware. The card and slot must be compatible; most are ISA (Industry Standard Architecture) or PCI (Peripheral Component Interconnect). Notebooks often take the credit card-like PCMCIA card (PC Memory Card International Association).

H. *Ports*

COM and LPT ports allow the PC to communicate with other devices. The type and configuration of the port will affect the operating speed. Expansion cards may incorporate extra ports for peripheral devices. The new USB (Universal Serial Bus) ports are much more flexible, allowing up to 127 peripheral devices to be connected to a PC via the same type of connector in a daisy chain or a star topology.

II. Input Devices

A. *Pointing devices*

One, two or three-button mice are used to select, move and resize items on the screen. The trackballs and mousepads on notebook PCs do the same job, but can be harder to control. Mice are not good for freehand sketches (a graphics pad is better). Light pens are used to point directly at the screen.

B. *Keyboards*

Notebooks normally have a condensed keyboard, which can be a problem if you make a lot of use of the numeric keypad. A curved keyboard or wrist support may help prevent repetitive strain injuries.

C. *Scanners*

Range from low-cost hand held devices that can scan a 3-4" strip as you roll the device over it, to high resolution, colour, flat bed scanners that scan a whole page at a time. Select a scanner when you know what you want to do with it.

D. *Other input devices*

Other popular devices include bar code readers, digital cameras (for stills and for video conferencing) and TV tuners.

III. Output Devices

A. *Monitors*

The standard monitor may need upgrading for very high-resolution graphics. It must be compatible with the PC's graphics card. A bigger, brighter display is more comfortable to look at for long periods. Check that a notebook's display can be viewed at an angle if necessary.

B. *Graphics cards*

Printed circuit boards that control the rate at which the monitor's screen is refreshed and the number of colours that can be displayed. At least 2 MB of RAM and an MPEG (Motion Pictures Expert Group) decoder are needed to display moving videos.

C. *Printers*

Range from low-cost low-quality dot matrix printers, ink or bubble jet printers which are intermediate in price and quality, to laser printers which are more expensive but faster and able to produce very high quality print. When buying a printer, check the cost of ink or toner cartridges and the number of pages they produce, and review your need to produce acetates and colour prints.

IV. Backing Up

A. *3.5" disk drive*

The standard floppy disk still provides an easy method for transferring relatively small files between PCs. File compression programs (such as WinZip) may be required to squeeze larger files, particularly images, onto a floppy disk.

B. *Zip and tape drives*

Zip drives back your data onto a 100-megabyte disk. Data can be retrieved from a zip disk as if it was a mini-hard drive. Tape drives back up to a cassette with a higher capacity, but in a much less accessible format.

C. *Optical drives*

The CD-ROM is now the standard medium for distributing software. Drives are specified by the rotation speed. Writeable CDs can be used to back up data, and are particularly useful where each backup is kept for a specified period.

V. General Software

A. *Word processors*

Specialist software for handling text, often with desktop publishing capabilities so that you can add drawings, tables and pictures. Usually feature a spell checker, mail merge facility and instant word count.

B. *Spreadsheets*

Number crunching software, usually with a range of built-in analytical functions and the facility to plot data in a range of formats.

C. *Presentation packages*

Provide a quick and easy way to prepare slide shows using pictures, charts and text imported from other applications. Usually feature animation effects for computer based presentations.

D. *Databases*

Relational databases can store everything from biochemistry data and dialysis machine parameters to clinic letters, x-rays and billing details. All the information is linked to minimize repetition and maximize flexibility. Usually feature facilities for generating reports.

E. *Office suites*

A package, such as Microsoft's Office, Lotus SmartSuite or Corel Office, containing a combination of the above applications. Allows a smooth transfer of text, tables, pictures etc. from one application to another.

F. *Program development*

When the software you want cannot be bought off-the-shelf you may have to develop your own. Commonly used languages include Fortran, C, Pascal, LISP, Prolog, Cobol, Basic, HTML and Java. They convert the task you want doing into machine code that the computer can execute. It may be possible to develop your application within a standard package, for example by writing 'macros' or user defined functions for a spreadsheet like Microsoft Excel. These techniques are described in more advanced tutorials and manuals.

G. *Virus checkers*

Can be set up to monitor every file you open for viruses. Most feature automatic updating of the virus encyclopaedia via the Internet.

VI. Dialysis Specific Software

A. *Machine software*

Most dialysis machines are controlled by microprocessors, usually with the means to download the data to a database. Some machines can share data with a PC using standard floppy disks or special cards.

B. *Renal data management packages*

Produced by several companies to collect clinical information, lab data and, where there are connections, data from dialysis machines and other devices such as scales or reprocessing units. The data is usually organized in a relational database and accessed via a customized user interface.

C. *Treatment prescription and audit*

Several companies have produced programs for assessing and planning dialysis prescriptions and anemia management. These work best if the data can be transferred directly from the clinical database to the program.

VII. Local Networks

A. *Local Area Networks (LANs)*

Can link a few computers sharing a printer or a complex arrangement covering a university or hospital site. Can be 'peer-to-peer' where no one computer has overall control, or 'file-server' where the server holds shared applications and data resources and provides it to other computers on the network as required. LANs are often used to provide local e-mailing. To create a LAN from a group of computers, they must be cabled together (see below) and fitted with a network interface card (NIC) and the software to control the network. A group of dialysis machines, electronic scales, blood pressure monitors and computers can also be connected in a LAN.

B. *Cables*

Twisted pair wiring, as used for telephone systems, is very easy to fit and can be used for distances up to 25m. It comes as unshielded (UTP) or shielded (STP). The shielded version is more expensive but less prone to interference. Coaxial cable is more difficult to connect up, but it is more robust and can be used for distances of up to 500m. For longer distances or environments with interference problems, fiber optic cables can be used. Making good connections with fiber optics is a skilled job, as the end of each fiber has to be carefully polished.

C. *Topology*

A star configuration has a central hub and satellites. A bus topology has the computers branching from a central wire or forming a ring. In some cases a combination of topologies may be needed.

D. *Transmission protocol*

'Ethernet' uses a protocol where the line is checked to make sure there is no activity before sending information, then rechecked to ensure that two computers didn't start sending information at the same time. If the system senses this it stops both senders and makes them wait for different times before trying again. The 'Token passing' protocols work by passing a kind of electronic permission slip round the network and computers wait till they get the token before sending information out. Token-ring, ARCNET and FDDI (Fibre Distributed Data Interface) all use token-passing. FDDI cabling gives the fastest transmission and is very secure, but it requires fibre optic cables.

VIII. Wide Area Networks and the Internet

A. Wide Area Network (WANs)

Networks of computers over a wider area, normally use telephone transmission lines to cover large distances.

B. Modem (Modulator-demodulator)

Modulation is used to convert digital information stored in the computer to an analogue signal that can be sent via a standard telephone line by changing the amplitude or phase of a carrier wave. Demodulation is the reconstruction of the original digital information at the other end. Modems can now transmit or receive at up to 57,600 bps (bits per second, about 7000 characters per second).

C. International Systems Digital Network (ISDN) adaptors

Allow faster transmission between devices in WANs (up to 128k bps), but require compatible phone lines.

D. The Internet

Emerged in 1973 when Vinton Cerf linked computer networks at US universities and research labs together in the ARPAnet (Advanced Research Projects Agency). Internet protocol was developed to control routing by 'gateway' computers. Transmission Control Protocol (TCP) that checks that information has arrived intact and if not sends it again. By early 1996 over 25 million computers were connected to the Internet.

E. Internet Service Providers (ISPs)

Provide a gateway to the Internet and an e-mail address book. May offer other facilities, such as technical support, parental control, and space for your own home page. Home page development software packages allow you to produce a home page without learning the details of HTML (HyperText Markup Language).

F. World Wide Web (WWW)

Developed in 1989 by Timothy Berners-Lee at CERN in Switzerland. Essentially a protocol for accessing information through 'web sites' which can include graphics, sound, animation and links to other sites. Sites are identified by the Uniform Resource Locator (URL) which gives the address of the computer that holds the information on the Internet and the file name of the site. For example, http://www.kidney.org/professionals/doqi takes you to the DOQI overview on the National Kidney Foundation's site.

G. Browsers

Software used to navigate the WWW and view HTML-encoded documents. Require frequent upgrading to cope with the rapid evolution of HTML.

H. Search Engines

The Yellow Pages for the WWW. Search engines and portals allow you to search for information by typing in key words or a question. A list of these sites is available at http://www.hotsheet.com. The search engine is normally only used as a spring board to find the first relevant site, on the WWW one good site normally leads to another!

I. Discussion groups

E-mail facilities allowing people sharing an interest (such as renal professionals) to share ideas, solve problems etc. E-mails sent by one member to a central address are automatically forwarded to all the other members of the group.

J. Bulletin boards

Another way for people to share ideas, this time without the need for an e-mail address. Participants visit the web-site and mail questions and comments directly to the board. There are discussion groups for various renal professions at http://www.renalweb.com.

Chapter 14
Required Basic Knowledge

Contributing Authors:

John A. Sweeny, BS, CHT, CBNT

Bill Hajko, CHT

Buz Womack, CHT, Chemistry

Ty Cobb, CHT, Physics

Kirk M. Lesher, CHT, Electronics

Chapter Outline

I. An Introduction to Basic Chemistry Concepts

A. Chemistry is defined as the scientific study of the properties, composition, and structure of matter. The concepts introduced below are intended to provide the dialysis technician with a basic understanding of the chemistry relating to dialysate and blood plasma. Please refer to the bibliography at the end of this section for additional texts available for further study.

B. An atom is the smallest part of an element that can enter into a chemical change. There are 92 elements that occur naturally in nature from the smallest, Hydrogen, to the largest, Uranium. Each atom has a structure consisting of a nucleus surrounded by a "cloud" of electrons that move around the nucleus. The nucleus contains small particles called protons and neutrons. The number of protons an atom has is referred to as its atomic number. Hydrogen has one proton, and Uranium has 92. There are larger manmade elements, which have as many as 109 protons. For each proton that has a positive charge, there is an electron with a negative charge orbiting about the nucleus. Chemistry deals with the interactions of the electrons between atoms. Only those electrons farthest from the atom's nucleus are available to form chemical bounds which involve the sharing of electrons between atoms. The other electrons are bound too tightly to the nucleus to enter into a chemical reaction. The elements are arranged on a chart called the Periodic Table by increasing atomic number. Generally, a one or two letter designation is used in chemistry to identify the different elements.

From the standpoint of dialysate chemistry there are only 8 elements that the technician need be concerned about. There are additional ones that come into play when water treatment is discussed, but this discussion will be limited to dialysate chemistry; the same principals presented below, however, apply to water chemistry. The elements with their chemical symbols found in dialysate are:

Sodium – Na	Potassium – K
Hydrogen – H	Oxygen – O
Calcium – Ca	Carbon – C
Magnesium – Mg	Chlorine – Cl

The two that are confusing are Sodium and Potassium. Sodium is Na because in the past it was called Natrium, and Potassium is K because it was Kalium. Even today, a condition of high Sodium or Potassium in a patient is referred to as hypernatremia or hyperkalemia.

C. Atomic weights are simply values that express the relative weight of an atom compared to a standard carbon atom. The atomic weight unit is called a Dalton. Carbon has an atomic weight of 12 Daltons. The weights in Daltons of other elements found in dialysate are:

Sodium = 23.00	Potassium = 39.10
Hydrogen = 1.00	Oxygen = 16.00
Calcium = 40.08	Carbon = 12.011
Magnesium = 24.30	Chlorine = 35.45

D. Elements combine to form molecules by sharing electrons. The molecular weight of a compound is the weight of all chemical species in a molecule. A good example is the number one molecule in dialysate: water. Water consists of one oxygen and two hydrogen atoms. Its chemical symbol is H_2O. The subscript after the H indicates that there are 2 atoms of Hydrogen in water. From the atomic weights listed above, we find that oxygen weighs 16 Daltons, and hydrogen weighs 1 Dalton; therefore, the Molecular Weight of water is $(2 \times 1) + 16 = 18$.

E. A Mole of any substance is that quantity of the substance that weighs (in grams) the same as its molecular weight. For example, molecular oxygen (O_2) has a weight of 32 (16 for each oxygen atom). One mole of oxygen weighs 32 g. A mole of a substance always contains the same number of molecules known as Avogadro's number. Avogadro's number is equal to 6.0221367×10^{23}. Said another way, the number of oxygen molecules (MW of 32) that it takes to equal 32 grams is $6.0221367 \times 10^{23} = 602,213,670,000,000,000,000,000$!

F. Atoms combine by sharing valence electrons. These electrons are found in the outermost energy level or shell of each type of atom. Almost all the elements would like to have 8 electrons in their outer shell. Hydrogen and Helium are the only exceptions: they want only two. Sodium only has one electron in its outer shell, but Chlorine has seven. By getting together, and sharing electrons both can effectively have 8. The compound formed, Sodium Chloride, is better known as simply table salt. Potassium has only one electron in its outer shell and combines with Chlorine to

Figure 14.1

Periodic Table of Elements

Period	GROUP 1 IA	2 IA	3 IIIA	4 IVA	5 VA	6 VIB	7 VIIB	8	9 VIII	10	11 IB	12 IIB	13 IIIB	14 IVB	15 VB	16 VIA	17 VIIA	18 IIIA
1	1 H 1.008																	2 He 4.003
2	3 Li 6.941	4 Be 9.012											5 B 10.81	6 C 12.01	7 N 14.01	8 O 16	9 F 19	10 Ne 20.18
3	11 Na 22.99	12 Mg 24.31											13 Al 26.98	14 Si 28.09	15 P 30.97	16 S 32.07	17 Cl 35.45	18 Ar 39.95
4	19 K 39.1	20 Ca 40.08	21 Sc 44.96	22 Ti 47.88	23 V 50.94	24 Cr 52	25 Mn 54.94	26 Fe 55.85	27 Co 58.47	28 Ni 58.69	29 Cu 63.55	30 Zn 65.39	31 Ga 69.72	32 Ge 72.59	33 As 74.92	34 Se 78.96	35 Br 79.9	36 Kr 83.8
5	37 Rb 85.47	38 Sr 87.62	39 Y 88.91	40 Zr 91.22	41 Nb 92.91	42 Mo 95.94	43 Tc 98	44 Ru 101.1	45 Rh 102.9	46 Pd 106.4	47 Ag 107.9	48 Cd 112.4	49 In 114.8	50 Sn 118.7	51 Sb 121.8	52 Te 127.6	53 I 126.9	54 Xe 131.3
6	55 Cs 132.9	56 Ba 137.3	57 La * 138.9	72 Hf 178.5	73 Ta 180.9	74 W 183.9	75 Re 186.2	76 Os 190.2	77 Ir 190.2	78 Pt 195.1	79 Au 197	80 Hg 200.5	81 Tl 204.4	82 Pb 207.2	83 Bi 209	84 Po 210	85 At 210	86 Rn 222
7	87 Fr 223	88 Ra 226	89 Ac ~ 227	104 Rf 257	105 Db 260	106 Sg 263	107 Bh 262	108 Hs 265	109 Mt 266	110 --- ()	111 --- ()	112 --- ()		114 --- ()		116 --- ()		118 --- ()

Lanthanide Series*	58 Ce 140.1	59 Pr 140.9	60 Nd 144.2	61 Pm 147	62 Sm 150.4	63 Eu 152	64 Gd 157.3	65 Tb 158.9	66 Dy 162.5	67 Ho 164.9	68 Er 167.3	69 Tm 168.9	70 Yb 173	71 Lu 175
Actinide Series*	90 Th 232	91 Pa 231	92 U 238	93 Np 237	94 Pu 242	95 Am 243	96 Cm 247	97 Bk 247	98 Cf 249	99 Es 254	100 Fm 253	101 Md 256	102 No 254	103 Lr 257

make Potassium Chloride that is used by people on a low salt diet (except ESRD patients!) and referred to as salt substitute. Another example is Magnesium. Magnesium has two electrons in its outermost shell, so it combines with two Chloride ions to form Magnesium Chloride. In the examples, Magnesium, Sodium and Potassium are donors of electrons, whereas Chlorine is an acceptor. Plus and minus symbols are used to indicate what each type of atom does with its electrons. A plus sign indicates a donor, and a minus sign indicates an acceptor. The number of pluses or minuses indicates how many electrons are either donated or accepted. It would take 3 Hydrogens (H^+) to join with one Nitrogen (N^{---}) to make NH_3, which is ammonia. Notice that when compounds are formed, the combination of pluses and minuses is always equal and hence, the total charge on the molecule is zero.

The charges on the dialysate elements are:

Sodium – Na^+	Potassium – K^+
Hydrogen – H^+	Oxygen – O^{--}
Calcium – Ca^{++}	Carbon – C^{++++}
Magnesium – Mg^{++}	Chlorine – Cl^-

Carbon can behave as if it has either 4 positive or negative charges and can bind with itself. This fact enables carbon to form an incredible number of complex compounds which are the building blocks for life. The study of carbon compounds is of primary concern in organic chemistry.

G. Ions are elements or molecules that were combined as a compound, but disassociated from their compound to form charged atoms in solution. A chemical that forms an aqueous solution that conducts electricity is an electrolyte. The more of the electrolyte there is, the more electricity the solution will conduct. Conversely, the less electrolyte, the less electricity is conducted.

For dialysate, there are two electrolytes that have not been mentioned yet, acetate and bicarbonate. These two ions are molecules with a single negative charge.

Acetate - CH_3COO^- Bicarbonate - HCO_3^-

In acetate dialysate, the acetate is present due to the dissociation of Sodium Acetate. For bicarbonate dialysate, the acetate ion is present from the breakdown of Acetic acid. Acetate dialysate contains no bicarbonate ions, but for bicarbonate dialysate, the bicarb is added in the form of Sodium Bicarbonate. Dextrose, a form of sugar is also present in dialysate, but it does not ionize in water.

We can determine if dialysate is prepared correctly by measuring the solution with a conductivity meter. Dialysis machines have conductivity meters that indirectly measure the total ion concentration of the dialysate during the dialysis treatment. It's important to note that these conductivity monitor systems cannot distinguish between electrolyte types, and only look at total conductivity effects. The use of an acid concentrate with a Potassium concentration of 2 mEq/L would not create a conductivity alarm if switched for an acid bath containing no Potassium. The net change would be too small to create an alarm condition. For this reason, it is extremely important to double-check all concentrates that are to be utilized by a machine to ensure they are of the proper formulation.

Figure 14.2

Molecular Weight Chart

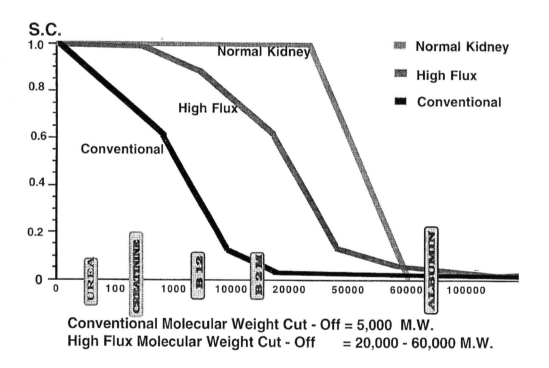

Conventional Molecular Weight Cut - Off = 5,000 M.W.
High Flux Molecular Weight Cut - Off   = 20,000 - 60,000 M.W.

This chart shows some of the common substances of concern in hemodialysis and their relative molecular weights. Note the cut-off pattern of the normal kidney compared to conventional membranes and then compared to high flux. Only the more permeable membranes have any significant capability to remove Beta 2 Microglobulin (The cause of Dialysis Associated Amyloidosis and Carpal Tunnel Syndrome.) Conventional membranes and High Efficiency membranes only remove the smaller molecules.

Reprinted from Althin Academy/Molecular Weight Chart

Sodium Chloride consisting of one atom of Sodium and one atom of Chlorine disassociates into an ion of Na^+ and Cl^-. Because the ions in a solution come from compounds that have a net charge of zero, any solution containing ions will always have an equal number of positive and negative charges.

If two electrodes are placed in a solution containing ions and a battery is connected to make one electrode positive (Anode) and the other negative (Cathode), the ions will move toward the electrodes based on their charge. The positively charged ions will move toward the negative cathode and the negative ions will move towards the positive anode. They follow the fundamental rule of nature that states that opposite charges attract. Because the positive ions collect at the cathode, they are called cations. The negative ions that collect at the anode are called anions.

The concentration of ions in a solution is measured in Equivalents per liter. One equivalent equals Avagadro's number (6.023×10^{23}) of pluses or minuses. If a liter of solution contained 1 mole of Sodium ions, that would be a concentration of one equivalent/liter of Sodium. Of course that same solution would also have to have the same concentration of a negative ions to balance the positive Sodiums. If the compound in the liter of solution was Sodium Chloride, then the solution would also contain one equivalent/liter of chloride ions. Calcium has a double charge, which means that you would only need a half mole of Calcium ions to make one equivalent of charge. When dialysate ion concentrations are given, they are generally expressed in mEq/L (milliequivalents/liter) because Eq/L is such a large amount.. The "milli" means divide by 1000. Normal saline contains 154 mEq/L of Sodium and Chloride ions. That's the same as a concentration of 0.154 Eq/L.

H. The density of a substance is defined as its mass divided by its volume and is expressed as grams/mL or grams/cc. With liquids, the term used is specific gravity. Water at a temperature of 4.0°C has a "density" of one gram per milliliter and is said to have a specific gravity of 1.000. Any water-based solution containing additional salt compounds will have a higher specific gravity. 36.83X acid concentrate, which is extremely salty, has a specific gravity of about 1.150. Dialysate has a specific gravity of about 1.007. This means that one liter of dialysate would weigh 1007 grams,

about 7 grams more than a liter of pure water. The specific gravity of urine is in the range of 1.003 to 1.030 gm/mL.

II. Basic Chemistry of Dialysate

A. Dialysis works by the process of diffusion. In fact, the term "dialysis" was first used by Thomas Graham, a Scottish chemist in a paper entitled "On Osmotic Force" in 1854. Graham was studying the diffusion of atoms across a membrane constructed from an ox bladder. If an electrolyte concentration is higher on one side of a membrane than the other, then the net effect is the transfer of the electrolyte from a higher concentration area to a lower one until equilibration takes place. For example, if the patient's blood has a Potassium level of 6 mEq/L and the dialysate contains 2 mEq/L of Potassium, then Potassium ions will move by diffusion from the blood to the dialysate and theoretically would equilibrate at 4 mEq/L if both volumes were equal. This action was exemplified by the early Batch Tank Systems in the 1950's. The larger the dialysate volume in the tank, the higher the reduction would be in the patient's blood plasma.

Because electrolytes such as Sodium and Potassium ions are only about 1 angstrom in diameter (10,000 angstroms = 1 micron), they can pass through the membrane of a dialyzer easily. Even for a standard membrane, the pore size on average is 25 to 50 angstroms. Without the use of dialysate within the dialyzer to match the electrolyte concentrations in the blood plasma, diffusion would quickly allow the electrolytes to be lost from the blood resulting in extensive

Figure 14.3

Blood Electrolytes vs. Dialysate

(values in milliequivalents/liter)

Electrolyte	Normal Blood	ESRD Blood	Dialysate
Sodium	136 – 148	127 – 140	132 – 150
Potassium	3.5 – 5.0	3.0 – 5.5	0.0 – 4.0
Calcium	4.25 – 5.25	4.25 – 5.50	2.5 – 4.0
Magnesium	1.5 – 2.5	2.0 – 3.5	0.5 – 1.5
Chloride	95 – 103	88 – 100	100 – 110
Bicarbonate	22 – 26	> 15	25 - 40
Acetate	0.0	0.0	3.0 – 4.0

hemolysis and possibly the demise of the patient. The table below compares the concentrations of electrolytes in normal blood to those in an end stage renal disease (ESRD) patient and typical bicarbonate dialysate.

B. In the early days of dialysis, dialysate was mixed by adding individual powered compounds into a known amount of water. Later, the process was simplified by concentrating the powdered compounds in water to form a liquid dialysate concentrate that could then be added to water to produce acetate dialysate. At these high ionic strengths, bacteria would not grow and preparing the final dialysate was much less labor intensive. 3.43 liters of concentrate diluted with water to a total volume of 120 liters is a 34:1 dilution. 3.43 liters of concentrate (1 part) + 116.57 liters of water (34 parts) = 120 liters of dialysate(35 parts). Today, the preparation of bicarbonate dialysate is more complex involving the use of two concentrates. Also, the bicarbonate concentrate utilized is not concentrated enough to be bacterio static and is difficult to keep bacteria free beyond a storage time of 24 hours.

Beginning in the 1980's, dialysis machines were designed to produce bicarbonate dialysate using a three-stream process. Two different dialysate concentrates are proportioned with water to prepare bicarbonate dialysate. The two concentrates are necessary because the bicarbonate ion will attach itself to either a Calcium or Magnesium ion if either are present in high concentrations. The two concentrates are referred to as acid concentrate and bicarbonate concentrate. The acid concentrate contains the Calcium and Magnesium ions, and the bicarbonate concentrate, as its name implies, has the bicarbonate ions. By diluting one concentrate in water prior to adding the second, precipitation of Calcium carbonate or Magnesium carbonate can be avoided. The mixing ratios in parts of acid concentrate, bicarbonate concentrate and water are shown below for various machines.

Figure 14.4

Mixing Ratios

Supplier	Acid Conc.	Bicarb Conc.	Water	Total
Cobe	1	1.72	42.28	45
Fresenius	1	1.225	32.775	35
Baxter/Althin	1	1.83	34	36.83

Dilution factors for acid and bicarbonate concentrates can be calculated from the data above by dividing the number of parts of the concentrate into the total. If this is done, the dilution factors are:

Figure 14.5

Dilution Factors

Supplier	Acid Concentrate	Bicarbonate Concentrate
Cobe	45X	26.16X
Fresenius	35X	28.57X
Baxter/Althin	36.83X	20.13X

Because dialysis machines are calibrated for use with a particular concentrate dilution, it's important to be familiar with these factors. Read the concentrate labeling carefully to ensure the proper concentrate is used.

The latest labeling utilizes geometrical shapes to aid in the identification of the concentrate types. The 45X will be enclosed in a triangle, the 35X will be inside a square, and the 36.83X will be inside a circle. Use of the wrong concentrate will create equipment alarms and prevent the initiation of the treatment.

C. In order for the final dialysate to have the proper ion concentrations, the quality of the water used by the machine is important. Low levels of electrolytes found in water can affect the final dialysate composition because the water is over 90% of the final volume of dialysate. Water requirements for hemodialysis have been established by the Association for the Advancement of Medical Instrumentation (AAMI). Refer to chapter five for information on these standards.

III. Concentrate Composition

A. Concentrate consists of a combination of salts that when diluted, creates a solution which is approximately of the same ionic composition as blood plasma. In the case of Potassium, Calcium and Magnesium, the final dialysate may contain slightly less of these electrolytes in order to help reduce their concentrations in the blood plasma.

The compounds used to prepare concentrate are:

Sodium Chloride	NaCl
Calcium Chloride	$CaCl_2$ $(2H_2O)$
Potassium Chloride	KCl
Magnesium Chloride	$MgCl_2$ $(6H_2O)$
Sodium Bicarbonate	$NaHCO_3$
Acetic Acid	CH_3COOH
Dextrose	$C_6H_{12}O_6$ H_2O

Both Calcium Chloride and Magnesium Chloride have water molecules associated with their compounds. These water molecules are a part of the crystalline structure of the compound. Both of these compounds are said to be hydrated. When either of these compounds exist without the water molecules, it is said to be in its anhydrous state. Dialysate concentrate can be manufactured using the anhydrous forms, but the hydrated salts are more common. Dextrose is added to the dialysate as a means of providing an influx of sugar to the patient. This function is especially important for the diabetic patient. The acid concentrate contains all of the compounds listed above except the Sodium Bicarbonate. All of the Sodium Bicarbonate is present in the bicarbonate concentrate. For the Baxter/Althin bicarbonate concentrate, some of the Sodium Chloride is also present.

2. After proportioning concentrate with water, dialysate composition is usually as follows:

Figure 14.6

Dialysate Composition

Chemical	Relative Amounts
Calcium – Ca^{++}	2.5 - 3.5 mEq/L
Potassium – K^+	0 - 4 mEq/L
Sodium – Na^+	132 - 150 mEq/L
Magnesium – Mg^{++}	0.5 - 1.5 mEq/L
Chloride – Cl^-	100 - 110 mEq/L
Acetate – CH_3COO^-	3 – 4 mEq/L
Bicarbonate – HCO_3^-	25 – 40 mEq/L
Dextrose	0 - 200 mg % (mg/dL)

IV. Concentrate Alteration

A. When a chemist talks about modifying a particular concentrate chemistry to customize the dialysate prescription for a treatment, there are three terms that will be used that all seem very similar. These terms are solute, solvent, and solution. The relationship between these terms is:

SOLUTE + SOLVENT = SOLUTION

Solute is the compound that will be dissolved by the solvent. The solvent is the dissolver. In our field of dialysis, the solvent is almost always water. Solution is the final mixture of the solute and solvent. When a manufacturer states that the bicarb powder (solute) in a bag makes 2.5 gallons of concentrate, the 2.5 gallons is a solution. If the powder is added to 2.5 gallons of solvent, the final solution will be greater than 2.5 gallons and the concentrate will be too dilute. The correct way to prepare the bicarb solution would be to start with about 2 gallons of water, add the powder, and then add additional water as the powder dissolves until the total is 2.5 gallons. With practice, the exact amount of water needed can be determined so the final water addition may not be necessary.

B. In order to determine the amount of a compound to add to a concentrate to produce a particular increase, there is a formula that can be used.

Desired change in mEq/L = (grams of solute)/ (milliEquivalent weight) x (liters of dialysate)

Example: Determine the amount of Calcium Chloride necessary to raise the dialysate level from 2.5 mEq/L to 3.0 mEq/L using 3.43 liters of 35X concentrate.

1) Calculate the mEq/L change desired.

3.0 mEq/L - 2.5 mEq/L = 0.5 mEq/L

2) Determine the total liters of dialysate by multiplying the quantity of concentrate by its dilution factor.

3.43 liters x 35 = 120.0 liters of dialysate.

3) Determine the molecular weight of Calcium Chloride. The formula for Calcium Chloride is: $CaCl_2$-$2H_2O$. Calcium Chloride comes with 2 water molecules attached. To get the total weight, all the atom's individual weights must be added together. The formulas for concentrate additives are found on the labels of most liquid concentrates. In many cases the weight of each compound used to make the concentrate is also given.

(40.08) + 2(35.45) + 2(2(1.00) + 16.00) = 40.08 + 70.90 + 2(18.00) = 146.98.

4) Divide the molecular weight by the number of charges on the Calcium ion. This will give a value that is the Equivalent weight for Calcium Chloride. By taking this answer and dividing by 1000, the answer becomes milliEquivalent weight for Calcium Chloride.

146.98/2 = 73.49 grams/equivalent = Equivalent weight.

73.49/1000 = 0.07349 grams/milliequivalent = milliEquivalent weight.

5) Substitute the values into the formula and solve:

(0.5 mEq/L) = (grams of solute)/ (0.07349 grams/mEq) x (120 liters)

or

Grams of solute = (0.5 mEq/L) x (0.07349 grams/mEq) x (120 liters)

Grams of solute = 4.41 grams of Calcium Chloride.

C. Potassium sometimes comes in liquid form in strengths of 3312 mEq/L or 3500 mEq/L. For these additives a dilution formula can be used to calculate the amount of needed additive.

(C1)(V1) = (C2)(V2)

Where: C1 = concentration of the additive in mEq/L

V1 = volume of additive required in mL

C2 = desired concentration increase in the dialysate in mEq/L

V2 = concentrate dilution factor times the concentrate volume in mL

The formula assumes that the amount of additive will be much less than the volume of concentrate.

For example, if you wish to raise the potassium from 2.5 mEq/L to 3.0 mEq/L in the final dialysate using a one gallon (3785 mL) of 45X concentrate, and the Potassium Chloride available has a concentration of 3312 mEq/L use the formula as follows:

C1 = 3312 mEq/L

V1 = volume of KCl needed.

C2 = 3.0 mEq/L – 2.5 mEq/L = 0.5 mEq/L

V2 = (45) x (3785 mL) = 170,325 mL

Solve for V1:

(3312 mEq/L) x V1 = (0.5 mEq/L) x (170,325 mL)

V1 = (0.5 mEq/L) x (170,325 mL)/(3312 mEq/L) = 25.7 mL.

V. Bicarbonate Precipitation

Anyone who has ever had to deal with bicarbonate dialysate has been made keenly aware of the problems that can result from precipitation occurring in the flow path of a dialysis machine. The McGraw-Hill Dictionary of Scientific and Technical Terms describes precipitation as "the process of producing a separable solid phase within a liquid medium." It also allows for gases becoming liquids, which certainly makes sense considering the fact that another common name for rain is precipitation.

Precipitation in a liquid occurs when the concentrations of ions that have an affinity for each other reach levels high enough to allow the ions to recombine to form solids. For a solid to form, two ions of opposite charge have to come together. Because dialysate contains multiple ion types in fairly high concentrations, the chances of this happening are fairly high.

In chemistry there is a concept called solubility product constant, (K_{SP}). This concept states that if you multiply the concentration of a particular positive ion by the concentration of a particular negative ion in a solution, the answer can predict if a solid will form. As long as the answer is below the solubility product constant number defined for the two ions involved, no precipitation will take place.

The ion causing the difficulty is the bicarbonate ion. A bicarbonate ion can combine with a water molecule to form a hydronium ion (H_3O^+ - the ion who's concentration is monitored by measuring pH) and a carbonate ion (CO_3^-). The equation looks like this:

$HCO_3^- + H_2O = H_3O^+ + CO_3^{--}$

Bicarb ion plus Water yields Hydronium ion plus Carbonate ion.

The real problem is that carbonate ions love to get together with Calcium and Magnesium ions to produce white precipitates of Calcium Carbonate and Magnesium Carbonate. That's why there's two concentrates necessary to produce bicarbonate dialysate. The acid concentrate has the Calcium and Magnesium ions and the bicarb concentrate has the bicarbonate ions. In a dialysate machine, they're allowed to get together only after one of the concentrates has first been diluted with water.

It doesn't take many Calcium or Magnesium ions in a solution with Carbonate ions to start a precipitation problem. If you tried to dissolve more than 106 milligrams of Magnesium Carbonate or as little as 16 milligrams of Calcium Carbonate in a liter of pure water, you'd find out you couldn't do it. On the other hand, you could dissolve over 500 grams of Magnesium Chloride or over 700 grams of Calcium Chloride in the same amount of water.

The chance that precipitation will occur is dramatically increased if hard water is used for dialysis. The concept of water being hard comes from the historical observation that when water was allowed to boil away in a pot, there remained a very hard substance in the bottom. What had actually happened was the ions became more concentrated as the water boiled away until the solubility limits were reached and precipitation occurred. Today, hardness is related to salts of Calcium and Magnesium. Carbonates, sulfates, bicarbonates, and chlorides of these two positive ions constitute the minerals, which we refer to as hardness. Hardness is measured in grains per gallon in the water industry. It takes 7,000 grains to make a pound. One grain equals 17.1 parts per million. Without water treatment, there would be very few areas in the United States that could do bicarbonate dialysis treatments.

To prevent Calcium Carbonate from precipitating in the machine's fluid path, we must reduce the concentrations of both the Calcium and Carbonate ions as much as possible. To minimize the Calcium concentration to only the amount supplied by the acid concentrate, we use a softener and a reverse osmosis machine to eliminate Calcium from the incoming water. What is done to reduce the carbonate ion is to add acid to the acid concentrate. The reason this works is rather interesting. Remember that carbonate ions form when bicarbonate ions break apart. If we add acid (Hydronium ions) to the dialysate bath to increase their concentration, they will combine with the carbonate ions to go back to being bicarbonate. This action reduces the carbonate ion concentration and hence helps prevent Calcium Carbonate precipitation. The same principals apply for Magnesium Carbonate as well. The acid used is Acetic Acid, which is why there are a few acetate ions in bicarbonate dialysate.

To prevent precipitation, there are several things that can be done. Properly prepared dialysate doesn't precipitate. After all, dialysate ion concentrations basically match the blood plasma ion concentrations and blood plasma doesn't have precipitation problems. The first thing you need to do is figure out what's causing the trouble. You don't want to spend your time having to rinse the machines of precipitate forever. Remember that precipitation occurs when ion concentrations are too high. Check your water supply to be sure your treatment system is functioning properly. Bicarbonate precipitation begins when the water to the machine exceeds a pH of 7.4. Make sure that the proper concentrates are being used and that the machines are set to properly proportion them. You may want to review bicarb mixing procedures with your staff to make sure the bicarbonate concentrate is being diluted properly. One of the most important things to keep in mind is that once precipitation starts, it can be a catalyst for further precipitation. Routine rinsing of your equipment with a weak acid such as white vinegar will ensure the machines stay precipitation free. It's easy to think that periodic rinsing isn't necessary if you haven't had a problem. ***Don't stop doing periodic rinsing.***

VI. Dialysis Related Physics

A. Fluid Dynamics

1. Background
   a) A dialysis machine uses a combination of pumps, valves and sensors to control the passage of a fluid (dialysate) through the dialysis machine. The dialysis machine controls the pressures and flow rate of the fluid as well as the dilution of various components of the dialysate. As this fluid comes in contact with the dialyzer, the fluid dynamics are also controlled by nature. The natural forces of diffusion and osmosis play out their role.

2. Definitions
   a) Fluid: A substance (liquid or gas) which changes shape at a steady rate when acted upon by a force.
   b) Dynamics: Deals with the motion and equilibrium of systems under the actions of forces.
   c) Solute: The substance dissolved in a given solution (the salt in salt-water).
   d) Solvent: A substance in a solution that dissolves another substance (the water in a salt-water solution).
   e) Solution: The mixture of substances (gas, liquid, or solid) without a chemical change.
      (1) Solvent + Solute = Solution

3. Topics
   a) Diffusion is a process whereby different fluids become mixed due to the continuous random motion of their molecules even if the solutions are separated by thin membranes. The movement of the solutes are from an area of greater concentration to an area of lesser concentration, until equilibrium is reached. At equilibrium the solute concentration is the same at all point in the solution.. An example is tea. Tea (solutes) diffuses through the tea bag (semipermeable membrane) into the surrounding water (solvent) and raises the concentration of the "tea" solution. It is the diffusion process that is the major cause of solute removal by a dialyzer.
   b) Osmosis is the movement of water across a semipermeable membrane from a lower concentration of solutes to a higher concentration of solutes. The natural forces

Figure 14.7

Diffusion

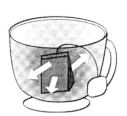
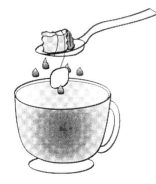

Source: NANT Core Curriculum for Reprocessing of Dialyzers, *p. 7, fig. 6.*

Figure 14.8

Convection

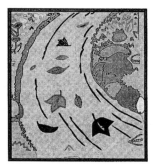

The Movement of Solute by Means of Water Currents

As water moves across the semi-permeable membrane, it pulls solute with it.

Reprinted with permission from Althin Academy/Basic Dialysis Theory (1)

at work here are trying to do the same basic thing as diffusion. Osmosis is diffusion with respect to the water molecules. The lower the concentration of solutes, the higher the concentration of water. The difference with osmosis is that the fluid in the tea cup is trying to creep back into the tea bag to make the solution within the tea bag more diluted. Diffusion and Osmosis can occur at the same time. For dialyzer membrane, water and electrolytes are so small with respect to the membrane pore size that the diffusion and osmosis process rates will be basically the same as if the membrane was not present. If an electrolyte were the size of a human being, the pores in a dialyzer would appear to be about 150 feet in diameter.

c) Osmosis can be easily identified when the solutes in a solution are too large to easily pass through a membrane. Consider a container separated into two compartments. One is pure water, and the other side is water with dissolved solute. The solute particles are too large to pass through the membrane, but the water can pass in either direction. The net flow will be water moving from the pure side of the membrane to the side with the dissolved particles in an effort to dilute them. Because the solute particles can not pass through the membrane, the concentrations of solute in the two compartments can never be equal. However, the water will not keep rising. The higher water level in the concentrated compartment will exert an

opposing hydrostatic pressure to eventually counterbalance the osmotic pressure.

The unit of measure of osmolality is the osmole. One osmole is the amount of osmotic pressure created by a solution with a solute concentration of one mole of particles per liter. One osmole of osmotic pressure is equivalent to a hydrostatic pressure of 17,000 mmHg. The osmolality of blood is 0.3 osmoles or 300 milliosmoles (mOsm). If blood was on one side of a dialyzer membrane, and pure water was on the other, the transmembrane pressure would be about 5,000 mmHg. Water would rush into the blood diluting the blood plasma and causing extensive hemolysis. Dialysate has an osmolality of approximately 290 mOsm. Because, dialysate has a slightly lower osmolality than blood plasma, a slight positive TMP is necessary in a dialyzer to create a net ultrafiltration rate of zero.

d) Convection is the transfer of heat and solutes by the physical circulation or movement of the parts of a liquid or gas. In dialysis; convective transport is also called solute-drag. As a fluid containing solutes crosses a semipermeable membrane, it drags along with it small molecular weight solutes. Even at relatively high ultrafiltration rates (2.0 kg/hr), convective transport will account for less than one tenth of the total solutes removed from a patient during a hemodialysis treatment.

e) Random motion of molecules in a fluid (liquid or gas) is possible because the molecules are more loosely bound together than in solids, the molecules tend to move around much more. This random motion of molecules increases as the temperature increases, and decreases if the temperature decreases. The motion of molecules is what makes osmosis and diffusion possible.

f) Pressure is defined as a force per unit area; i.e., PSI (pounds per square inch). Consider a gas contained in a box. The gas particles move in random directions and some of them hit the wall of the box. If more particles hit the wall, the net force (or pressure) on the wall increases.

(1) During dialysis various pressures are monitored. Venous and Arterial monitors measure the pressures in the bloodlines. The pressure in the dialysate compartment of the dialyzer is also monitored. The Transmembrane Pressure (TMP) is the pressure difference (pressure gradient) between the positive blood compartment pressure and the less positive (or negative) pressure in the dialysate compartment.

(2) The pressure gradient determines the direction of fluid movement in the dialyzer.

(a) If the blood side pressure is greater, the fluid moves to the dialysate compartment.

(b) If the dialysate pressure is greater, the fluid moves into the blood compartment.

(c) If the pressure is equal, fluid does not cross the membrane.

(d) It is common to see the pressure gradient in the dialyzer change from one end to the other, i.e., fluid moves from the dialysate compartment to the blood compartment on the venous end while fluid moves from the blood compartment to the dialysate compartment on the arterial end.

g) Flow Rate is the speed (volume to time ratio) of a given fluid moving through a vessel. In dialysis we measure the flow rate of blood or dialysate as milliliters per minute (mL's/min).

B. Thermodynamics

1. Background

a) Thermodynamics is the study of the relations between heat and other forms of energy. Internal energy is the total potential and kinetic energy between the particles of a substance. These particles include molecules, ions, atoms, and subatomic particles. If a substance is heated (given more energy) these particles will move more rapidly. For example, a gas that is heated will expand if possible; if not, its pressure will increase. In a solid such as a metal rod, the rod will increase in length if heated. If the substance is cooled (less internal energy) the particles of the substance will move less, i.e., the pressure of a gas will decrease and the volume of a solid will contract. This phenonmenon is evident everywhere in life. The expansion joints of a highway are but one example of a way to allow for natural expansion and contraction of the concrete to prevent damage to the highway. In dialysis one example is that heated dialysate is offered plenty of internal energy for the particles of the dialysate to move freely.

2. Definitions

a) Internal Energy is the measure of all the energy, potential and kinetic, possessed by molecules in a system.

3. Topics

a) Laws of heat movement show that energy added to a system can increase the system's temperature (increase its internal energy) and/or allow the system to do more work.

C. The Gas Laws

1. Background

a) Matter can exist in three different physical forms called states. Matter is classified as being either a gas, liquid, or solid. In the Gas State, the molecules move rapidly and are far apart from each other. Because only weak intermolecular forces exist, gaseous substances have the ability to expand to fill any volume and take on the shape of their container. Gases are easily, though not infinitely, compressible. All gases display similar behavior and follow similar laws regardless of their molecular formula. The state of a gaseous sample is generally defined by four variables: pressure (P), volume (V), temperature (T), and the number of moles (n). Volume is generally expressed in liters (L) or milliliters (mL). The temperature of a gas is usually expressed in Kelvins (K).

2) Definitions

a) Temperature: A physical property of an object, which determines the direction of heat flow when, placed next to another object. It is measured using an absolute temperature scale (Kelvin) with the triple point of water (where water exists as a gas, liquid and solid at the same time) defined as 273.16 kelvins. In 1967 the International System changed the term from degrees Kelvin to simply kelvin.

b) Atmosphere (atm): Refers to the average atmospheric pressure at sea level. 1atm = 760 mmHg = 14.7 PSI.

c) Standard Temperature and Pressure (STP): Used as base conditions when studying or measuring gas volumes and densities. Standard temperature is 0°C (273.16 K) and standard pressure is 1 atm. At STP, one mole of a gas will occupy 22.4 liters.

3. Topics

a) Boyle's Law

(1) Experiments performed by Robert Boyle in 1660 led to the formulation of Boyle's law which states that if a gas sample is held at constant temperature (isothermal) conditions, the volume of the gas is inversely proportional to its pressure. If the pressure increases, the volume will decrease.

(a) $(P_1)(V_1) = (P_2)(V_2)$
where P_1 = original pressure, V_1 = original volume, P_2 and V_2 = the new pressure and volume.

b) Charles' Law

(1) Charles' Law was developed during the early 19th century. The law states that at a constant pressure, the volume of a gas is directly proportional to its absolute temperature (expressed in Kelvin). In English, if a gas is heated, its volume will increase, if the pressure can remain constant.

(a) $\dfrac{(V_1)}{(T_1)} = \dfrac{(V_2)}{(T_2)}$
where V_1 = volume at temperature T_1, V_2 = volume at temperature T_2

c) Combination Gas Law

(1) In order to remember one formula, the gas laws above can be combined.

(a) $\dfrac{(P_1)(V_1)}{(T_1)} = \dfrac{(P_2)(V_2)}{(T_2)}$

A good example of the application of Boyle's Law is in the deaeration systems in dialysis machines. Most of the air dissolved in water is in the form of small microbubbles. At room pressure, these bubbles are small enough to be bounced around by the water molecules and stay in solution. By applying a high negative pressure to the water, Boyle's law states that these gas bubbles will increase in size. With increased size, the bubbles will displace more water and hence increase their buoyancy causing them to rise to the top of their container. Also, because the bubbles are larger, they have a high chance of colliding with other bubbles to form even larger bubbles. The air that collects at the top of the container can be pulled away by a vacuum pump freeing the water of air.

D. Temperature Measurements

1. Background

a) Commonly, temperature is the relative measure of how hot or cold something is. When studying temperature, however, we must measure it quantitatively on a defined scale. There are four scales used to make these measurements of temperature on a thermometer: The Fahrenheit (°F), the Celsius (°C), the Rankine (°R), and the Kelvin (K) scales. In order to measure temperature accurately, we use two natural events, that always occur at the same temperature. The freezing (solid/liquid phase)point and the boiling (liquid/gas phase) point of water at 1 atm pressure (sea level) are such fixed points. The interval between these points is divided into a fixed number of equal degrees. Two other reference points used for higher temperatures are the melting (solid/liquid phase) points for silver (960.8°C) and gold (1063.0°C).

2. Definitions

   a) Absolute zero: The temperature at which all-molecular motion stops and the material has zero thermal energy. 0 K or –273.15°C.

   b) Fahrenheit: The temperature scale typically used in engineering and household measurements.

   c) Celsius: Formerly called the centigrade scale. This scale is typically used for scientific measurements.

   d) Rankine: The absolute Fahrenheit scale. 0°R = Absolute zero = -460°F

   e) Kelvin: The absolute Celsius scale. 0.0 K = Absolute zero = -273.15°C. Note that Kelvin temperature is typically not referred to as degrees Kelvin or °K, only as K.

3. Topics

   a) Temperature Scales:

Figure 14.9

Temperature Scales

Situation	K	°C	°F	°R
Absolute zero	0	-273	-460	0
Freezing point of water	273	0	32	492
Normal human body temperature	310	37	98.6	558.6
Boiling point of water	373	100	212	673

   b) Conversion Formulas

   (1) Fahrenheit to Celsius °C = 5/9(°F - 32)

   (2) Celsius to Fahrenheit °F = (9/5) °C + 32

   (3) Celsius to Kelvin K = °C + 273.15

   (4) Fahrenheit to Rankine °R = °F + 460

VII. Dialysis and Electronics

The field of dialysis has become more dependent on electronics with each passing year. Automated equipment, electronic monitors, and personal computers have made a basic understanding of electronics a real necessity. The following is a brief introduction to the basic principals of electronics with attention paid to their dialysis applications.

A. Electricity

Electricity has three basic elements that are important when discussing its flow through an electrical circuit. Those elements are VOLTAGE, CURRENT, and RESISTANCE. Electricity must have a complete circuit to flow through, that is, it must have a conductive path that allows it a complete round trip between two poles of a power supply, such as a battery or power outlet. Voltage is the force that causes electricity to flow through the complete circuit. Current is the quantity of electricity that is flowing through the circuit. Resistance is the obstruction that the circuit offers to the flow of electricity. All circuits exhibit these characteristics. Water is a popular analogy to relate to electricity. Voltage is like pressure in the water analogy. Current is the quantity of water that flows through the pipe. Resistance is the pipe diameter, or the restriction that prevents water from flowing at its maximum rate. Voltage is measure in volts, current is measured in amperes, and resistance is measured in ohms.

B. Conductivity

In dialysis, a common form of measurement is *conductance*. Conductance is the measurement of a circuit's ability to conduct electricity, and is measured in Siemens. In the past, the unit of measure for conductance was ohm spelled backwards or "mho". It was derived from the fact that conductance is the reciprocal resistance. If an electrical component has a resistance of 50 ohms, then it also has a conductance of 1/50 Siemens which equals 0.02 Siemens or 20 milliSiemens. It is important to realize that pure water is almost a perfect insulator. It is only when impurities are added to water that it becomes capable of any conduction of electricity. As more impurities are added to water, its ability to conduct electricity increases. A consequence of that is that sea water would be more conductive than tap water. This fact makes conductivity an important measure of water purity. Tap water will have a relatively high conductivity, while treated water will have a much lower conductivity. This fact is used to assess the effectiveness of a water treatment system at any given time, without having to do an expensive series of chemical analysis and wait for lab results. This is not to infer that lab analysis is never required, but that conductivity tests are useful when an immediate result is desired. Lab analysis need to be performed less frequently. An increase in conductivity of treated water which was formerly known to be of good quality would require investigation to determine why the conductivity had increased.

In addition to water quality, conductivity tests are essential to determining whether dialysate has been properly prepared. Nearly all dialysate in the U.S. is prepared by combining concentrates with purified water. Conductivity tests are performed to assure that those components are mixed in the proper proportions.

Since pure water of very low conductivity is utilized, any detected conductivity must be from the chemicals in the concentrates. Because the proportions of chemicals in the concentrates are very precisely controlled during manufacture, the conductivity is a good assurance of the proper chemical proportions in the final dialysate solution. Too low of a conductivity indicates not enough concentrate; and conversely, too high a conductivity would indicate too much concentrate. This sensitive measure is an industry standard in assuring the quality of the dialysate solution before treatment. Modern dialysis equipment has constant monitoring of conductivity to assure safety throughout the treatment procedure.

All dialysis machines that measure conductivity also measure the temperature of the dialysate near the same point where the conductivity is measured. This is done because temperature affects the actual conductivity reading. A change of 1°C will cause a change of about 1.8 % in a conductivity reading. Most conductivity circuits use a conductivity cell and thermistor to determine the conductivity of the dialysate. The actual conductivity as seen by the cell is adjusted by the circuit using the thermistor's temperature reading to give the equivalent conductivity at a temperature of 25°C. When a bicarb concentrate is said to have a conductivity of 14.0 mS/cm, the value is for 25°C. At a body temperature of 37°C, that same solution will have a conductivity of about 17.0 mS/cm. All conductivity circuits, even the older handheld devices took temperature measurements and adjusted the conductivity results to the equivalent value at 25°C.

The calculation of actual solution conductivity is an extremely complicated process. Each ion type conducts electricity differently. A Potassium ion will have a much larger affect on conductivity than a bicarbonate ion even though both have a single charge because the bicarb ion is larger and moves more slowly in solution. Temperature as mentioned above also affects the final answer. Dextrose doesn't ionize, but because it's in the dialysate, it blocks the movement of the ions and actually reduces the conductivity. Another complication is the interaction of the ions with each other. As the concentration of ions is increased, each addition will have less of an effect on the conductivity value. This characteristic can be demonstrated using a dialysate machine that does fixed proportioning. Allow the machine to proportion only acid concentrate and read the conductivity. For an acid that is proportioned 36.83X, the answer will be about 10.0 mS/cm. Next allow the machine to proportion only the bicarb

concentrate (20.13X). The result will be about 5.0 mS/cm. If both concentrates are now proportioned, the expected result of 15.0 mS/cm will not occur. The actual answer will be only 14.0 mS/cm.

Most manufacturers publish conductivity data for properly proportioned concentrates. Proper proportioning of concentrate and water to obtain accurate values requires the use of laboratory instruments such as volumetric flasks and pipettes. There are many simplified formulas which can be used to estimate the expected conductivity for a given formulation. These simplified formulas tend to work because all dialysate is basically the same. Remember that one of the purposes of the dialysate is to maintain ion equilibrium of the patient's blood plasma ions as the blood passes through the dialyzer. Because all blood plasma is the basically the same, all dialysate is similar as well.

C. Electrical Leakage

As a safety measure, medical equipment is periodically tested for electrical leakage. This is a measure of how much current is present on the external chassis during normal operation, with the ground wire disconnected from the wall power outlet. An elevated level of leakage current may be indicative of a possible electrical problem. As machines age, there is a tendency for electrical leakage to increase as the insulation begins to deteriorate. In normal operation, the ground wire would be attached, shunting any leakage current to ground and preventing an electrical shock. For the dialysis patient, the standard needs to be much higher because the patient's skin is punctured by two metal conductors (typically 14 gauge needles) that are in an electrolyte (blood plasma) which leads directly to the heart.

For dialysis machines, the maximum allowable electrical leakage risk current is 100 microamperes for the machine chassis and 50 microamperes for the patient connection as defined by the American National Standard Safe Current Limits for Electromedical Apparatus – Document 2.3. This standard is referenced in the Association for the Advancement of Medical Instrumentation (AAMI) Standards and Recommended Practices – Dialysis Volume 3. Components that would contribute to elevated electrical leakage would include motors, heaters, and transformers. Qualified persons are required to isolate the faulty component and rectify the problem.

For human beings, the skin when dry provides resistance against electrical shock. The feeling of slight tingling begins at about one milliampere (1,000 microamperes) for an a/c current at 60 hertz. The shock increases as the current increases. At around 20 milliampere, the current is high enough that the muscles will effectively freeze, and a person will be unable to release themselves from the electrical source. At levels of 100 milliamperes, the heart can be effected directly. To protect against electrical shock, ground fault interrupters (Gfis) are used to monitor the electrical current entering and exiting electrical devices. If the difference exceeds 5 milliamperes, the Gfi will act as a circuit breaker and switch off the power to the instrument.

D. Isolation Transformers

Isolation transformers get their name from their ability to isolate electrical circuits from each other. The transformer doesn't reduce leakage current by reducing voltage, but by making it more difficult for the electrons to leak away from the individual components. For a perfectly insolated dialysis machine, all the electrons would enter the machine through the black "hot" wire in the power cord, and exit through the white "neutral" wire. The black wire will be at 120 volts a/c and the white wire will be at 0 volts. There would be no electrons moving in the green "ground" wire and hence, no leakage current.

To explain how an isolation transformer works, we will use a model that looks at the transformer from the viewpoint of an electron. The electrons are given energy when they visit the power company. This gain in energy is generally measured in volts. Although the voltage at the power company may be hundreds of thousands of volts, the energy is stepped down to lower energy at substations so that by the time the electrons reach the wall outlet, they are down to the familiar 120 volts. When a machine is plugged into the outlet, the electron energy is then available to operate electrical components when the machine is switched on. One of the first components the electrons will encounter when they enter the machine is an isolation transformer. Like all transformers, the isolation transformer has a primary coil of wire and a secondary coil of wire. One of the laws of electricity states that if electrons pass through a coil of wire and lose energy, that energy will be passed to the electrons in the secondary coil. All transformers work on this principal. In fact, the voltage (energy) lost by electrons in the primary coil can be raised or lowered by increasing the number of turns of wire in either coil. If the secondary has fewer turns, the output voltage will be lower, and if it has more turns, the voltage will be higher. For the isolation transformer in this discussion, the coils will be equal so that the voltage in will equal the voltage out.

The electrons coming from the power company want to go back to the power company because mother nature always wants a balance of charge. In other words, just like in an electrolyte solution, the number of positive charges must equal the number of negative charges. For every electron that leaves the power company, the power company needs to get one back. The electrons that are going to make the round trip pass through the primary of the transformer losing energy and then return "home." The energy lost by the Power Company electrons is transferred to the electrons in the transformer's secondary, which gives them the ability to energize the various dialysis components so they can do their particular jobs.

As far as the dialysis components are concerned, they couldn't care less whether the electrons which give them energy come from the power company or somewhere else as long as they get the energy they need to function. Since the primary voltage was 120 volts from the wall, the secondary provides the same voltage to keep the components happy. Power supplies in the machine can change the voltages and convert the alternating current to direct current for the various circuits, but they are still dependent on energy from the secondary of the isolation transformer. Also, the electrons from the power supply will want to return to the power supply because the power supply needs to maintain its balance of charge. To keep things simple, lets assume that the isolation transformer runs all the components directly. In other words, the secondary electrons will go to the various components, give up their energy to make them function, and then return to the transformer to get charged up again.

Unfortunately, just like in real life, not all the electrons play by the same rules. There is a rule in nature called the principle of least action. The rule says effectively: Electrons will always take the easy way out. Electrical components aren't perfect. Some of the electrons find that it's easier to get back to the transformer by not passing through the entire component. They take a "short cut through the pass" by going through the component's insulation to the chassis of the machine. Although this works great in cowboy movies, it's not the thing to do in dialysis equipment. The electrons which leave the components early create what is called the leakage current, just like water which leaves a pipe before it gets to do its job is called a leak. If these electrons had come from the power company, they would have two ways to get back to their starting point. One way is through the ground wire, and the other, if the ground wire is gone, is through someone touching the machine. Once someone touches the unit, the electrons can pass through that person into the earth and return to the power company, which is also touching the earth. When this happens, the individual that provided the path feels a shock.

Machines with isolation transformers make this situation very difficult to do. The reason is that the electrons running the electrical components don't come from the power company, they come from the isolation transformer's secondary. Once they get to the chassis of the machine, the only way back to the secondary is to go to the isolation transformer mounted on the chassis and try to get back into the secondary. Their problem is that the transformer has <u>isolated</u> the secondary from the primary and the ground. Not only that, but remember what mother nature said about balance of charge. If an electron wants to leave the components attached to the secondary, there has to be an electron to take its place. Since this is now extremely difficult to do, the leakage current is greatly reduced and hence also the shock hazard.

The leakage current considered safe by the American Association of Medical instrumentation (AAMI) is 100 microamperes (one ten thousandth of an ampere). The isolation transformer also gives an added advantage in that, even as the electrical components age, the leakage current will not increase because even though more electrons might consider leaving the components, the path back to the transformer won't be any easier.

In the event of total electrical failure, the leakage current will still remain unchanged. The only way the leakage could increase is through breakdown of the isolation transformer. Obviously, this is a principal factor taken into consideration when the transformer is designed.

A final word on equipment in general that contain isolation transformers. Some equipment does not have total isolation, which means some critical components are not operated off the transformer. Those components that use the most power, such as heaters and motors, tend to leak the most eletrons. As a result, a large isolation transformer is required and the larger the transformer the higher its cost. Therefore, just because an instrument has an isolation transformer, don't assume you can't get shocked. Also, remember that the primary of an isolation transformer is operated by power company electrons, so care should always be taken when working around the incoming power.

E. Electronic Components

1. Resistors

Resistors are components that limit flow of electricity. They are used to reduce current flow in electronic circuits, and also to reduce voltage level to a useful value in a particular circuit. Resistors have two basic characteristics: resistance value, measured in ohms, and power rating, measured in watts. Resistance values up to several million ohms are not uncommon. Very low resistance values often are used in high current applications, such as main power supplies, and are designed to handle high wattage. These devices will dissipate large amounts of heat, so they are made of a high temperature ceramic material, and are located to prevent heat transfer to other components. Typical resistors that are used on circuit cards are rated at a fraction of a watt.

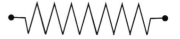

Symbol of a resistor

2. Capacitors

Capacitors are devices which pass alternating current while blocking direct current. They are primarily used in two applications. Large capacitors, called electrolytic capacitors, are used as filters in power supply circuits to remove fluctuations in direct current. Small value capacitors are mostly used to pass specific frequencies of alternating current, while filtering out other frequencies. The unit of capacitance is the farad, but since it is such a large and impractical unit, the microfarad is the common unit seen.

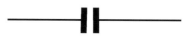

Symbol of a capacitor

3. Diodes

A diode is the simplest semiconductor device. Semiconductors today are almost exclusively made of silicone. A diode will pass electric current in one direction, while blocking the current in the reverse direction. The characteristics which define diodes are voltage and current ratings. Small and large voltage diodes look similar, but large current diodes are larger than low current devices due to the amount of heat they must dissipate. Large current diodes are often called rectifiers. Diodes are quite useful in logic circuits, and rectifiers are mostly used in the conversion of ac to dc voltage in power supply circuits. A variation of diode, called a zener, is used to set a precise voltage level, such as in a voltage regulation circuit. Another useful variation on the diode is a Light Emitting Diode, or LED, which produces a small amount of light. These are often used in indicator panels in place of light bulbs due to their much longer life expectancy.

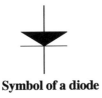

Symbol of a diode

4. Thermistors

Thermistors are devices which exhibit a predictable change in resistance in response to temperature changes. This makes them an ideal remote temperature sensor in dialysate systems, oral thermometers, motor speed controls, and many other applications where a rapid report of temperature is required. These devices are produced in various ways, carbon systems and semiconductor devices being two common types. Thermistors are not interchangeable due to different characteristics -some devices increase resistance due to temperature increases, others decrease resistance in the same conditions.

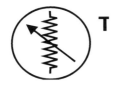

Symbol of a thermistor

5. Transistors

Transistors are probably the best known semiconductors. Who has not heard of a transistor radio, for instance? A transistor is an electrical "gate" which can regulate a large range of current flow by using a small amount of control current. In most applications, this principal is used to produce amplification of a small signal to a larger signal. Transistors vary in their physical size and mounting style depending on how much current they are asked to regulate. Voltage and wattage are important characteristics of transistors. They are also classified by their gain, or amplification ability. Specialized transistors, called phototransistors, can respond to light variations. This makes them useful in dialysis equipment for blood leak detection.

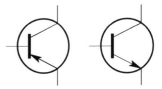

Symbol of a pnp and npn transisitor

6. Integrated Circuits

After the development of semiconductors, the integrated circuit is probably the most important step. These are devices, which use a process similar to microfilm to produce microscopic electronic devices on silicon wafers, or chips. In addition to their very small size, these devices are remarkable in the great amount of components they offer at very low price. An amplifier on an integrated circuit can have hundreds of transistors and other support components while costing as much as a couple of single transistors! These devices are much more stable and durable than circuits made of individual components, and can be easily replaced by qualified technicians. Circuits today are much more precise due to the inclusion of many integrated circuits, while space and power dissipation are much smaller than identical circuits made of individual components. Due to their small size, integrated circuits generally do not handle large amounts of power, since they are damaged by large amounts of heat. The increase in features that are offered in modern dialysis equipment is made possible in part by the use of integrated circuits.

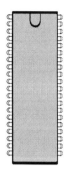

Integrated Circuit Chip

7. Voltage Regulators

Formerly made of individual components, integrated circuits have made complicated forms of voltage regulation possible using very little space. Keeping a constant supply voltage is important in electronic circuits; voltage regulators can compensate for changing conditions and keep supply voltages within close tolerances. Systems which require large amounts of current will use integrated circuit voltage regulators to control large power transistors on heat sinks to keep the voltage regulator from damaging high temperatures.

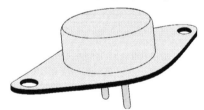

Voltage Regulator

8. Microprocessors

The zenith of today's electronic technology would have to be the microprocessor. In a miniaturization many times more fantastic than mentioned above, instead of hundreds of transistors a microprocessor such as a Pentium would contain over 4 million transistors. Powerful computers no longer occupy

rooms, but a space on a desktop. In addition to personal computers, microprocessors are becoming common in numerous applications where logic and controlled reactions to various circumstances is desirable. Modern dialysis equipment would be economically unfeasible without microprocessors to control the various treatment parameters physicians request, such as sodium and ultrafiltration modeling. Microprocessors can handle logic with incredible speed. They can be controlled with memory circuits that may be rigidly set to follow a specific behavior, or readily programmed to allow much control and flexibility.

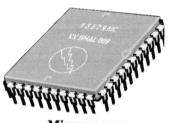

Microprocessor

Microprocessors require a protected environment to operate correctly. They must be kept dry, cool, and have a well regulated, constant supply voltage. Due to the microscopic nature of their individual components, microprocessors are quite susceptible to damage from static electricity. A static spark, which a person may find unpleasant when touching a doorknob, could destroy the individual circuit elements of a microprocessor.

9. Memory

Microprocessors require instructions to know how to operate. These instructions are stored in memory circuits that are read and understood by the micro-processor. Memory circuits come in many types. Read Only Memory, or ROM is a form that has instructions permanently formed into it. It cannot be changed. Many pieces of dialysis equipment have ROM memory, and when an upgrade to new instructions is desired, new ROM chips must be obtained and installed. Random Access Memory, or RAM is memory which can easily be changed, such as the memory in my computer which stores the keystrokes used in typing this document. RAM memory is quite useful, but a brief interruption of power will cause its information to be lost, where as RAM memory would maintain it's information. Either form of memory, like any microcircuit, is damaged by static electricity.

The Resistor Color Code

The resistor color code was developed many years ago as a simple way to label resistors so that their resistance could be determined easily in spite of their size or mounting position on a printed circuit board. The use of numbers made determining their individual values difficult, especially for resistors with a resistance of millions of ohms. Also, care had to be taken when mounting the resistors to ensure that the resistance could still be read. By using color bands that circle the resistor, identification of resistor size can be done easily.

The color code assigns a particular color to each of the numbers between 0 and 9.

0 = Black	5 = Green
1 = Brown	6 = Blue
2 = Red	7 = Violet
3 = Orange	8 = Gray
4 = Yellow	9 = White

The resistance of a resistor is determined by reading the color of the bands and converting the colors to numbers. The color bands are placed on the resistor close to one end. The color bands are then read in order from that end. In order to limit the number of color bands, the third band is used as a multiplier in much the same way as using scientific notation. A fourth band is also used to give a tolerance value. The color gold is used for 5% accuracy, silver for 10% accuracy, and if there is no fourth band, the tolerance is 20%. For resistors with very tight tolerances of 1% or finer, the actual number value will be labeled on the resistor.

The illustration and table below show how the code functions.

Figure 14.10

Resistor Color Code

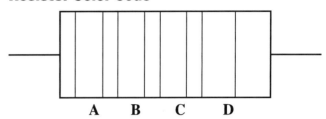

Color	A	B	C	D
Black	0	0	1	-
Brown	1	1	10	-
Red	2	2	100	-
Orange	3	3	1,000	-
Yellow	4	4	10,000	-
Green	5	5	100,000	-
Blue	6	6	1,000,000	-
Violet	7	7	10,000,000	-
Gray	8	8	100,000,000	-
White	9	9	-	
Gold	-	-	0.1	+/- 5%
Silver	-	-	0.01	+/-10%
No band	-	-	-	+/-20%

Here are some examples of the color code and its conversion into numerical values.

1. YELLOW GREEN RED GOLD = 4500 ohms +/- 5%

This first example is straightforward. Yellow is 4, Green is 5 and the multiplier is 100. Another way to look at the multiplier is to just think red equals 2 and add two zeros after the 4 and 5. The gold band gives a tolerance of 5 percent. Instead of writing 4500 ohms, the value could be stated simply 4.5 kilo-ohms or 4.5 K ohms.

2. BROWN BLACK RED GOLD = 1000 ohms +/- 5%

In this next example, Brown is 1, Black is 0, and again, the multiplier is 100. The result is 1K ohms. 1,000 can't be done by using only a brown and orange to yield one and three zeros. The rules require that three colors be used for each number to avoid confusion.

3. RED RED GREEN = 2,200,000 ohms +/- 20%

The answer using two twos and multiplying by 100,000 (or just adding 5 zeros) has no fourth band. As a result, the tolerance is +/- 20%. The answer could be written as 2.2 megohms.

4. BLUE VIOLET GOLD GOLD = 6.7 ohms +/- 5%

Example four takes advantage of the gold band in position three. Instead of multiplying, the 67 is divided by 10 to yield 6.7 ohms.

Being able to determine the value of a resistor can be very helpful when troubleshooting a printed circuit board. Today, although most printed circuits are too complicated to troubleshoot without special equipment, it is still possible to test a circuit by looking at its input and output signals to see if the circuit is responding properly. By using a circuit schematic diagram to identify a resistor on the board which is directly connected to a particular input or output that needs testing, the test point can be found by finding the resistor with the value stated on the schematic.

If the resistor has a value of 10,000 ohms, the first two colors would be brown and black. This leaves three zeros, which is the color orange. The resistor to look for will have the colors: brown, black, orange. The fourth band for tolerance is generally not needed in the identification process. It may be that there are more than two resistors on a board with the same value. In those cases, identifying a second resistor or another circuit component connected to the first resistor may be necessary.

Suggested Readings

AAMI (1996), *AAMI Standards and Recommended Practices,* 1996 Edition, Arlington: Association for the Advancement of Medical Instrumentation.

Dickson, T.R. (1971), *Introduction to Chemistry,* John Wiley & Sons, Inc. New York, London, Sidney, Toronto.

King, Coldwell, Williams (1972), College Chemistry, Sixth Edition, Glen Miller, Professor of Chemistry, Santa Barbara, Canfield Press, San Francisco.

Miller, Glen (1972), Principles of College Chemistry, Canfield Press, San Francisco.

Barron's Educational Series:

Downing, Douglas (1989), *Algebra, the Easy Way,* Second Edition.

Leheman, Robert L. (1990), *Physics, the Easy Way,* Second Edition.

Mascetti, Joseph A. (1984), *Chemistry, the Easy Way,* Second Edition.

Miller, Rex (1988), *Electronics, the Easy Way,* Second Edition.

Texts referenced in the preparation of information for the Chemistry, Physics, and Electronics section:

McGraw-Hill Dictionary of Scientific and Technical Terms; 2nd Edition; Daniel N. Lapedes, Editor in Chief; Copyright 1978, McGraw-Hill; ISBN 0-07-045258-X.

Concise Dictionary of Physics and related subjects; 2nd Edition; James Thewlis; Copyright 1979, J. Thewlis;Pergamon Press; ISBN 0 08 023048 2.

CRC Handbook of Chemistry and Physics; Robert C. Weast, Editor; Copyright 1977, CRC Press Inc.; ISBN 0-8493-0458-X.

Chemistry, A Textbook for Colleges; William McPherson, William Edwards Henderson, Edward Mack Jr., W. Conard Fernelius; Copyright 1940, Ginn and Company.

Hemodialysis for Nurses and Dialysis Personnel; 6th Edition; C. F. Gutch, Martha H. Stoner, Anna L. Corea; Copyright 1999, Mosby Inc.; ISBN 0-8151-2099-0.

Handbook of Dialysis; 2nd Edition; John T. Daugirdas, Todd S. Ing; Copyright 1994 John T. Daugirdas, Todd S. Ing; Little, Brown, and Company; ISBN 0-316-17383-5.

AAMI Standards and Recommended Practices, Volume 3 Dialysis; Copyright 1995; Association for the Advancement of Medical Instrumentation; ISBN 0-910275-50-5.

Allied Electronics Data Handbook; 4th Edition; Nelson M. Cooke, Editor; Copyright 1963 Allied Radio Corporation; Library of Congress Catalog No. 62-21444.

University Physics; Francis Weston Sears, Mark W. Zemansky; Copyright 1949 Addison-Wesley Press, Inc; Library of Congress Catalog No. 49-48255.

Physics for Students of Science and Engineering; David Halliday, Robert Resnick; Copyright 1960, John Wiley and Sons, Inc.; Library of Congress Catalog No. 60-6455.

Dorland's Illustrated Medical Dictionary; 27th Edition; Elizabeth J. Taylor, Editor; Copyright 1988 W. B. Saunders Company; ISBN 0-7216-3154-1.

Chapter 15

DOQI

NKF – Dialysis Outcomes Quality Initiative Clinical Practice Guidelines

Compiled by:

Philip M. Varughese, BS, CHT

Philip Andrysiak, BS, MBA, CHT

Chapter Outline

I. Hemodilaysis Adequacy

II. Peritoneal Dialysis Adequacy

III. Vascular Access

IV. Anemia Management

Introduction

What follows is an overview of the National Kidney Foundation (NKF) Dialysis Outcomes Quality Initiative Clinical Practice Outcomes. This is only intended as an overview. For a full description of the guidelines please read the NKF Guidelines. While these tools are very useful remember that they do not replace Continuous Quality Improvement (CQI). They are good starting points but all health care practitioners should always look for ways to continuously improve the quality of care. In practicing this technique, it is important to have consistency. Everyone does everything the same way. This is the only way that results can be compared. DOQI guidelines are based either on evidence or on opinion. Some are based partly on evidence and opinion.

The guidelines address four main areas: HD adequacy, PD adequacy, vascular access and treatment of anemia from chronic renal failure.

I. Hemodialysis Adequacy

A. Hemodialysis Dose

B. Consisting of 16 guidelines

C. All patients receiving hemodialysis in the same dialysis facility should have the delivered dose of hemodialysis measured using the same method. (Guideline #3)

D. Kt/V and URR

Dialysis care team should deliver a Kt/V of at least 1.2 (Single-pool, variable volume) for both adult and pediatric hemodialysis patients. For those using the URR, the delivered dose should be equivalent to Kt/V 1.2, or an average URR of 65%, however URR can vary substantially as a function of fluid removal. (Guideline#4)

E. Prescribed Dose of Hemodialysis

Should be Kt/V 1.3 or URR of 70% in order to prevent the delivered dose of dialysis from falling below the recommended minimum dose. A variety of factors may result in the delivered dose of hemodialysis falling below the prescribed dose, including:

1. Compromised urea clearance

2. Actual treatment time less than the prescribed treatment time

3. Laboratory or blood sampling errors.

F. Acceptable methods for BUN sampling

1. Blood samples for BUN measurement must be drawn in a particular manner

2. Pre-dialysis BUN samples should be drawn immediately prior to dialysis, using a technique that avoids dilution of the blood sample with saline or heparin.

3. Post dialysis BUN samples should be drawn using the Slow Flow/Stop Pump Technique that prevents sample dilution with recirculated blood and minis the confounding effects of urea rebound.

G. Stop pump technique:

1. At the completion of hemodialysis, turn off the dialysate flow and decrease the ultrafiltration rate (UFR) to 50ml/hr, or the lowest transmembrane pressure (TMP)/UFR setting, or off. If the dialysis machine does not allow for turning off the dialysate flow, decrease the dialysate flow to its minimum setting. Purpose: Stop the hemodialysis treatment without stopping the blood flow completely decreases the blood flow to 50-100ml/min for 15 seconds. To prevent pump shut-off as the blood flow rate is reduced, it may be necessary to manually adjust the venous pressure limits downward. The purpose is to fill the arterial needle tubing and the arterial bloodline with non-recirculated blood (in case there is any access recirculation) by clearing the dead space in the arterial needle and the arterial bloodline.

2. Immediately stop the blood pump

3. Clamp the arterial and venous bloodlines. Clamp the arterial needle tubing.

4. Blood for post-dialysis BUN measurement may be sampled by needle aspiration from the arterial sampling port closest to the patient. Alternatively, blood may be obtained from the arterial needle tubing after disconnection from the arterial bloodline and attaching a vacutainer or syringe without a needle.

5. Blood is returned to the patient and the patient disconnection procedure proceeds as per unit protocol Slow Flow Technique: follow the above step up to 2 and 3 and then proceed with 6.

6. With the blood pump still running at 50-100 ml/min, draw the blood sample for post dialysis BUN measurement from the arterial sampling port closest to the patient. Purpose: Drawing the blood from arterial sampling port ensures the post dialysis BUN measurement is performed on un-dialyzed blood. Stop the blood pump and complete the patient disconnection procedure as per dialysis unit protocol.

7. If a hollow fiber dialyzer is to be reused, the total cell volume (TCV) of that hemodialyzer should be measured prior to its first use. Batch testing and/or use of average TCV for a group of dialyzers is not an acceptable practice. (Guidelines #11) During each reprocessing, the total cell volume of reused dialyzers should be checked. Dialyzers having a total cell volume <80% of original measured value should not be reused.

H. Optimizing patient comfort and compliance

1. Without compromising the delivered dose of hemodialysis, efforts should be undertaken to modify the hemodialysis prescription to prevent the occurrence of intradialytic symptoms adversely affect patient comfort and compliance. (Guidelines #15)

2. Strategies to Minimize Hypotensive Symptoms.

   Without compromising the delivered dose of hemodialysis, efforts should be undertaken to minimize intradialytic symptoms that compromise the delivery of adequate dialysis, like hypotension and cramps. These efforts may include one or more of the following:
   a) Avoid excessive ultrafiltration
   b) Slow the ultrafiltration
   c) Perform isolated ultrafiltration
   d) Increase the dialysate sodium concentration
   e) Switch from acetate to bicarbonate-buffered dialysate.
   f) Reduce the dialysate temperature
   g) Correct anemia
   h) Optimize patient behavior

II. Peritoneal Dialysis Adequacy

A. There are 32 recommended guidelines outlining PD Adequacy.

Adequacy is measured through Kt/V and creatinine clearance calculations. If the patient is on CAPD, their Kt/V should be at least 2, with a creatinine clearance of 60 liters. If the patient is on CYCLER, their Kt/V should be at least 2.1 with a corresponding creatinine clearance of 63 liters. Further recommendations regarding PD Adequacy can be found in the DOQI guidelines. For the purpose of this chapter, the focus is on hemodialysis issues only.

III. Vascular Access

A. Consisting of 38 guidelines

1. Timing of access placement:

   Patient should be referred for surgery to attempt construction of a primary AV fistula when their creatinine clearance is <25 ml/minute, their serum creatinine level is > 4mg/dl. (Guideline #8)

2. A new primary fistula should be allowed to mature for at least 1 month, and ideally for 3 to 4 months, prior to cannulation.

3. Dialysis AV grafts should be placed at least 3 to 6 weeks prior to dialysis.

B. Types of vascular access (Guideline #3)

C. The order of preference for placement of AV fistulae in patients requiring chronic hemodialysis is:

1. A wrist (radial-cephalic) primary AV fistula
2. An elbow (brachial-cephalic) primary AV fistula
3. An arteriovenous graft of synthetic material
4. A transposed brachial-basilic vein fistula
5. Cuffed-tunneled central venous catheters should be discouraged as permanent vascular access.

D. Monitoring access (Guideline #10)

1. Dynamic Venous Dialysis Pressure Monitoring Protocol.

2. Establish a baseline by initiating measurements when the access is first used.

E. Measure venous dialysis pressure from the hemodialysis machine at QB 200ml/ min during the first 2 to 5 minutes of hemodialysis every hemodialysis session.

1. Use 15 gauge needles (establish own protocol for different needle size)

2. Assure that the venous needle is in the lumen of the vessel and not partially occluded by the vessel wall.

3. Pressure must exceed the threshold three times in succession to be significant

4. Assess at same level relative to hemodialysis machine for all measurements.

F. Interpretation of results

1. Three measurements in succession above the threshold are required to eliminate the effect of variation caused by needle placement. Hemodialysis machines measure pressure with different monitors and tubing types and lengths. These variables, as well as needle size, influence venous dialysis pressure. The most important variable affecting the dynamic pressure at a blood flow of 200 ml/min is the needle gauge. It is essential to set thresholds for action based on machine manufacturer, tubing type, and needle gauge.

2. Using 15- gauge needles, the threshold that indicates elevated pressure (and therefore the likely presence of hemodynamically significant venous outlet stenosis) for Cobe Century 3 machines is a pressure of 125 mmHg, whereas the threshold of Gambro AK10 machines is a pressure of 150 mmHg. Data for Baxter, Fresenius, Althin and other dialysis machines are not available but are likely to be similar to those of the Cobe Century 3 if the same gauge venous needle is used.

3. Trend analysis is more important than any single measurement. Upward trends in hemodialysis pressure over time are more predictive than absolute values. Each unit should establish its own venous pressure threshold values. For this reason trend charts for each patient is recommended. If you program allows for it, a trend line should also be included. This is a quick method to see what direction the measurements are moving.

4. Patients with progressively increasing pressures or those who exceed the threshold on three consecutive hemodialysis treatments should be referred for venography.

G. Measurement of access recirculation

1. Recirculation should be measured using a nonurea-based dilutional method or by using the two-needle urea based method. The three-needle peripheral vein method of measuring recircualtion should be used.

H. Skin preparation technique for permanent AV accesses

1. A clean technique for needle cannulation should be used for all cannulation procedures (Guidelines #14).

2. Locate and palpate the needle cannulation sites prior to skin preparation.

3. Wash access site using an antibacterial soap or scrub and water

4. Cleanse the skin by applying 70% alcohol and / or 10% povidone iodine using a circular rubbing motion. Start at the cannulation site and scrub with concentric circles moving away from cannulation site.

I. Needle insertion technique

1. Use approximately 45-degree angle of insertion for AV graft and approximately 25-degree angle for AV fistula.

J. Needle removal technique

1. Remove needle at same or similar angle to the angle of insertion, and NEVER APPLY PRESSURE BEFORE THE NEEDLE IS COMPLETELY OUT.

IV. Anemia Management

A. Total guidelines consisting of #28

B. Anemia in patients

The primary cause of anemia in patients with CRF is insufficient production of erythropoietin (EPO) by the diseased kidneys. Additional factors which may cause or contribute to anemia include: iron deficiency, either related to or independent of blood loss from repeated laboratory testing, needle punctures, blood retention in the dialyzer and tubing, or gastrointestinal bleeding; severe hyperparathyroidism; acute and chronic inflammatory conditions; aluminum toxicity; folate deficiency; shortened red cell survival; hypothyrodism; and underlying hemoglobinopathies.

Recombinant human erythropoetin has been used in the treatment of the anemia of CRF since 1986. Iron is also essential for hemoglobin formation. The iron status of the patient with CRF must be assessed and adequate iron stores should be available before Epoetin therapy is initiated.

C. Epoetin alfa (Epogen®), is the only approved recombinant human erythropoietin (rHuEPO) product available in the United States manufactured by Amgen Inc. Amgen uses ovary cells of the Chinese hamster to make Epogen.

D. Initiation of anemia work-up

An anemia work-up should be initiated in-patients with chronic renal failure when the: (Guideline #1&2)

1. Hct is <33% (Hg <11 g/dl) in pre-menopausal females and pre-puberty patients

2. Hct is <37% (Hg <12 g /dl) in adult males and post-menopausal females. Evaluation of anemia should consist of measurement of at least the following: Hematocrit (Hct) and /or Hemoglobin (Hgb)

E. Anemia evaluation

1. Hematocrit and /or Hemoglobin

2. Red blood cell (RBC) indices

    (a) Reticulocyte count

3. Iron parameters

    (a) Serum iron

    (b) Total Iron Binding Capacity (TIBC)

    (c) Percent transferrin saturation (serum iron x 100 divided by TIBC) TSAT

    (d) Serum ferritin

4. A test for occult blood in stool.

    (Hemoglobin: The part of the red blood cells that carries oxygen (11 and 12 gm/dl)

    Hematocrit: The proportion of blood that is comprised of red cells (33% -36%)

    Ferritin: Measures the amount of iron stored in the body for long term use (100ng/ml)

    Transferrin: Transferrin saturation is a measure of the iron that is available to bone marrow for red blood cell production. (at least 20%)

F. Administration of epoetin:

1. Epoetin should be administered subcutaneously (SC) in pre-dialysis and peritoneal dialysis patients.

2. The preferred route of Epoetin administration is SC in hemodialysis patients. Studies have indicated that Epoetin requirements are , on average, about 15% to 50% less with SC than with IV dosing.

3. When Epoetin is given SC to adult patients, the dose should be 80-120 units/kg/wk in two to three doses per week.

4. When Epoetin is given IV for hemodialysis patients, the dose should be 120-180units/kg/wk, given in three divided doses.

Conclusion

DOQI guidelines are current recommendations for renal disease management. Implementation of these guidelines allows the practitioner to administer optimum care to patients. By the end of this year, a new set of guidelines Kidney Disease Outcomes Quality Initiative (K-DOQI), will be initiated to expand DOQI and include all phases of kidney disease. K-DOQI will standardize the assessment of renal disease in its' various stages of progression. There will also be the final publication of the NKF-DOQI guideline on nutrition and updates on many of the original guidelines including hemodialysis and PD. K-DOQI will also recommend specific treatments for patients stratified into specific subsets based on progression of disease, and other risk factors.

Reference

DOQI Guidelines 1997, National Kidney Foundation

Chapter 16
Peritoneal Dialysis

Contributing Authors:

Migdalia Rosario, BS, RN, CPDN

Ruth Stallard, BSN, RN, CNN

Chapter Outline

I. Historical Perspectives

1923: Ganter described peritoneal dialysis in uremic animals and reported the first use of peritoneal dialysis for uremia in a human.

1959: Commercially available sterile peritoneal dialysis solution.

1964: Boen developed the first closed automated delivery system.

1964: Palmer designed a Silicone catheter for chronic use.

1965: Weston and Roberts designed an acute stylet catheter.

1967: Tenchhoff designed the Silicone double cuff catheter.

1976: Papovich and Moncrief described continuous ambulatory peritoneal dialysis technique.

1978: FDA approved peritoneal dialysis solution in polyvinyl bag for use in the USA.

1981: Diaz-Buxo et al. described continuous cycling peritoneal dialysis.

1980s: New CAPD systems, cycling machines, and catheter designs.

1994: Seventeen per cent of the USA dialysis population is on PD.

II. Anatomy and Physiology

A. Normal Peritoneum

1. The peritoneum consists of serous membrane with a size of 1-2 square meters.

2. In an adult, the surface area of the peritoneal membrane approximates the body surface area.

3. The peritoneum lines the abdominal wall and covers the abdominal organs.

4. The dialyzing membrane consists of the vascular wall, interstitium, mesothelium, and adjacent fluid films.

5. In females, the ovaries and fallopian tubes open into the peritoneal cavity.

6. In males, the peritoneum is closed and continuous.

B. Blood Supply

1. The superior mesenteric artery supplies the visceral peritoneum.

2. The intercostal, epigastric, and the lumbar arteries supply the parietal peritoneum.

Figure 16.1

Cross-Section of Peritoneal Cavity (shaded) and Internal Organs

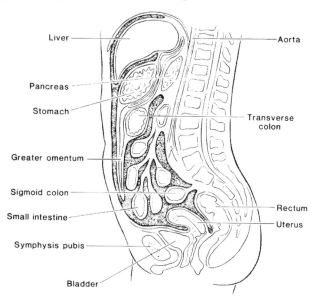

Source: **ANNA** Core Curriculum, *Third Edition, p. 285, fig. XI.1*

3. Blood from the visceral peritoneum converges and enters the portal vein.

C. Peritoneal Lymphatics

1. From the peritoneal cavity, lymphatic drainage is achieved through specialized lymph stomata that are found in the subdiaphragmatic peritoneum.

2. The initial or terminal lymphatics are the smallest lymphatic vessels. Their purpose is to collect fluid and materials from the blood and interstitial tissue.

3. Excess intraperitoneal fluid and protein are returned to the systemic circulation from the lymphatics that drain the peritoneal cavity.

4. Lymphatic flow rate is influenced by several factors: respiratory rate, intra-abdominal pressure, body posture, and peritonitis.

5. The lymphatics contribute to host defenses of the peritoneum by removing any foreign bodies that might enter the peritoneal cavity.

6. In CAPD, the average lymph absorption rate is approximately 0.5 – 1 ml/minute.

7. The average daily lymph absorption is at least one liter.

Figure 16.2

Osmonic Ultrafiltration

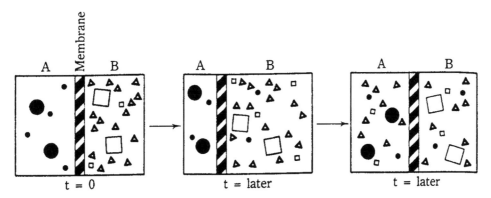

Solution A represents the blood and solution B the dialysate. The open triangles represent the osmotically active solute (e.g., glucose). Small squares and circles represent large, nonpermeable solutes (e.g., proteins). As shown, an osmotic water shift takes place early *(middle panel)*, tending to equalize the total particle concentration on either side of the membrane. However, as the glucose is absorbed *(right panel)*, the water shift reverses to restore the water content on either side of the membrane back to the initial state.

Source: Handbook of Dialysis, *p. 249, fig. 13.2*

D. Kinetics

1. Semi-Permeable Membrane

   The peritoneal membrane is a semi-permeable membrane that allows small solutes and water to pass through but retains large particles like proteins and blood cells.

2. Diffusion

   a) Definition - Movement of solute across the peritoneal membrane from an area of higher solute concentration to an area of lower concentration.

   b) In peritoneal dialysis, diffusion is the principal mechanism for removal of waste products.

   c) The two solutions in peritoneal dialysis are the blood and the dialysate. They are separated by the peritoneal membrane.

   d) The blood perfuses the capillaries which are adjacent to the peritoneal membrane. The dialysate is in the abdomen.

3. Factors Influencing Rates of Diffusion

   a) Concentration gradients between blood and dialysate

   b) Molecular weight of the solute

   c) Peritoneal membrane permeability

   d) Peritoneal membrane size or surface area

   e) Peritoneal blood flow

   f) Dialysis solution volume

   g) Dialysate solution temperature

4. Factors that Enhance Diffusion

   a) Increased Blood flow to the Peritoneum.

   (1) The rate of solute delivery to the membrane can be increased by increasing the blood flow to the peritoneum.

   (2) During peritoneal dialysis, blood flow is near maximal levels.

   (3) Infusion of fresh dialysis solution causes peritoneal blood flow to increase.

   b) Increasing the Volume of the Dialysate.

   (1) Clearances will be greater with the use of higher volumes of dialysate.

   (2) The volume of dialysate can be increased by increasing the infusion volume or the number of exchanges.

   c) Temperature of the Solution

   (1) Prewarmed dialysate enhances diffusion.

   (2) Solution that is cooler than body temperature will initially slow the rate of diffusion until the dialysate warms to body temperature.

   d) High Concentration Gradient

   (1) The net solute transport will approach zero when the concentration difference between the solution decreases.

   (2) To maintain the concentration gradient between blood and dialysate, the dialysate in the abdomen requires changing at prescribed intervals.

5. Osmosis
   a) Definition – The movement of water across the peritoneal membrane from an area of lower solute concentration to an area of higher solute concentration.
   b) Ultrafiltration is the mechanism whereby fluid is removed in peritoneal dialysis.
   c) A substantial percentage of total solute removal can be accounted for by ultrafiltration.
   d) The principal mechanism whereby fluid moves from blood to dialysate in peritoneal dialysis is osmotic ultrafiltration.

6. Ultrafiltration
   a) Definition - The bulk movement of water along with permeable solutes through a semi-permeable membrane.
   b) Ultrafiltration is the mechanism where by fluid is removed in peritoneal dialysis.
   c) A substantial percentage of total solute removal can be accounted for by ultrafiltration.
   d) The principal mechanism whereby fluid moves from blood to dialysate in peritoneal dialysis is osmotic ultrafiltration.

7. Principles of Ultrafiltration
   a) Glucose in the dialysate generates a high osmotic pressure, which induces ultrafiltration.
   b) Ultrafiltration rate is higher at the beginning of the exchange when glucose concentration gradient is at its highest.
   c) As glucose concentration decreases, the ultrafiltration rate declines.
   d) Ultrafiltration amounts will vary depending on the glucose concentrations of the dialysate.
   e) The use of 1.5% dialysis solution will result in minimal or zero fluid removal.
   f) The use of 2.5% or 4.25% dialysate solutions that are hypertonic will result in increased ultrafiltration.
   g) Ultrafiltration volume will peak at about two to three hours.
   h) Shortened dwell time will increase ultrafiltration volume, as the glucose gradient is maintained at a high level.
   i) Reabsorption of water occurs if the dialysate is allowed to dwell past osmotic equilibration.
   j) Persistent use of hypertonic dialysis solution may cause excessive fluid removal.

E. Drug Transport

1. Effect of Medications on Dialysis
   a) Systemic vasodilators that increase blood supply to nearby capillary beds may increase clearances.
   b) Medications that cause a decrease in blood flow from the abdomen will decrease clearances.

2. Effect of Dialysis on Medications
   a) Medications that are administered intraperitoneally may enter into the systemic circulation.
   b) A dosage increase may be required for medications that are removed by peritoneal dialysis.
   c) Dosage decrease may be required for medication that are poorly removed by peritoneal dialysis, or are normally excreted by the kidneys.

3. Heparin
   a) For acute peritoneal dialysis, heparin (200-500u/L) is usually added to the solution to prevent obstruction of the catheter by fibrin clots.
   b) For episodes of infectious peritonitis, or other intraperitoneal inflammatory conditions, the addition of heparin (250-1000u/L) to the dialysis solution is recommended.
   c) Heparin is not absorbed through the peritoneum. The addition of low doses of heparin does not cause systemic heparinization.

4. Insulin
   a) Regular insulin can be added to the dialysis solution of each exchange.
   b) Regular insulin can be administered by the intraperitoneal route.
   c) Insulin administered intraperitoneally enters the systemic circulation via the hepatic portal system.
   d) Insulin binds to the solution bags, thereby necessitating an increase in the insulin dosage required.
   e) Incomplete absorption of insulin from the dialysis solution will require an increase in dosage.

III. Solutions

1. To enhance ultrafiltration, the osmolarity of the dialysate is increased by the addition of dextrose.

2. Dialysis solutions are available in various dextrose concentrations: 1.5g%, 2.5g%, and 4.25%.

3. Normal serum levels are simulated in the electrolyte concentration of the solution.

4. Lactate (sodium lactate) is the most common buffer used.

5. Solutions are available in 2.5 mEq/L and 3.5 mEq/L calcium. Elevated serum calcium levels would be an indication for the use of low calcium solutions.

IV. PD Catheter Access

A. Catheter Types

Most common catheter types are shown in Figure 17.4 (from *ANNA Core Curriculum*, 3rd edition, pg 291, Figure XI.6)

1. Most catheters are made of flexible silicone. Polyurethane is also used.

2. The catheter can be divided in three segments.

a) Intraperitoneal segment

  (1) Contains tiny side holes and an end port for infusion and drainage of dialysate.

  (2) The tip of the catheter may be straight or curled (pigtailed).

  (3) Length of this section ranges from 11cm to 15cm.

b) Intermural segment

  (1) The mid-section of the catheter contains an anchoring device such as dacron polyester or velour cuffs, beaded flanges or balloon disks.

  (2) Most commonly used are two dacron polyester or velour cuffs that promote tissue in growth and create a physical barrier to the peritoneum.

  (3) The cuffs prevent bacterial infections and tunnel leaks.

  (4) Tissue growth into the cuffs provides catheter stability preventing the catheter from sliding within the catheter tunnel.

c) External segment

  (1) Connects to a transfer set using a titanium or plastic adapter that connect to either a transfer set or the disposable PD system set.

Figure 16.3

Composition of Solutions for Peritoneal Dialysis

	Standard Solutions	Low Magnesium Solutions	Low Calcium Solutions
Sodium (mEq/L)	132	132	132
Calcium (mEq/L)	3.5	3.5	2.5
Magnesium (mEq/L)	1.5	0.5	0.5
Chloride (mEq/L)	102	96	95
Lactate (mEq/L)	35	40	40
pH	5.2 – 5.5	5.2 – 5.5	5.2 – 5.5
Osmolarity (mOsm/L)			
1.5% Dextrose	347	346	344
2.5% Dextrose	398	396	394 - 395
3.5% Dextrose	448	447	445
4.25% Dextrose	486	485	483

Source: ANNA Core Curriculum, *Third Edition, p. 290, table XI.1*

Figure 16.4

Chronic Peritoneal Dialysis Catheters

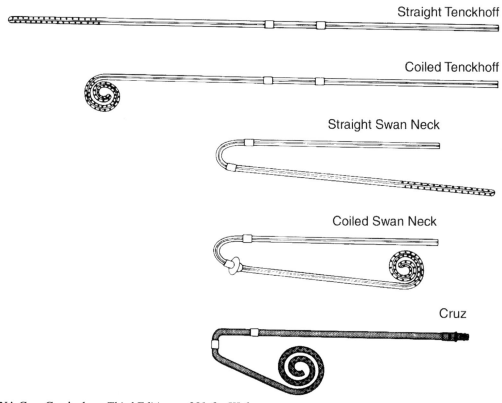

Straight Tenckhoff

Coiled Tenckhoff

Straight Swan Neck

Coiled Swan Neck

Cruz

Source: **ANNA** Core Curriculum, *Third Edition, p. 291, fig. XI.6*

B. Catheter Placement

1. The catheter position is evaluated with the patient in both the supine and sitting positions prior to surgery.

2. The catheter should exit the skin either above or below the belt line, avoiding skin folds or scars.

3. The optimum catheter placement is with the external segment of the catheter oriented in the down and lateral position.

   a) The downward orientation prevents the exit site from collecting debris and moisture.

   b) The lateral position minimizes contamination from the pubic area.

4. Midsection of the catheter is tunneled through the abdominal muscle wall and subcutaneous fat layers exiting through the skin.

5. The intraperitoneal segment rests in the lower portion of the pelvis.

C. Catheter Complications Post Insertion

1. Slow Drain

   a) An average of 200cc of solution/minute is expected to drain from a functioning catheter.

   b) If slow drain is noted, the location of the intraperitoneal segment may not be in the optimal position for adequate drain or the intraperitoneal catheter segment may be kinked.

Figure 16.5

Healthy Catheter Exit Site

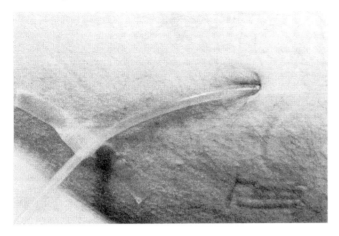

Source: ANNA Core Curriculum, *Third Edition, p. 298, fig. XI.8*

2. Tight Catheter Tunnel due to the use of snug sutures at the exit site does not allow drainage of necrotic tissue and results in skin sloughing.

3. Large Tunnel allows excessive movement of the catheter with in the tunnel thus prolonging healing around the exit site.

D. Exit Site

1. Qualities of a Healthy Exit Site
   a) The skin color encircling the exit site may present as natural, darkened, light pink, or have a dark purplish discoloration.
   b) There should be an absence of external drainage.
   c) There should be no presence of crust at the exit site, but minimal crust may be considered acceptable.
   d) Epithelium should partly cover the visible sinus.
   e) Visual sinus should be dry, but a small amount of clear or thick drainage may be exhibited.
   f) There should be an absence of granulation tissue or proud flesh externally.

2. Maintaining a Healthy Exit
   a) The goal is to prevent infections of the exit site.
   b) Routine exit site care consists of washing the exit site with antibacterial non-irritating liquid soap on a daily basis during showering.

c) The exit site should not be submerged in bath water.
d) The exit site should be cleaned if the site gets dirty or moist.
e) Dressings are worn over the exit site until well healed. Once healed the patient may or may not wear a dressing.
f) All catheters should be anchored to the abdomen by taping in such a manner that the catheter does not pull at the exit site.

V. Patient Selection

A. Contraindications to Peritoneal Dialysis

1. Hypercatabolism – Inability of peritoneal dialysis to adequately remove the uremic metabolites.

2. Inadequate transfer surface area due to multiple adhesions and scarring as a result of the following:
   a) Multiple surgeries
   b) Previous peritonitis
   c) Sclerosing peritonitis

3. Patent opening between peritoneal and pleural cavities.

4. Mental or physical disabilities in the absence of an assistant.

B. Patient Selection for Self Care

1. The PD Candidate should be motivated to do self-care.

2. The severity of the patient's illness should not be such that it would interfere with the ability to perform the exchange in a responsible manner.

3. Visual, motor or muscular function should be adequate in order for the patient to safely perform the exchanges.

4. Availability of Family/Community Resources
   a) Is family support available for patient's decision or be available for assistance?
   b) Availability of proper nutritional resources.

5. Patient physical environment should include access to electricity and water supply and an adequate area to perform aseptic procedures/exchanges.

VI. Peritoneal Dialysis Process

A. *The Exchange or Cycle*

1. Definition: The exchange begins with draining out dialysate that has been infused into the peritoneal cavity through the PD catheter and allowed to dwell for a predetermined amount of time. The drain, dwell, and infusion phases are repeated the prescribed number of times throughout a 24 hour period.

2. Drain

   a) The dialysate solution containing the uremic toxins plus the ultrafiltrate is drained from the peritoneal cavity by gravity or under gravity like pressure.

   b) This phase can take from 15 to 30 minutes depending on the amount of infused volume.

   c) The patient can usually recognize when most of the PD solution has been drained, as they will feel empty, or have a slight pulling sensation in their abdomen.

   d) The drain phase can be impeded by fibrin blockage within the catheter, constipation, or by migration of the catheter out of the normal lower pelvic area.

3. Infusion Phase

   a) Warmed dialysis solution flows into the peritoneal cavity by gravity or under gravity like pressure through the PD catheter.

   b) The infusion can be done manually using a bag of dialysate solution hung on an IV pole, or by automation using a cycler device or exchange device.

   c) This phase takes approximately 10 minutes and depends on the volume of solution to be infused.

4. Dwell

   a) The dwell phase is where the dialysate solution is allowed to remain in the peritoneal cavity for a predetermined period of time to allow for diffusion of solutes (urea, creatinine, phosphorus and other uremic toxins) and ultrafiltration of fluid to take place.

   b) The time the solution dwells in the peritoneal cavity determines how efficiently the toxins are removed. The optimum dwell time is individualized for each patient and may range from approximately 2 hours to 5 hours (overnight (CAPD) or long day (CCPD) dwell phase may exceed the optimal dwell time).

   c) The Peritoneal Equilibration Test (PET) and the Peritoneal Function Test (PFT) are the tests that determine whether a shorter or longer dwell time is more efficient for clearing uremic toxins and excess fluid for the patient.

B. *Aseptic Technique*

1. Definition: Medical aseptic or clean technique is the practice that limits the number of microorganisms and prevents their spread from one place or person to another.

2. Critical element of peritoneal dialysate exchanges is maintenance of aseptic technique

3. Sterility of the bag-catheter connection and system must be maintained.

   a) Methods used to decrease the risk of infections

      (1) Good handwashing technique using disinfectant soaps to remove or destroy pathogenic organisms is considered one of the most effective infection control measures.

      (2) Use of a facemask when performing an exchange or making a connection prevents the organisms from sneezing, coughing, or exhaling from contaminating the connections during the exchange.

      (3) Turning off ceiling or floor fans, window air conditioners, and closing doors decreases the flow of air, dust and possible contaminates while performing the exchange.

      (4) Removing pets from the room while performing an exchange prevents accidental contamination by the pet.

C. *The Connection/Transfer Set*

1. Description

   a) The transfer set, a 6 to 8 inch length of tubing with a clamp, leur locks to the titanium or plastic adapter of the catheter and connects to the disposable PD system

   b) The transfer set is changed every six months or when it accidentally becomes contaminated or damaged.

2. Purpose of the transfer set is to prevent direct contamination of the implanted catheter when accidental contamination occurs and to prevent tugging and twisting at the catheter exit site when the connections are made.

VII. Modalities

A. *Manual Therapies*

1. Continuous Ambulatory Peritoneal Dialysis (CAPD)

   a) CAPD is a manual form of peritoneal dialysis where the patient performs his/her exchange without the aid of a dialysis machine.

   b) The patient may use an assist device to aid in performing a safe connection but the patient controls the infusion procedures, the drain procedures and the time the exchanges are done.

   c) Patients generally perform 4 or 5 exchanges per day.

   d) The exchanges generally occur before or after breakfast, lunch, and dinner, and just prior to going to bed. The medical personnel can tailor the exchange time to accommodate the patient's activity.

2. Daytime Ambulatory Peritoneal Dialysis (DAPD)

   a) Treatment is received during the day for 12-16 hours, when the patient is ambulatory. No treatment is received during the night.

   b) The solution is drained out prior to going to bed and the peritoneal cavity is dry during the night.

   c) DAPD is beneficial for the patient who reabsorbs fluid during the long nighttime dwell.

   d) An extra exchange may be added during the day to improve clearances.

3. Systems and Assist Devices

   a) Y-Set Systems

      (1) The PD system has a Y shaped configuration.

      (2) The short end of the Y is connected to the patient's catheter.

      (3) One arm of the Y is the drain line, which may be pre-attached to a drain bag, or the patient may need to attach a drain bag.

      (4) The patient attaches the dialysate solution bag to the other arm of the Y.

      (5) This type of set requires 2-3 sterile connections to be made by the patient.

   b) Twin Bag Systems

      (1) The PD system is Y shaped as above but the dialysate solution bag and the drain bag are pre-attached.

      (2) The need to connect a dialysate bag is eliminated thus decreasing the chance for contamination.

      (3) These systems require the patient to break a plastic cone or frangible to allow fluid to flow from the dialysate bag.

   c) Connection Assist Devices

      (1) Aids the patient to safely connect the dialysate solution bag to the Y-Set to prevent contamination.

      (2) Can assist the patient in making a safe connection between the patient's catheter and the disposable PD system.

      (3) Assist devices can be used by patients with limited eyesight, decreased dexterity or coordination, or decreased strength.

   d) Ultra-Violet Connection Assist Devices (U-V Flash)

      (1) The device makes the bag connection and/or the patient connection under bacteriocidal doses of ultra-violet light.

B. *Automated Peritoneal Dialysis (APD)*

1. Automated Peritoneal Dialysis

   a) APD is defined as peritoneal dialysis using a machine or cycler to perform all or most of the dialysis exchanges.

   b) APD requires a prescribed amount of time connected to the PD machine or cycler usually while the patient sleeps.

   c) APD includes Continuous Cycling Peritoneal Dialysis (CCPD), Intermittent Peritoneal Dialysis (IPD), Nightly Intermittent Peritoneal Dialysis (NIPD), and the use of a night-time exchange device with CAPD.

2. Continuous Cycling Peritoneal Dialysis (CCPD)

   a) A cycler or machine performs all exchanges.

   b) 3 to 5 exchanges (cycles) or as prescribed by the physician are done each night.

   c) The machine fills the peritoneum with fresh dialysate just prior to disconnection in the morning.

Figure 16.6

HomeChoice® PRO

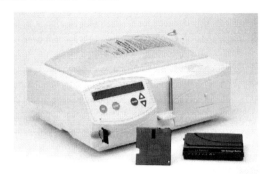

The HomeChoice® does not depend on gravity for flow. It is small and light weight making travel relatively easy. A patient data card allows for reprogramming prescription changes via modem or by the clinician in the clinic.

Reprinted with permission of Baxter Healthcare Corporation

Figure 16.7

Freedom Cycler

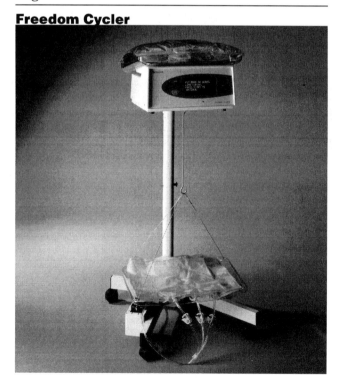

The Freedom Cycler uses gravity flow. It can be easily disassembled for travel.

Reprinted with permission of Fresenius Medical Care North America

d) This last dialysate fill dwells all day until the patient connects to the cycler for the next night's treatment.

e) The dialysate solution that dwells all day is then drained out as the first step of the night treatment.

3. Intermittent Peritoneal Dialysis (IPD)

a) IPD refers to an APD dialysis regimen that has a period off dialysis >10% of the total time.

b) May be used while waiting for a new catheter or hernia repair to heal or for a leak to resolve.

c) Not commonly prescribed, as adequate clearances and ultrafiltration are very difficult to achieve.

4. Nightly Intermittent Peritoneal Dialysis (NIPD)

a) NIPD indicates that the patient may receive dialysis for 8-12 hours at night.

b) The treatment ends with a full drain of the peritoneal cavity and the patient's peritoneal cavity remains dry for a prescribed time during the day.

c) The NIPD treatment starts by connecting to the cycler at night at the fill phase of the cycle.

d) May be beneficial to patients who reach equilibration quickly during the exchange.

e) Beneficial while recovering from hernia repairs or leaks, as the peritoneal cavity is dry during the day when patient is ambulatory.

f) May be used in patients with diminished appetite due to feeling full. These patients may have some improvement in their appetite by having their peritoneal cavity dry during the day.

C. Combination Therapies

One of the methods of increasing the dose of dialysis is combining different therapies. The combination of automated (cycler) and manual therapies are done to increase clearance and ultrafiltration.

1. CCPD with 1 or 2 CAPD or cycler exchanges during the daytime period.

a) Three to four exchanges may be performed while on the cycler.

b) Depending on the patient needs, two manual or cycler exchanges may be performed during the day.

c) The patient may receive 4 to 6 exchanges in a 24 hour period.

2. CAPD Using a Night Exchange Device

    a) A simple device is used to perform one of the CAPD exchanges during the night.

    b) The device is used to add an additional exchange if needed to increase clearances.

D. CAPD vs. APD

CAPD and APD are appropriate therapies for most patients. There are certain factors that may influence the selection of one method over the other.

1. Major Factors in Selecting the Method of Peritoneal Dialysis

    a) Patient's peritoneal membrane transport characteristics may determine the length of dwell times needed to achieve adequate clearances.

        (1) CAPD is preferable for patients who need long dwell times.

        (2) APD/CCPD is preferable for patients needing shorter dwell times to prevent reabsorption of uremic toxins and fluid.

    b) Patient's lifestyle and personal preferences.

        (1) Work schedules, family responsibilities may influence the choice of method.

        (2) Comfort level with learning and trouble-shooting devices, may influence choosing CAPD which is less technical to learn.

        (3) Preferring not to be connected to a machine or device for a set time at night.

        (4) The need for assistance in performing the therapy may influence the choice of method.

VIII. Prescription

A. Membrane Characteristics

1. Peritoneal Equilibration Test (PET) or Peritoneal Function Test (PFT)

    a) The PET or the PFT is done to determine how quickly solutes pass through the membrane.

    b) The PET or PFT may be used to determine appropriate treatment modality and prescription.

    c) Each patient's membrane is unique in its ability to filter the uremic toxins from the blood.

    d) The patient will fall into one of four categories of permeability: High Transporter, High-Average Transporter, Low- Average Transporter, and Low Transporter.

    e) The permeability of the membrane changes over time.

Figure 16.8

Peritoneal Membrane Characteristics According to the Peritoneal Equilibration Test

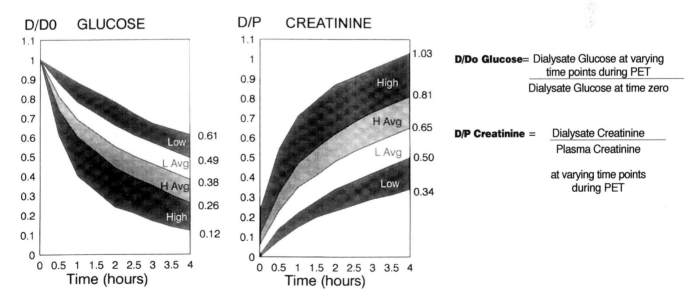

Source: ANNA Core Curriculum, *Third Edition, p. 288, fig. XI.5*

2. Transport Characteristics or Membrane Permeability

  a) High Ttransporters do well APD or CCPD with shorter dwell times as solutes and fluid pass quickly through the peritoneal membrane.

    (1) Higher dextrose solutions are needed to ultrafiltrate.

  b) High Average Transporters do well on all modalities, and will have a choice of CAPD or CCPD.

    (1) Solutes clear well and ultrafiltration is maintained.

  c) Low Average Transporters do best on CAPD with longer dwell times as solutes pass more slowly through the peritoneal membrane.

    (1) These patients ultrafiltrate easily using 1.5% and 2.5% dextrose concentrations.

  d) Low Transporters are best on CAPD as solutes are very slow to cross the peritoneal membrane.

    (1) Ultrafiltration occurs easily.

    (2) These patients have difficulty reaching the recommended adequacy targets and are at risk for failure of the therapy.

B. Adequacy

Guidelines for adequacy levels have been proposed by the National Kidney Foundation's Dialysis Outcomes Quality Indicators (DOQI) Peritoneal Dialysis Work Group. The goal of the adequacy guidelines is to maintain optimal clinical and laboratory parameters.

1. Clinical Indicators of Adequate Peritoneal Dialysis

  a) Patient feels well.

  b) Fluid balance is maintained.

  c) Maintains good nutritional state with body weight maintained.

  d) Blood pressure is well controlled.

  e) Patient does not experience uremic symptoms; nausea, vomiting, loss of appetite or loss of sleep.

2. Laboratory Tests to Determine Adequacy

  a) Urea Kenetics - Kt/V_{urea}

    (1) **K**= clearance of urea, **t** =Time, **V**= volume of total body water

    (2) Kt/V measures removal of urea (the product of protein catabolism) from the blood, indicating the clearance of small solutes during peritoneal dialysis.

    (3) The PD Kt/V is usually reported as a weekly clearance rate, unlike HD where the reported Kt/V refers to the urea clearance per HD treatment.

    (4) Total Kt/V includes both the urea clearance from the peritoneal dialysis exchanges (pKt/V) and the urea clearance from the residual renal function (rKt/V).

  b) Creatinine Clearance – CrCL

    (1) Creatinine clearance measurement indicates the amount of creatinine cleared by peritoneal dialysis from the blood over a specific time.

    (2) Creatinine clearance is measured in liters of serum cleared per week or L/week.

    (3) Total creatinine clearance includes creatinine removed by peritoneal dialysis and creatinine removed through urine the patient produces.

3. DOQI – Dialysis Outcomes Quality Indicators

The DOQI Adequacy Guidelines recommend the following targets. The targets represent the total clearances of urea and creatinine from both dialysate and urine.

  a) Weekly CAPD target

$$KT/V - 2.0$$
$$CrCl - 60. \text{ L/week}$$

  b) Weekly CCPD target

$$KT/V - 2.1$$
$$CrCl - 63 \text{ L/week}$$

  c) Weekly NIPD target

$$KT/V - 2.2$$
$$CrCl - 66 \text{L/week}$$

4. Methods to Increase Dialysis Dose

  a) CAPD

    (1) Increased Exchange Volume.

      (a) Increasing from 2 L to 2.5L increases clearances by 25%.

      (b) The maximum exchange volume currently used is 3000cc.

      (c) Larger exchange volumes may be tolerated better in the supine position and can be started with the bedtime exchanges in CAPD patients.

    (2) Increased number of exchanges

      (a) The number of exchanges can be increased from 4 to 5 during the 24 hour period.

(b) A device may be used to perform an additional exchange during the night.

(3) The type of membrane permeability characteristic and the patient lifestyle influence whether an increased exchange volume or an increased number of exchanges is appropriate for the patient.

b) CCPD

(1) Increased Exchange Volume

(a) Larger exchange volumes may be tolerated better in the supine position while the patient is on the cycler at night.

(b) The maximum exchange volume currently used is 3000cc.

(2) Increased Number of Cycler Exchanges

(a) The increased exchange cycles will decrease the total number of hours each exchange will dwell while the patient is on the cycler.

(b) Treatment time on the cycler can be increased so that the dwell time for each exchange is lengthened to increase solute removal.

(3) Addition of Midday Exchange

(a) A midday exchange decreases the amount of solutes and fluid reabsorbed during the long day dwell of CCPD therapy.

(b) A midday exchange performed either manually or by connecting to the cycler increases the number of exchanges performed in 24 hours.

c) NIPD

(1) Increase Exchange Volume

(2) Increase Number of Cycler Exchanges

(3) Increased Treatment Time on Cycler

IX. Complications of Peritoneal Dialysis

A. Peritonitis

1. Definitions

a) Peritonitis – Inflammation of the peritoneum.

b) Infectious Peritonitis - Inflammation of the peritoneum related to microorganisms

c) Recurrent Peritonitis – Reappearance of symptoms within two weeks of the completion of antibiotic therapy. Organisms and sensitivities must be identical.

2. Risk Factors for Peritonitis

a) Patients younger than 20 and older than 60 years of age.

b) Diabetes Mellitus

c) Patients on immunosuppressive therapy.

d) History of diverticulitis.

e) Persistent or chronic exit site/tunnel infections.

f) Staph aureus nasal carrier.

3. Potential Modes of Entry of Microorganism

a) Intra-Luminal (Transluminal)

(1) Breach in technique, allows bacteria to enter the peritoneal cavity through the catheter.

(2) Contamination occurs at the connection site during the exchange procedure.

b) Peri-Catheter (Exit Site/Tunnel) Introduction of bacteria from the skin into the peritoneal cavity by way of the catheter track.

c) Transmural – Bacteria normally found in the intestinal region enter the peritoneal cavity through the bowel wall.

(1) The presence of multiple intestinal organisms in the peritoneal fluid may be indicative of fecal leak.

(2) Diverticulosis is a major source of fecal peritonitis.

d) Transvaginal- An ascending infection occurs, when organisms from the vagina reach the peritoneum via the uterine tubes.

e) Hematogenous -Bacteria enter the peritoneum via the bloodstream from a distant site for example infections that could be related to dental procedures.

4. Organisms

a) Gram Positive Organisms

(1) The most common Gram positive organism is Staph Epidermidis, with Staph. Aureus seen frequently.

(2) Approximately 75% are related to normal skin and nasal flora.

b) Gram Negative Organisms

(1) Pseudomonas, acineotobactec, and enterobacter species are the most common Gram negative organisms.

c) Mixed Gram Positive and Negative Organisms

(1) The presence of mixed organisms is usually indicative of a gastro-intestinal source.

d) Fungi – Yeast are most common

e) Other – Mycobacterium Tuberculosis

5. Incubation period

a) Incidents involving touch contamination have and incubation period of 24-48 hours.

b) Incubation periods of 6-12 hours have occasionally been noted.

6. Peritonitis Rates – the average peritonitis rate is now under one episode per patient year.

7. Signs and Symptoms may be present in various combinations.

a) Cloudy effluent due to increase in WBC and fibrin.

b) Abdominal pain and/or tenderness

c) Rebound tenderness

d) Fever

e) Nausea and/or vomiting

f) Chills

g) Diarrhea

8. Clinical Diagnosis

a) To establish a clinical diagnosis, the presence of two of the following criteria is required in any combination.

(1) Abdominal pain

(2) Cloudy dialysis solution containing white blood cell count > 100/mm^3, with a differential >50% neutrophils.

(3) Presence of organism on Gram Stain or culture.

9. Culturing of Dialysate

a) Culturing of the effluent is important in order to establish the appropriate antibiotic therapy.

b) Specimen and culture should be done on the first cloudy bag.

10. Treatment of Peritonitis – Adapted from the AD HOC Committee, Keane WF et al. PD International Update 1996

a) Initial Treatment

(1) To remove products of inflammation and to alleviate pain, 1 to 3 rapid exchanges may be performed.

(2) Cephalosporins, Aminogylcosides, and Heparin would be added to the patient's routine exchanges until the Gram stain or culture results are available.

b) Treatments for Gram Positive Organisms

(1) Treatment may be initiated with first generation cephalosporins.

(2) Vancomycin can be used as an alternative therapy to first generation cephalosporins.

NOTE: In view of reports of Vancomycin resistant organisms it has been advised that Vancomycin should be utilized for organisms that are not sensitive to other recommended therapies.

c) Gram Negative Organisms

(1) Gentamycin or Tobramycin are the recommended antibiotics.

(2) Gentamycin and the combination of Gentamycin and Vancomycin have been associated with the development of ototoxicity.

(3) Second and third generation Cephalosporins should be considered to reduce the risk of ototoxicity.

d) Mixed Organisms: Gram Positive and Gram Negative are found on the culture. A combination of gram positive and gram negative therapies are instituted.

e) Fungal Peritonitis

(1) The most common organism is yeast.

(2) Risk factors associated with fungal peritonitis include prior antibiotic therapy, bowel perforation, and immune suppression.

(3) Anti-fungal treatment can be administered orally, intravenously, or intraperitoneally.

(4) Systemic treatment is recommended.

(5) Prompt catheter removal is recommended by most experts.

(6) Fungal peritonitis has been associated with increase morbidity and mortality.

f) Mycobacterium TB Peritonitis

(1) Patient usually has a positive history of tuberculosis.

(2) Treatment for mycobacterial peritonitis consists of catheter removal, and appropriate TB drug therapy.

g) Heparin

(1) Heparin is used to inhibit the formation of fibrin and to prevent subsequent adhesions formation.

(2) Dosing schedule is 500 – 1000u/L to dialysate until effluent is clear.

11. Indications for Catheter Removal
    a) An episode of peritonitis that has not resolved after 4 days of appropriate antibiotic treatment may be an indication for catheter removal.
    b) Presence of tunnel infection.
    c) Fecal peritonitis
    d) Fungal peritonitis that has not responded to therapy after four to seven days.
    e) Mycobacterium peritonitis

12. Complication Related to Peritonitis
    a) Temporary loss of ultrafiltration capacity that results in fluid weight gain.
    b) Protein losses during peritonitis are increased thereby compromising nutritional status.
    c) Temporary decrease in solute clearances.
    d) Adhesion formation
    e) Catheter loss
    f) Transfer to Hemodialysis
    g) Death

B. Exit Site Infection

1. Definition - Inflammation of the catheter exit site with the presence of purulent drainage.
   NOTE: Positive culture of the exit site in the absence of inflammation does not indicate infection.

2. Most common organisms responsible for exit site infection are Staphylococcus aureus and Staphylococcus epidermis.

3. Risk Factors
   a) Trauma to the exit site such as excessive twisting or pulling of catheter, or external pressure from belts, tight clothing, or seat belts may result in infection of the exit site.
   b) Cuff Extrusion - Recurrent trauma caused by pulling, twisting, or tugging of the catheter may result in external extrusion of the cuff.
   c) Staph Aureus Nasal Carriers are at a higher risk of developing staph aureus exit site infection.
      (1) Prophylactic treatment to prevent exit site infection infections may be instituted with either oral antibiotics or topical application of antibiotic ointment to the nose.
   d) Wet Exit Site or moisture due to excessive perspiration or submersion of catheter presents a risk factor for exit site infection.
   e) Skin breakdown around the exit site.

4. Characteristics of an Infected Exit Site

   An infected exit site may present with a variety of combinations of signs and symptoms.
   a) Color- may present as red or bright pink.
   b) Swelling around exit site
   c) Drainage
      (1) External drainage may be visible, with or without compression of the sinus.
      (2) External drainage is purulent or may present as bloody drainage.
   d) Tenderness, pain, or soreness may be noted.
   e) Proud flesh- the presence of proud flesh and or exuberant granulation tissue may be noted around the exit site or visible sinus.

5. Diagnosis
   a) Culture and gram stain of the drainage is needed to determine antibiotic choice.
   b) A positive culture on its own is not indicative of clinical infection.
   c) Sero-sanguinous discharge alone does not indicate clinical infection.
   d) Diagnosis can be based on clinical signs and symptoms.

6. Treatment
   a) Oral, intraperitoneal, intravenous antibiotic therapy or a combination may be instituted.
   b) Use of topical antibiotics may be initiated if the drainage is minimal.
   c) The frequency of exit site care should be increased.
   d) If the cuff of the catheter has completely extruded, the cuff can be shaved to the harboring of organisms.

7. Complications of Exit Site Infections
   a) Tunnel Infections
   b) Catheter removal – Exit site infections is the predominant cause of catheter removal.
   c) Peritonitis – Approximately 20% of the exit site infections are associated with future episodes of peritonitis with the same organism.

C. Tunnel Infection

1. Most common organism is staphylococcus species.

2. Risk Factors
   a) Contamination occurs when the catheter is placed.

b) Severe traumas such as a hard pull on the catheter.

c) Exit site infection.

d) Wound healing is delayed.

e) Presence of dialysate leak from exit site.

f) Extrusion of the external cuff of the catheter at the exit site.

3. Signs and Symptoms

a) Pain and tenderness along the tunnel tract.

b) Abscess area over the catheter tunnel.

c) Thickening along the subcutaneous tunnel.

d) Redness over the tunnel segment.

e) Copious amounts of purulent drainage. Despite the presence of copious amount of purulent drainage the exit site may not exhibit any other signs of infection.

f) Exit site infection and/or peritonitis may occur with the same organisms.

4. Diagnosis of Tunnel Infection

a) Visual assessment and palpation of track may be used in the diagnosis of tunnel infection.

b) Although ultrasound has been recommended, its effectiveness as a diagnostic tool for tunnel infection is not high.

5. Treatment

a) Cure for tunnel infections are rare.

b) Antibiotic treatment may be attempted.

c) Catheter removal is often required.

6. Complications

a) Cellulitis of the abdominal wall

b) Peritonitis

c) Temporary transfer to hemodialysis until a new catheter can be inserted.

D. Non-Infectious Complications

1. Increased Intra-Abdominal Pressure

a) Dialysate volume instilled into the peritoneal cavity increases the pressure within the abdomen.

b) Excessive coughing, straining, or lifting heavy objects also increases intra-abdominal pressure.

c) Intra-abdominal pressure is greatest in the sitting position followed by the standing then supine position.

d) The incidence of complications related to increased intra-abdominal pressure is lower in CCPD or NIPD patients due to the patient dialyzing in the supine position.

2. Complications related to Increased Intra-Abdominal Pressure

a) External Dialysate Leaks

(1) Usually occurs around the catheter at the exit site or along the midline incision.

(2) May result from creating a tunnel or catheter tract that is too large or using the catheter prior to complete healing and tissue ingrowth in the cuffs takes place.

(3) Previous abdominal surgeries may increase the risk of external leaks.

(4) Assessment of the clear fluid around the exit site or incision for the presence of glucose determines if fluid is dialysate or exudate.

b) Internal Dialysate Leaks

(1) Dialysate fluid leaks into the subcutaneous tissues can result in abdominal wall edema, perineal edema, or penile edema.

(2) A dialysate leak through an inguinal hernia can result in scrotal edema.

(3) Assessment includes monitoring for increased abdominal girth, flank edema, and decreased exchange volume.

c) Interventions for Dialysate Leaks

(1) PD may need to be temporarily discontinued and the patient can be maintained on HD until the leak resolves.

(2) If PD is continued, the patient is dialyzed in the supine position with smaller fill volumes, until the leak is resolved.

(3) If the leak persists, the catheter surgical intervention may be indicated to correct a large catheter tract or to replace the catheter.

(4) Assess for peritonitis and exit site infections as the patient is at greater risk for developing these complications.

d) Hernias can occur as a result of increased intra-abdominal pressure

(1) The instillation of dialysate, and activities such as coughing, straining, or lifting are associated with increasing the intra-abdominal pressure.

(2) Anatomical abnormalities or weak abdominal muscles may contribute to the formation of hernias.

(3) Most common sites for hernia development are incisional, umbilical, inguinal, ventral and hernias that develop at the catheter insertion site.

(4) Left untreated, hernias may result in incarceration, pain, or bowel entrapment.

e) Intervention

(1) Significant hernia requires surgical repair.

(2) Postoperatively the patient may be maintained on HD until PD can be resumed.

(3) If necessary, PD may be continued using small fill volumes with the patient in the supine position.

f) Other complications related to Increased Intra-Abdominal pressure

(1) Cardiopulmonary compromise – cardiac output is decreased with increased intra-abdominal pressure.

(2) Gastrointestinal symptoms, decreased appetite, feeling full, gastrointestinal reflux and hemorrhoids can occur.

3. Hydrothorax is the rapid accumulation of fluid in the pleural spaces that results from congenital weaknesses or hernias in the diaphragm.

a) Usually occurs shortly after initiation of PD.

b) Occurs more commonly in females.

c) Patient displays symptoms of dyspnea, chest pain, weight gain and/or respiratory failure.

d) Intervention

(1) Resolution of pleural effusions is accomplished by discontinuing PD.

(2) Defect may seal with time, or can be corrected by pleurodeses using talc, or fibrin glue.

(3) Can be regarded as a contraindication to PD.

4. Peritoneal Catheter related Complications

a) Catheter Malfunction

(1) Inability to drain or infuse due to kinking along the subcutaneous tunnel or in the intra-peritoneal segment.

(a) Fibrin or blood clot obstruction may be occluding the lumen or distal holes of the catheter.

(b) Catheter may be clamped or kinked externally.

(c) Constipation may cause pressure on the catheter from neighboring organs

(2) Catheter Migration Out of Pelvis

(a) Solution may infuse without difficulty but will not drain.

(b) Catheter may have moved due to peristalsis.

(c) Catheter may have become wrapped in omentum.

(d) Fluid gets trapped in pockets that cannot be drained by the migrated catheter.

(e) Intervention

i. Abdominal x-rays will verify catheter location or the presence of kinking.

ii. Alleviating constipation or inducing peristalsis may reposition the catheter correctly.

iii. Ambulation and activity may also help to reposition the catheter.

iv. Surgically removing the omentum if the cause of drain problems may be indicated.

(3) External Catheter Cuff Extrusion

The catheter cuff is visible at the skin exit site.

(a) Occurs when the catheter attempts to straighten or resume its original curve if, on insertion, the tunnel does not follow the natural shape of the catheter.

(b) Will occur if the tunnel is shorter than the subcutaneous segment.

(c) Will occur if the placement of the external cuff is too close to the skin surface or the exit site is too large.

(d) Excessive tugging or pulling on the catheter may cause the external cuff to extrude.

(e) Chronic exit site infection, tunnel infection or peritonitis may result from a cuff that has extruded.

(4) Rectal or Suprapubic Pain may be the result of pressure of the catheter on the rectum or bladder area when the peritoneal cavity is drained.

(a) Occurs when the intraperitoneal segment is too long.

(b) May be relieved when fluid is infused.

(c) May be prevented by leaving a small volume of dialysate in the peritoneal cavity at the end of the drain phase or end of the APD treatment to float or cushion the catheter.

5. Complications related to Peritoneal Dialysis

a) Back pain

(1) The presence of dialysate in the abdomen causes an alteration in the normal center of gravity by moving it forward which effects body posture.

(2) Weak abdominal muscles, multiple abdominal surgeries and poor posture can contribute to back pain.

(3) Neuromuscular diseases such as degenerative spinal diseases and bone diseases may be aggravated by the weight of the dialysate in the abdomen.

(4) Fill volumes may need to be decreased temporarily, Shoulder pain is referred pain from the diaphragm.

b) Shoulder pain

(1) Can be caused by the infusion of air into the peritoneal cavity.

(2) A malpositioned or migrated catheter can exert pressure on the diaphragm during the infusion of dialysate and can cause the referred pain to the shoulder.

(3) A perforated bowel may also create pressure on the diaphragm and cause the referred pain to the shoulder area.

(4) Mild analgesics to treat the symptoms may alleviate the pain.

c) Bleeding or Blood Tinged Dialysate

(1) As little as 2 ml of blood/liter will result in blood-tinged dialysate.

(2) Transient and benign bleeding can occur in menstruating females before menses or during ovulation.

(3) Ruptured kidney or ovarian cysts, endometriosis, cholecystitis, and minor trauma to the abdominal wall may also cause blood-tinged dialysate.

(4) The bleeding can also occur with peritonitis, pancreatitis, visceral ruptures, and tumors. Bleeding has also been reported after colonoscopies and enemas.

(5) In many cases, the bleeding resolves without intervention.

(6) Heparin may be added to the dialysate to prevent clotting and fibrin formation in the catheter.

(7) Rapid exchanges can be done at room temperature to stop the bleeding.

d) Peritoneal Eosinophilia

(1) Although not an infectious peritonitis the patient presents with cloudy dialysate. No other symptoms of peritonitis are present.

(2) Thought to be allergic response to dialysate solution, plasticizers, sterilizing agents, intraperitoneal medications, heparin or other foreign materials.

(3) Usually resolves spontaneously without treatment or residual effects.

(4) The patient must be monitored closely. If dialysate does not clear reassessment of cause should take place.

X. Nutrition

Requirements differ from hemodialysis requirements. Generally dietary restrictions are not required depending on the ability to adequately control fluid balance with the different solution glucose concentrations. In some cases, increased intake of specific nutrients is encouraged to maintain a healthy nutritional state.

A. Protein

1. Increased protein intake is recommended and encouraged, protein and amino acids are lost across the peritoneal membrane with each exchange.

2. Average daily protein loss ranges from 8-10 gm/day, but can vary from 5-15gm/day.

3. Fifty percent of protein intake should come from high biological value protein.

4. Protein and amino acid loss increases during peritonitis.

5. Recommended protein intake to prevent malnutrition – 1.2 to 1.5 gm/kg of ideal body weight per day. During peritonitis the requirement increases to 2.0 gm/kg.

6. Protein intake may be inadequate due to decrease appetite related to the increased glucose load in the dialysate solutions.

7. Protein and amino acid supplements are prescribed if adequate intake of protein can not be maintained.

8. Decreases in albumin, the protein used to measure nutritional status is associated with an increased risk of morbidity and mortality.

B. Calorie Intake

1. Glucose absorption from the dialysis solution contributes significantly to the total caloric intake.

2. The use of hypertonic high glucose solutions effect blood glucose and plasma insulin levels.

3. Absorption from the PD solutions may make up 20%-30% of daily caloric requirements.

4. 1.5% dextrose solution
   a) Contains 1.3 gm glucose
   b) Provides 60kcal/L.
   c) Approximately 70% of the glucose is absorbed from each exchange.

5. 4.25% dextrose solution
   a) Contains 3.76 gm glucose
   b) Provides 170 kcal/L
   c) Approximately 60% of the glucose is absorbed from each exchange.

6. Appetite can be suppressed by the absorption of glucose in undernourished patients.

7. Weight gain is can be seen due to the absorption of glucose from the dialysate.

C. Fluid Control

1. Usually no restrictions on fluid or sodium intake are needed.

2. Fluid balance is usually easily maintained by varying the use of 1.5%, 2.5% and 4.25% solutions.

3. Average fluid removed per each type of dextrose solution
   a) 1.5% - 200-250 cc per 4 hour dwell
   b) 2.5% - 500-700 cc per 4 hour dwell
   c) 4.25%- up to 1000 cc per 4 hour dwell

D. Phosphorus

1. High phosphorus levels are a problem in PD patients as the recommended increase in protein intake results in increased phosphorus levels.

2. Phosphorus levels are controlled by restricting oral intake of high phosphorus foods and by the use of phosphate binders.

E. Potassium

1. Restrictions are not usually necessary due to the easy and continual loss of potassium with each exchange.

2. Increase in potassium rich foods may be encouraged if potassium levels decrease.

F. Vitamins

1. Daily supplements are prescribed to replace the water-soluble vitamins lost with each exchange.

2. Supplements do not include the fat-soluble vitamins A, E or K as these vitamins are not removed by dialysis.

G. Lipids

1. Hypertriglyceridemia can be a problem in PD patients, with approximately 50-70% of patients having elevated triglyceride levels.

2. HDL may be decreased and LDL and VLDL cholesterol fractions are increased.

3. Weight reduction and reduced intake of saturated fats and carbohydrates may be indicated.

4. Limit the use of high dextrose dialysate solutions.

5. Eliminate other risk factors such as smoking, alcohol consumption and inactivity.

6. Lipid lowering medications may be indicated.

XI. Patient Technique Survival

1. During the period between 1994 and 1998, the percentage of US dialysis population on PD has been 15-17%.

2. The percentage of PD patients has leveled off in recent years (1998-1999).

3. The trend has been a movement of patients from CAPD to APD.

4. Currently, 57% of the PD population is on CAPD and 43% are on APD.

5. Fifty percent of the patients in the US are switching from CAPD to APD.

6. As of 1999, 50% of prevalent PD patients still have not met DOQI targets.

7. Inadequate dialysis dose is associated with poor patient survival in PD (CANUSA Study).

8. Inadequate dialysis is directly responsible for at least 10% of the transfer to HD.

References and Suggested Readings

Advisory Committee on Peritoneal Management of the International Society for Peritoneal Dialysis. Keane, W.F., et al. (1996). Peritoneal Dialysis – Related Peritonitis Treatment Recommendations: 1996 Update. *Peritoneal Dialysis International, 16:6, 557-573.*

Baxter Healthcare Corporation (1998). *Peritoneal Dialysis Catheter & Complications Management,* Baxter Healthcare Corporation, Renal Division, Deerfield: Illinois.

Diaz-Buxo, J. A. (1999). Prospects for Peritoneal Dialysis in the Future. *Nephrology News and Issues,* 13:2, 12-14.

Dougirdas, J.T., (Ed.). (1994). *Handbook of Dialysis,* (2nd ed.) Boston: Little, Brown and Co.

Gokal, R., & Kolph, K. D., (Eds.). (1994). *Textbook of Peritoneal Dialysis.* Dordrecht, Netherlands: Kluwer Academic Publications.

Khanna, R., Nolph, K. D., Oreopoulas, D. G., (1993). *Essentials of Peritoneal Dialysis,* Dordrecht, Netherlands: Kluwer Academic Publications.

Lancaster, L., (1995). *ANNA Core Curriculum for Nephrology Nursing,* third edition, Pitman, New Jersey: Anthony J. Jannetti, Inc.

Luzar, M. A. (1991). Exit Site Infection in Continuous Ambulatory Peritoneal Dialysis A Review. *Peritoneal Dialysis International, 11, 14-21.*

NKF – Dialysis Outcome Quality Indicators Clinical Practice Guidelines for Peritoneal Dialysis Adequacy. (1996). National Kidney Foundation.

Nissenson, A. R., & fine, R. N. & Gentile, D. E., (Eds.). (1995) *Clinical Dialysis,* (3rd ed.) (Chapters14-19). Norwalk, Connecticut: Appleton & Lange.

United States Renal Data Systems (1998). *Annual data report.* Bethesda, MD: National Institutes of Health.

Chapter 17
Renal Transplantation

Contributing Author:

Jenny Orsini, MSN, RN, CNN

Chapter Outline

I. History and Statistics

   A. Historical Events

   B. Statistics

   C. Data Source of Renal Replacement Therapies

II. Immunological Aspects

   A. Functions of the Immune System

   B. Innate System

   C. Acquired Immune System

   D. Major Histocompatibility Complex

III. Evaluation of Potential Kidney Transplant Recipient

   A. Recipient blood typing and histocompatibility

   B. Medical and social evaluation

IV. Evaluation of Potential Kidney Transplant Donor

   A. Cadaver Donation

   B. Living Donation

   C. Summary of Compatibility Testing

V. Pre/Peri/Post-operative Issues

   A. Pre-operative Care

   B. Recipient Surgery

   C. Post-operative Concerns

VI. Complications of Renal Transplantation

   A. Non-surgical

   B. Surgical

VII. Long Term Concerns

   A. Recurrence

   B. Chronic Rejection

   C. Malignancies

   D. Steroid

   E. Hypertension

   F. Ulcers

   G. Cataracts

   H. Bone Disease and Destruction

VIII. Commonly Prescribed Medications

   A. Immunosuppressives

   B. Antirejection/induction

   C. Antimicrobials

I. History and Statistics

A. Historical events

1. 1954-first successful kidney transplant between identical twins

2. 1972-Public Law passed to fund medical care for dialysis and transplantation in End Stage Renal Disease patients
   a. patient had a right to equitable care
   b. patient must be offered three options if not medically contraindicated

3. 1986-United Network of Organ Sharing (UNOS)
   a. responsible for establishing membership standards for organ procurement organizations (OPO) and transplant centers
   b. monitors distribution of organs in US
   c. developed point system for distribution of organs
      1) ABO match
      2) HLA match
      3) Time waiting
      4) Preformed antibody (PRA) level
      5) Medical necessity
      6) Age - Waiting time
         infant - 5 yrs old-6months
         6-10 yrs old - 12 months
         11-17 yrs old - 18 months

4. 1980s - cyclosporine began a new era of increased success rates due to specificity of immunosuppressive effect, soon followed by many others such as: OKT3, Prograf, Cellcept

5. 1990s - newer medications such as Thymoglobulin, Simulect, Rapamycin

6. Improved surgical techniques for donors - laparascopic nephrectomy

B. Statistics

1. cadaveric-80-85% patients -1 year graft survival

2. Living Related Donor (LRD)- 90-95% patients - 1 year graft survival

3. Non-Related Living Donor (NRLD)- 85-90% -1year graft survival

4. Pediatric transplantation also had significantly improved rates due to newer medications and improved morbidity and mortality rates in children with renal failure

C. Data sources of renal replacement therapies

1. US Renal Data System - USRDS

2. United Network of Organ Sharing Scientific Registry - UNOS

3. North American Pediatric Transplantation Cooperative Study – NAPRTCS

4. European Dialysis and Transplantation Association Registry - EDTA

II. Immunological Aspects

A. Functions of the immune system - consists of millions of cells - capable of performing three functions:

1. Defense - specific or non-specific
   a. resistance to invasion by foreign antigens
   b. destruction of invading organisms
   c. memory-remember foreign antigens

2. Homeostasis of immune system
   a. protection of self
   b. destruction of self - autoimmuneity anaphylaxis
   c. removal of senescent or dead immune cells

3. Surveillance - recognition of foreign antigens (ie: lymphocytes seek out cancer cells)

4. Organs of the immune system-bone marrow, thymus, lymph nodes and vessels, spleen, tonsils appendix, Peyer's patch.

B. Innate system (non-specific, natural response)

1. Anatomical barriers
   a. skin - maintains proper pH (acid), temperature, and moisture to inhibit bacterial growth
      Langerhans cells - contain and release APC (antigen presenting cells) which activate the specific immune response
   b. mucous membranes - also have a barrier of protection that limits bacterial growth
   c. ciliated epithelium - respiratory tract removes bacteria

2. Chemical barriers

   a. GI, GU and conjunctiva mucosa all secrete protective immunoglobulins called IgA

   b. Gastric acid possesses a low pH, which prevents bacterial growth

   c. Interferons - proteins that are secreted by virally invaded cells and lymphocytes interfere with viral replication and activate natural killer cells

3. Leukocytes (myeloid or lymphoid type)

   a. Myeloid type - back bone of innate system neutrophils, basophils, eosinophils, macrophages-increase in response to infection, allergic or anaphylactoid reaction

   b. Phagocytosis-innate system reaction ingestion and digestion of the foreign cells

     1) carried out by phagocytic cells referred to as RES (reticuloendothelial system)

     2) essential for the initiation of the acquired response - cellular and humoral

   c. Inflammation

     1) body's attempt to restore homeostasis

     2) initial reaction to injury, 1st step of healing

     3) cellular & systemic reactions that localize and destroy the offending antigen, maintain vascular integrity and limit tissue damage

     4) circulatory effects are vasodilation, increased blood flow, increased vascular permeability which allows movement of immune cells from the circulation to the tissues resulting in pain, edema, tenderness or swelling

     5) phagocytes migrate to site

     6) dying phagocytes release pyrogens that stimulate the hypothalamus to produce fever

     7) bone marrow is then stimulated to release more leukocytes

C. Acquired (lymphoid) immune system

1. Lymphocytes-lymphoid type
Primary defenders of acquired immune system, recognize specific antigens

   a. B - cells

     1) humoral response

     2) produce antibodies-memory for several months

     3) defend against infections & transplanted organs (hyperacute rejection)

   b. T- cells

     1) cell mediated response

     2) helper T cells facilitate the differentiation of B-cells into plasma cells

     3) suppressor T cells feedback to inhibit differentiation of B- cells & decrease antibody formation by plasma cells

     4) cytotoxic T cells, (killer cells)

       a) receptors bind with antigens to cause irreversible damage

       b) attack transplant cells unless cell surface is identical to host

       c) also identify & attack malignant cells

     5) memory T cells

       a) sensitize and clone to remember foreign antigen

       b) memory retained for several years

2. Acquired immune response

   a. all cells have identifying cell surface antigens

   b. through specific receptors B & T cells recognize foreign antigens, differentiate, proliferate, clone & destroy

   c. specific genes are responsible for the uniqueness that allows recognition of foreign antigens, major histocompatibility complex (MHC)

D. Major Histocompatibility Complex

Determines specific cell surface identity or antigen -Human Leukocyte Antigen (HLA)

1. Facilitates distinction between self and non-self

2. Present on most cells in the body (leukocytes, platelets, tissues & organs, not on erythrocytes)

3. Genetic complex located on sixth chromosome

4. Class I antigens - A, B, C

   a. Located on almost all nucleated cells in the body

   b. Cytotoxic T cells have receptors that recognize class I antigens and will be activated

   c. B cells will be activated and antibody production will be initiated

   d. The most significant loci in this class are A & B

5. Class II antigens - DR, DP, DQ

   a. Limited distribution in body cells

b. Activate interaction among macrophages, B cells & activated T cells

c. The most significant loci in this class is DR

6. Inheritance

   a. There are six HLA loci on the 6th chromosomes HLA-A, HLA-B, HLA-C, HLA-DR, HLA-DQ, HLA-DP

   b. Each loci has a pair identified as a letter & a number, (A5, A9 on the HLA-A locus)

   c. Each individual inherits 6 pairs, one set or haplotype from - each parent, (A5 maternal, A9 paternal from HLA-A locus)

   d. There is a 25% chance of inheriting the same HLA as a sibling, 25% chance of total dissimilar HLA as a sibling, and 50% chance of sharing one haplotype with a sibling

7. Histocompatibility

   a. Rejection of a transplanted organ or tissue is the normal protective host immune response

   b. H LA testing is one way to decrease the potential for rejection

   c. Antibody testing is performed to detect preformed antibodies as a result of repeated infusions, prior transplantation or multiple pregnancies. Usually tested monthly.

   d. ABO testing is also necessary to limit the potential for rejection- ABO antigens are present on most body tissues as well as on RBC's, must be compatible.

III. Evaluation of Potential Kidney Transplant Recipient

A. Recipient blood typing and histocompatibility

1. Blood typing (ABO) *(see figure 18.1)*

   a. ABO compatibility testing must be performed (antigens found on erythrocytes or red blood cells (RBC)

   b. One gene for blood type is inherited from each parent to determine blood type

   c. Types-ABO, A and B are codominant, O is recessive

   d. A and B have antigens, O type has no antigen. This means that any one can accept blood type O kidney (see table) for recipient versus donor for blood type compatibility

e. Rh is the other antigen expressed on erythrocytes; however in kidney transplantation, it is not of significance

2. Human leukocyte antigen (HLA) testing *(see figure 18.2)*

   a. HLA testing is performed. The greater the amount of matching antigens, the greater the chances of long term success which may ultimately have an effect on the amount of immunosuppressive medication necessary (HLA are found on all cells except erythrocytes)

   b. Half inherited from each parent, three from each parent for total of six which are the most important in transplantation HLA-A, HLA-B, HLA-DR (see table) labeled as a letter and number more than 100 have been identified to date

   c. Siblings have 25% chance of being HLA identical, 25% chance total mismatch and 50% chance of half match means three out of six referred to as haplotype match

B. Medical and social evaluation

1. Social

   a. must be able to give informed consent (or guardian)

   b. must understand the long term responsibility and side effects of immunosuppressive medications

   c. psychosocial evaluation to look at patient's expectations, understanding, compliance, coping mechanisms, support systems, insurance issues, possible living donors, history or evidence of drug abuse and potential need for psychological or psychiatric therapy

2. Medical

   a. must be in good condition to undergo surgery safely, receive immunosuppressive medications with minimal risk to self

   b. history of blood transfusions, past transplants and /or pregnancy can increase the risk of exposure to antigens and hence increase the number of preformed antibodies in the recipient

   c. primary disease must be under control (i.e.: diabetes, hypertension or autoimmune diseases) diabetic may be able to receive pancreas transplant to avoid re-occurrence of disease in transplanted kidney

d. infections
1) patient must be free of all infections (ear, chest, urinary tract, sinuses, dental- all work must be completed before transplant)
2) virology and serology testing must be done (CMV, EBV)
3) Hepatitis and HIV screening
4) in children all immunization must be up to date, especially live vaccine can not be administered after transplant
5) PPD testing or other screening for tuberculosis should be performed

e. malignancies
1) those with history of malignancies that have been resected or treated may safely undergo transplantation
2) incurable malignancies are contraindicated

f. nephrectomy/parathyroidectomy
1) nephrectomy-only is such cases as: hypertension (uncontrolled with antihypertensives), high grade ureteral reflux, recurrent pyelonephritis, massive sized polycystic kidneys
2) parathyroidectomy- in cases of severe bone disease

g. cardiovascular
1) elderly, diabetics and dialysis patient have a high incidence of arteriosclerosis and vascular disease-transplantation also places the patient at great risk, history must be carefully reviewed
2) patient must be able to tolerate surgical procedure, EKG would normal part of evaluation, stress test as well as other diagnostic studies may be indicated if cardiac function is questionable
3) all corrective cardiac surgery if indicated must be performed prior to transplant

h. genitourinary tract/gynecological
1) VCUG must be performed in patients with repeated UTI to rule out any obstructions or ureteral reflux
2) patients with neurogenic bladders may require ileal conduit or self catheterization after transplant

3) any repair for reflux or need for nephrectomy should be performed prior to transplant
4) females-Pap smear and exam, mammogram > 40 yrs old
5) male >40 yrs old -prostate specific antigen (PSA) screening

i. gastrointestinal system
1) patient with peptic ulcer needs repair or treatment prior
2) hx of gallbladder warranting cholecystectomy also must be performed prior to transplant
3) liver abnormalities must be thoroughly investigated due to risk of side effects of immunosuppressive medications

j. pulmonary system
1) chest x-ray is normal procedure for evaluative purposes of infection or any chronic disease; pulmonary function tests will follow if indicated
2) all immunizations should be up to date and any all viral titers drawn

IV. Evaluation of Potential Kidney Transplant Donor

A. Cadaver donation is major source of kidney donation for adult population

1. neurological evaluation-must meet criteria of brain death
a. cerebral unresponsiveness
b. brain stem unresponsiveness
c. no activity on EEG or absence of blood flow
d. absence of toxic drugs which may contribute to neurological state

2. medical evaluation
a. age infant to 70 yrs old
1) small children (<3 yrs old) that are donors present technical difficulties-usually both kidneys are removed and transplanted together
2) donors over 55 yrs old are carefully evaluated

b. history
   1) long term hypertension or diabetes mellitus
   2) systemic disease or infections affecting the kidneys
c. medical
   1) virology, serology studies
   2) normal kidney function-BUN, creatinine, good urine output since admission

3. donation process
   a. declaration of brain death responsibility of donor medical team
   b. consent obtained from next of kin by designated individuals of hospital
   c. organ recovery and preservation
      1) upon removal, cold solution in flushed through kidneys to minimize the ischemia time between 0-5 minutes
      2) they are then preserved either by cold storage which is dry ice (most common and easily facilitated) or via a perfusion machine which continually infuses the kidney with the cold solution and oxygen (allows longer storage time)
      3) storage can be maintained up to 72 hrs; however delayed graft function increases after 24 hours for any type storage

B. Living donation

1. related donors-parents, siblings, and extended family members, immediate family members are usually the first to be considered

2. non-related-spouse, friends, adoptive and step parents, related donors are generally preferred over non-related donors

3. donor's age must be 18 yrs old or older, minors may require court approval for consent and generally used

4. only in exceptional situations

5. social evaluation
   a. must be able to give informed consent
   b. must understand the risks of surgery and nephrectomy
   c. psychosocial evaluation to look at donor's reasons for donation and that donation is without coercion; donor recipient relationship and dynamics must also be evaluated

d. insurance issues- payment is covered by recipient insurance
e. time required in hospital and recuperation time

6. medical
   a. ABO and histocompatibility testing
   b. Complete history and physical-must be in good condition to undergo surgery and nephrectomy
   c. No history of diabetes, hypertension, renal calculi, anemia or malignancies which may place the donor at future risk of renal failure or affect function of donated kidney
   d. Normal kidney function-diagnostic tests will be performed to evaluate kidney function and renal arteriography is performed to detect problems with vasculature and confirmation of two kidneys
   e. Absence of any infections which can be transmitted to recipient
      1) virology and serology testing must be done (CMV, EBV)
      2) Hepatitis and HIV screening

7. Nephrectomy
   a. open nephrectomy –traditional method
      1) hospital stay usually 5-7 days and recuperation 4-6 weeks
      2) flank incision-generally results in more post operative pain than recipient, pain management is major concern post-operatively
      3) post-operative -usually have urinary catheter, IV and sometimes central line, sometimes epidural catheter is placed for pain management
   b. laparoscopic nephrectomy
      1) hospital stay 2-3 days, recuperation 2-3 weeks
      2) less pain experienced than open nephrectomy
      3) selection for laparoscopic nephrectomy is dependent on physical body structure and complexity of vasculature is a surgical decision

C. Summary of compatibility testing

1. ABO must be compatible (not identical) between donor and recipient

2. HLA need not be identical or match, but the more antigens that match perhaps may add to longevity of transplanted kidney

3. Mixed lymphocyte culture (positivity) is not an absolute contraindication to transplant performed as part of the HLA testing to determine severity of disparity in non-identical HLA donor recipient pairs

4. Final cross match (cytotoxic T cell crossmatch) performed as last step prior to transplantation is used to detect preformed antibodies-if positive, is an absolute contraindication to transplantation between donor and recipient

V. Pre/Peri/Post-operative Issues

A. Preoperative care - cadaveric/LRD

1. in cadaveric donation final cross match is done ASAP for patients on waiting list specimen is sent from dialysis unit or MD office monthly to always have current sera for final cross match this expedites the process and minimizes storage time of kidney while identifying potential recipient

2. final cross match for LRD performed week before scheduled Tp

3. labs, EKG, chest x-ray, dialysis as needed

4. IV line placed to facilitate administration medications pre-op

5. NPO 6-8 hr pre-op

6. Prophylactic antibiotics

7. IV steroids on call to OR

8. LRD-oral immunosuppressive therapy usual started 2-7 days prior to scheduled Tp depending on type of medications administered

9. additional immunosuppressive medications may be utilized in patients who are at high risk for rejection referred to as induction therapy (ie: prior tp, cadaveric, small children)

B. Recipient surgery

1. urinary catheter is placed in bladder to facilitate healing of ureteroneocystostomy usually removed 4-5 days post-op

2. central venous catheter placed to facilitate central venous pressure readings and to assist in accurate fluid management

3. transplanted kidney (graft) is placed in the extra-peritoneal iliac fossa which facilitates

   a. access to iliac vessels-renal artery anastomosed to internal iliac artery and renal vein to external iliac vein

   b. access to bladder-transplant ureter anastomosed to recipient bladder (ureteroneocystostomy)

   c. allows ease of physical assessment of graft

4. in small children kidney may be placed intraperito-neally attached to aorta and inferior vena cava

5. length of surgery generally 2-4 hours

6. storage time in LRD is minimal due to simultaneous scheduling of surgery in adjoining OR rooms

7. ischemia time between removing the kidney from the ice and attachment and unclamping of vessels in recipient ideally should be between 25- 45 minutes

C. Post-operative concerns

1. respiratory system

   a. deep breathing, coughing, early ambulation, incentive spirometers

2. circulatory system

   a. frequent monitoring of patient-temperature, BP, central venous pressure monitoring

   b. pulses-pedal, popliteal, femoral

3. fluid and electrolytes

   a. strict I/O, daily weights

   b. fluid replacement as per orders

   c. blood work as per orders

   d. assessment of fluid balance

4. infection

   a. monitor for fever

   b. meticulous aseptic technique for dressing changes-wound and lines

   c. avoid persons with active bacterial or viral infections

   d. patient education concerning proper physical and oral hygiene

5. Patient education

   a. physical limitations 4-6 weeks avoidance of heavy lifting

b. no contact sports forever

c. medications-purpose, dose, side effects

d. signs/symptoms of rejection and infection

e. dietary restriction

    1) no concentrated sweets, no added salt

    2) fluid intake must be sufficient to avoid dehydration, output plus insensible losses

f. B/P, temperature, weight or glucose monitoring at home

g. follow-up visits,

h. how and when to call in case of emergency

VI. Complications of Renal Transplantation

A. Non-surgical

1. Rejection-immune system recognizes foreign tissue (ie: transplanted kidney) there is then an attack and attempt to destroy the foreign tissue

    a. hyperacute rejection-occurs minutes to hours after transplant due to binding of preformed antibodies to antigen site of new kidney or ABO incompatibility

        1) pain, fever, chills, tenderness, inflammation over graft, anuria

        2) scan will show no perfusion, graft must be removed immediately

    b. acute rejection - creates risk 2 to 12 weeks after transplant due to primarily cytotoxic cell formation and some antibody response

        1) pain, fever, chills, tenderness over graft site, rise in creatinine, BUN, decrease urine output

        2) may be seen on scan, renal biopsy can be done to differentiate other cause of non-functioning kidney, treatment includes antirejection medications, dietary and fluid restrictions and dialysis as necessary

    c. chronic rejection-occurs > 3 months post transplantation due to HLA disparity, prior sensitization or inadequate immunosuppression

        1) slow, progressive graft dysfunction, increase proteinuria, hypertension, rising creatinine and BUN

        2) renal biopsy will assist with this diagnosis and no treatment is indicated, will not respond to immunosuppressive medications, patient will progress to ESRD can take years

2. Infection

    a. symptoms: fever, pain over graft or other site of collection if localized leukocytosis or burning on urination in urinary tract infection (see long term effects for other infectious disease concerns)

    b. causes: due to surgical procedure and immunosuppressive medications patients are at higher risk for infections

    c. intervention: antibiotics

3. Acute Tubular Necrosis (ATN)-referred to as early non-function of transplanted kidney, more common in cadaveric donation

    a. symptoms: elevated BUN, creatinine and other lab values, no or low urine output, generalized edema and hypertension

    b. cause: prolonged cold or warm ischemia time during harvesting and transplantation process

    c. intervention/dx: may be seen on scan, dietary and fluid restrictions, antihypertensives if B/P is elevated, dialysis as needed

B. Surgical

1. Bleeding-mild hematuria is normal due to surgery will resolve without intervention

    a. symptoms: tachycardia, hypotension, falling hematocrit

    b. causes: Heparinization used for patients at high risk for thrombosis may contribute to bleeding, leaking at vascular anastomosis may be a cause of bleeding

    c. intervention/diagnosis (dx): may be seen on ultrasound, may require protamine if heparin is contributing factor and surgical exploration

2. Arterial thrombosis

    a. symptoms: anuria, tenderness

    b. causes: may be due to hypercoagulopathy or surgical technique

    c. intervention/dx: may be seen on ultrasound or scan, thrombectomy and surgical exploration will be necessary to salvage kidney

3. Venous thrombosis

    a. symptoms: decreased urine output, swelling of graft, affected thigh or leg, hematuria

    b. causes: hypercoagulopathy, rejection

    c. intervention/dx: may be seen on Doppler ultrasound, treated with anticoagulation

4. Renal artery stenosis

   a. symptoms: bruit over graft, hypertension

   b. causes: torsion of artery, intimal hyperplasia or arterial sclerosis from rejection

   c. intervention/dx: may be seen on ultrasound, arteriography or doppler ultrasound, balloon angioplasty, antihypertensives

5. Urine leak

   a. symptoms: may include drop in urine output, labial or scrotal edema, leaking of clear fluid at wound, pain around site or increase in size of abdomen, palpable collection around wound, may lead to infection

   b. causes: may include leaking at surgical of surgical anastomosis of ureter, necrosis due to ischemia from rejection impeding blood supply to ureter

   c. intervention and dx: may be seen on ultrasonography or scan, sometimes drainage via percutaneous nephrostomy to relieve pressure otherwise surgical intervention is necessary to re-implant or reconstruct the ureter

6. Vesicoureteral reflux

   a. symptoms: increase in creatinine, may cause infection

   b. cause: ureteroneocystostomy is allowing urine to back up from bladder to ureter and possibly up to transplanted kidney

   c. intervention/dx: may be seen on voiding cysto-ureterogram (VCUG), suppressive antibiotics are necessary and for repeated infections-surgical revision of ureteroneocystostomy

7. Ureteral stenosis-narrowing of ureteroneocystostomy

   a. symptoms: rise in creatinine

   b. causes: surgical anastomosis will naturally have tendency to narrow

   c. intervention/dx: may be seen on ultrasound, balloon dilatation, stent or surgical reconstruction and reimplantation

8. Lymphoceles, urinomas, hematomas may cause compression or blockage of flow of urine

   a. symptoms: may result in rise in creatinine or decreased urine output

   b. leak of lymph, urine or blood around graft site

   c. intervention/dx: may be seen on ultrasound, surgical intervention or percutaneous drainage may be performed if large leak, other times if small may resolve spontaneously

VII. Long Term Concerns

A. Recurrence of primary disease in transplanted kidney

1. Membranoproliferative glomerulonephritis - MPGN II

2. MPGN I

3. Focal Segmantal glomerosclerosis - FSGS

4. IgA Nephropathy

5. Sickle cell anemia

6. Multiple myeloma

7. Amyloidosis

8. Oxalosis

9. Diabetes mellitus

10. Hemolytic Uremic Syndrome - HUS

B. Chronic rejection

C. Malignancies due to long term immunosuppressive therapy

D. Steroid or prograf induced diabetes

E. Hypertension, cardiovascular disease

F. Ulcers, liver disease, cholecystitis, pancreatitis

G. Cataracts

H. Bone disease and destruction

VIII. Commonly Prescribed Medications

A. *Immunosuppressives (see Fig. 17.3)*

B. *Antirejection/induction (see Fig. 17.3)*

C. *Antimicrobials*

Immunosuppressed patients are highly susceptible to opportunistic viral, bacterial and fungal infections.

1. Antivirals
   Used for opportunistic viruses such as: Cytomegalovirus (CMV), herpes (HSV-1 & HSV-2), and contact with any of the communicable diseases could be fatal if patient is not immune. Prophylactic antiviral medications may be prescribed for 3-6 months post transplant.
   a. Gancyclovir (cytovene) used to prevent and treat CMV, EBV
   b. Acyclovir (zovirax)- used to prevent and treat HSV I & II, varicella zoster

2. Antibiotics
   Used for bacterial infections such as: urinary tract and upper respiratory infections. Prophylactic antibiotics may be prescribed for a period of time after transplantation. As well as prior to going to surgery
   a. trimethoprim and sulfamethoxazole (TMP-SMX), Bactrim, Septra
   b. ciprofloxacin (Cipro)
   c. cephalosporines (Cefotan, Ancef)

3. Antifungals
   Used for fungal infections such as: Candidiasis-oral thrush, vaginal infections
   a. Nystatin (Mycostatin)
   b. clotrimazole troche (Mycelex)
   c. fluconazole (Diflucan)

4. Antihypertensives
   Steroids and immunosuppressive medications can cause hypertension early in post op period when doses are high. Some common antihypertensives used for transplant patients are as follows:
   a. Nifedipine (Procardia)
   b. Diltiazem (Cardiazem)
   c. Isradipine (Dynacirc)
   d. Lobetolol (Normodyne)

5. Ulcer prophylaxis and therapy
   Steroids and other immunosuppressive medications can cause increased acidity and gastritis and predispose the patient to peptic ulcers. Anti-ulcer medications may be used prophylactically in the early post-op period.
   a. Ranitidine (Zantac)
   b. Cisapride (Propulsid)

6. Diuretics
   Steroids can cause sodium and water retention contributing to hypertension sometimes medications such as diuretics are used to excrete excess fluid.
   a. furosemide (Lasix)
   b. Bumetanide (Bumex)

Figure 17.1

ABO COMPATIBILITY FOR KIDNEY TRANSPLANT

DONOR	RECIPIENT
A, O	A
B, O	B
A, B, O, AB	AB (EXCEPTIONS APPLY ie: IF PT HAS A1, A2 ANTIBODIES)
0	O

Figure 17.2

CONDENSED VERSION OF IDENTIFIED HLA TYPES

HLA-A	HLA-B	HLA-DR
A1	B5	DR1
A2	B7	DR2
A3	B8	DR4
A9	B21	DR7
A11	B18	DR9

Figure 17.3

Medications in Renal Transplantations

Medication	Purpose/action	Administration	Side effects
Steroids Prednisone – po Prednisolone – po Methylprednisolone – IV	Prevent or treat rejection Prevent release interleukin 1 thus prevent T-cell activity, antiinflammatory	IV for (6 doses) 0-2 POD PO - 2mg/kg/D to 0.15 mg/kg/D tapered	cushingoid syndrome, increased appetite, obesity, Na/water retention GI disturbances, mood swings, steroid induced diabetes, avascular joint necrosis, cataracts, acne, fungal infections
FK-506-Prograf Tacrolimus	Prevent acute rejection Inhibits T cells, helper and cytotoxic	*IV only if NPO, is very nephrotoxic po 0.5, 1 & 5 mg capsules-used instead of neoral, 0.15 mg - 0.30 mg/kg/D	Tremors, HTN, nephrotoxic, diabetes, neurotoxic less cosmetic side effects than neoral
Cyclosporine Neoral or sandimmune – po liquid or pills cyclosporine- IV	prevents rejection interferes with T cell activation and growth	*IV only if NPO, is very nephrotoxic, over 24 hours Neoral po form always preferred route, comes in 100, 25 mg capsules or po liquid 100 mg/ml, 5 -10 mg/kg/D	nephrotoxicty, hirsutism, gum hyperplasia, hypertension, hepatoxicity, hand tremors, seizures, flushing, GI disturbances, leukopenia
Cellcept Mycophenolic acid	prevent rejection inhibits proliferation of T & B cells suppresses antibody formation	po capsules in 250 mg capsules or liquid 200 mg/ml 1 Gm B id	GI disturbances, diarrhea, vomiting, and abdominal pain, anemia, leukopenia, Herpes. CMV more prevalent
Rapamune Sirolimus	Prevents rejection Inhibits T-lymphocyte activation and proliferation	Oral solution 1mg/ml daily Dose can be from1-5mg/day starting with a loading dose approx. 3x daily	High cholesterol and triglycerides, HTN, rash, acne, anemia, joint pain, diarrhea, hypokaleima, thrombocytopenia
Simulect Basiliximab	prevents rejection inhibits interleukin-2 activation of lymphocytes	IVSS (20mg/ml)-12 mg/m2 for max. of 20 mg in 50ml over 20-30" 2 doses given, (1st) 1-2 hrs pre-op and (2nd) on POD # 4	GI upset, headaches, tremors, hypertension Increased risk of infection, malignancies and leukopenia.
Thymoglobulin Monoclonal antibody ATG from rabbit	Anti-rejection as well as induction therapy	1.5 mg/kg for 7-14 days high flow vein and .22 micron filter for IV infusion of 4-6 hours, **must pre-medicate tylenol, steroids, benadryl**	**First 2 doses may cause** flu like symptoms, high fever, chills, pain, headache, diarrhea long term side effects-viral infections, lymphoma
OKT3 Muronab, monoclonal antibody from mice	Treat ATN or acute rejection when unresponsive to steroids, Inhibits proliferation of T cells and lysis of transplant cells Removes T cell infiltrates from rejection site	IV only 2.5 mg <30 kg child, 5 mg >30 kg (5mg/ml) 7-14 days/ rejection, **must premedicate with tylenol, steroids, benadryl: make sure pt is not fluid overloded**	**first 2 doses will cause** flu like symptoms, high fever, chills, tremors, N/V, dyspnea, pulmonary edema, wheezing, chest pain long term side effects-viral infections, lymphoma
Imuran Azothiaprine	Prevent rejection interferes with synthesis of leukocytes, inhibits B & T cells Blocks antibody production	can be given IV or PO, sometime used for those unable to take cellcept or neoral 1 - 3 mg/kg/D	Bone marrow suppression, anemia, thrombocytopenia, bleeding, leukopenia, hair thinning, infections, GI disturbances, mouth ulcers, hepatotoxicity, hepatitis
ATG-antilymphocyticglobulin Atgam, polyclonocal antibody from horse	treat rejection decreases activity of T cell, forms antigen-antibody complex	IV infusion slowly in central line only, premedicate with benadryl, tylenol-used in place of OKT3 10 -15 mg/kg/D x 7-14D	Hypersensitivity, generalized rash,tachycardia, dyspnea, chills, fever, chest pain, back pain, hypotension, anaphylaxis

Suggested References

Cecka, J.M. & Terasaki, P.I. (2000), *Clinical Transplants 1999*, LA, CA: UCLA Immungenics Center

Flye, M.W. (1989), *Principles of Organ Transplantation,* Philadelphia: W.B. Saunders

Hariharan, Sundaram, *Recurrent and DeNovo Diseases after Renal Transplantation.* Seminars in Dialysis 13:195-199, 2000

Lancaster, L., (1995), *ANNA Core Curriculum for Nephrology Nursing,* 3rd edition, Pitman, New Jersey: Anthony J. Janetti, Inc.

Meyer, M. Norman, D.J., Danovitch,G., (1992) *Handbook of Renal Transplantation,* edited by G. DanovitchBoston: Little Brown & Co.

Sollinger, Hans & Pirsch, John, (1996), *Transplantation Drug Pocket Reference Guide,* 2nd edititon, Georgetown, Texas: Landes

UNOS - United Network of Organ Sharing offer a wealth of information on the web site www.unos.org.

Chapter 18
Proper Monitoring and Disinfection of Dialysis Delivery System

Contributing Authors:

Diane Dolan, CWSV

Philip M. Varughese, BS, CHT

Chapter Outline

I. Importance of Monitoring and Disinfection

A. Hemodialysis is the most common renal replacement therapy for patients with end stage renal disease (ESRD). Normally patients receive dialysis treatments three times a week, and during that time, they can be exposed to many toxins that can diffuse across the nonselective dialysis membranes.

B. Municipal water is treated and purified before it is used in dialysis; malfunction or human error during the purification process can cause fatalities. Municipal water can contain many known or unknown chemical and bacterial contaminants.

C. Developments in membrane technology, e.g. high flux and high efficiency dialyzers warrant more stringent purification standards to ensure the safety of dialysis patients.

D. The major reason for this is because High Flux and High Efficiency dialyzers use larger pore sizes which can cause back filtration which would force water from the dialysate compartment back to the blood compartment.

E. With ever increasing treatments involving dialyzer reuse, the risk of blood leaks significantly increases. During a blood leak, the dialysate can mix with the blood which may be toxic to the patients.

F. In dialyzer reuse, during the cleaning and disinfection process, treated water is used to fill the blood compartment of the dialyzer. Because the water is in the blood compartment, the protective mechanism of the membrane is no longer in place, allowing the patient to be exposed to any contaminants present in the water. Therefore, AAMI has stricter guidelines for dialyzer reuse by requiring stringent testing of endotoxin levels.

G. The mixing of bicarbonate dialysate facilitates bacterial proliferation, which in return, demands higher standards for water purification.

II. Water Testing Methods

A. AAMI Analysis, Measures Trace Elements

1. AAMI Analysis is a test for chemical contaminants, which should be performed at least yearly on the product water for dialysis; more often if there are problems. Effective August 2001, three additional contaminants were added to the AAMI standards due to changes in the Safe Drinking Water Act. They are Antimony, Beryllium and Thallium.

2. If problems are occurring with the quality of water from the RO or DI treatment system, then an analysis should also be performed on the tap water.

3. Tap water quality changes will cause a difference in the product water and there may need to be an adjustment made to the water treatment system.

B. Plate (Colony) Count

Measures live bacteria even in well designed water treatment systems, enough nutrients remain in treated water to sustain microbial growth. Colony counts determine the number of living bacteria in a defined volume of fluid. Various techniques are used to determine the growth organisms. New AAMI Standards, effective August 1, 2002 require product water used to prepare dialysate or concentrates from powder at a dialysis facility or to reprocess dialyzers for multiple use should contain a total viable microbial count of less than 200 CFU/ml, with an action level of 50 CFU/ml.

1. Membrane Filtration Technique A defined sample volume is filtered, and bacteria are collected and cultured on the filter. This filtration also removes substances in the sample that may inhibit growth and artificially lower counts.

2. Dipstick Devices Sample is drawn through a pore in the dipstick by capillary action, wetting a dehydrated bacterial growth medium and inoculating the membrane simultaneously. This is a qualitative test with less specificity.

3. Pour Plate Technique A defined volume of fluid is spread over the growth medium and cultured. A disadvantage of this technique is that heat from the melted medium can kill organisms and artificially lower counts.

4. Preferred Method Micro biologic assay of the samples should be by means of the spread- plate technique, or membrane filtration.

   a) When the spread-plate technique is used, the sample must be quantitatively measured with a pipette, not a calibrated loop. By means of a pipette, 0.1 to 0.5 ml of the sample is placed directly onto the culture medium; the sample is spread evenly across the surface by means of a sterile spreader. Because the calibrated loop places such a small amount of sample on the culture plate (0.001 ml or 0.01 ml), it cannot provide sensitivity needed for culturing dialysis fluids. It can not reach the required sensitivity below 10 CFU/ml.

b) The culture medium should be trypticase soy agar (AAMI). Previous standards and guidelines have included blood agar and standard plate count agar. However, these media do not optimally recover the types of micro-organisms that are associated with bicarbonate concentrate based fluids. It has been shown that the culture medium needs to contain some NaCl. Trypticase soy agar does, and the others do not.

c) The cultures should be incubated at 35°C to 37°C, and the colonies counted after 48 hours.

d) At present AAMI recommends plate counts of <2000 units for dialysate.

C. LAL (Limulus Amebocyte Lysate), Measures Endotoxin

Endotoxin concentrations should be determined by the Limulus Amebocyte Lysate (LAL) assay at least monthly. LAL assays are based on the observation that the blood of horseshoe crabs (Limulus) clots when mixed with endotoxin. Clotting is due to an enzymatic reaction between endotoxin and a protein in Limulus amebocyte. LAL assays are very sensitive and may be enhanced or inhibited by components in dialysate or other solutions. Results of a given test are compared to those obtained using reference samples with known amounts of endotoxin. Results are reported in endotoxin units per milliliter (EU/ml).

1. The LAL assay measures endotoxin units/ml

2. Endotoxin are the toxic compounds released by living bacteria and the decomposition of dead bacteria

3. As bacteria lives, it sheds it's skin, which is the source of the endotoxin. When bacteria die, the residue left behind is also an endotoxin.

III. Testing of Microbial and Endotoxin

A. A colony count measures the amount of living bacteria in the water. In this test, a defined amount of water is placed on culture media. After a 48 hour incubation, the number of colonies that grow are counted.

B. An endotoxin test (LAL) measures the strength of the by-products of living bacteria, and the residue of the dead bacteria...endotoxin. Endotoxin are created

when bacteria is killed. Endotoxin is not alive, so it cannot be killed. This makes it difficult to remove.

C. Since it is very possible to have bacteria-free water with high levels of endotoxin, both a colony count and LAL test must be performed.

IV. Importance of LAL and Endotoxin Testing

A. When a sufficient amount of endotoxin are present, they cause pyrogenic reactions in dialysis patients, ie. unexplained fever or chills. Tap water can have very high levels of endotoxin, but pyrogenic reaction only occurs when endotoxin enters the blood stream.

B. Ways that endotoxin can enter the bloodstream include:

1. High levels of endotoxin in dialysate
   a) High-flux membranes are more permeable than regular membranes, which may allow more endotoxin to cross the membrane.
   b) Some studies suggest that high-flux membranes absorb more endotoxin than conventional membranes.
   c) Because it can be broken down into different sizes, endotoxin can cross through any membrane (high flux or conventional).

2. Rinsing of dialyzers in reuse. Endotoxin can bind to the membranes and release during dialysis.

C. Endotoxin are created by:

1. Improper disinfection. If a complete "burn out" is not done, with very adequate rinsing, endotoxin may be created.

2. Ultra-Violet light. UV is excellent for killing bacteria, but it is actually an endotoxin generator. When bacteria is killed, endotoxin is created.

V. What's a Safe Level?

A. The Association for Advancement of Medical Instrumentation (AAMI) have set new standards for water bacteriology. Several investigations have shown that pyrogenic reactions are caused by endotoxins that are associated with gram-negative bacteria, and gram-negative bacteria multiplies rapidly in treated water for hemodialysis, dialysis and dialysate.

B. Bacterial endotoxins are able to cross dialysis membranes, either intact or as fragments.

C. New AAMI standards require that endotoxin levels for water used to prepare dialysate or concentrates, or for reprocessing dialyzers for multiple use contain an endotoxin concentration of less than 2 EU/ml, with an action level of 1 EU/ml.

D. Properly maintained water treatment equipment will usually show an endotoxin level below .05 endotoxin units.

VI. LAL Sampling

The LAL test replaced the rabbit Pyrogen test for all the water monographs in the United States Pharmacopeia (USP) in 1983.

A. Locations for Taking Your LAL Sample.

1. Final product water after RO or DI system. If the main water treatment device is contaminated with bacteria, endotoxin will be in the product water. Monitoring at this point will prevent the entire system from becoming contaminated.

2. Re-use area If endotoxin are present, they will plate onto the inside plastic fibers of the dialyzer when it is flushed. When the patient's blood flows through the membrane fibers, releases the endotoxin causing pyrogenic reactions.

3. Dialysis machine The pores in the membrane are of a size where it would be difficult for endotoxin to pass through, but it has been shown that endotoxin will cause "sympathetic" reaction across the membrane wall during the dialysis process. If a membrane should have a slight tear, endotoxin will pass into the patient's bloodstream.

4. Bicarbonate mixing station If liquid bicarbonate concentrate is formulated from a pre-packaged powder mix, the concentrate should be prepared immediately prior to patient use. It's very important to monitor and prevent water with high bacteria levels and endotoxin from being used to make up the solution.

5. Return water from the recirculation loop Any contamination in the water treatment system or the plumbing loop will show up here.

B. Proper LAL Sampling Procedure - Sending to Outside Lab

Most outside labs perform LAL testing by using a Chromogenic or Kinetic procedure. These methods are accepted by the FDA as an alternative to the gel clot method and provide exact endotoxin levels rather than a positive or negative. By having exact levels and trending, problems can be eliminated before they occur.

1. Disinfect the sample port by filling a container with chlorine, soaking the port for one minute. When not in use, the port is warm and damp which makes an excellent place for bacteria to grow. It's important to sterilize this port to avoid a false reading.

2. Flush the port for at least two minutes. This is necessary because residual chlorine and bacteria can cause inaccurate LAL test results. The more thoroughly the port is flushed, the more accurate the results will be.

3. Clean catch the specimen in a sterile tube. Fill the tube a little over halfway, leaving room for water expansion if it freezes.

4. Prepare for shipment/testing
   a) Place frozen cold pack over sample immediately and ship by next day air to sampling location. Be sure to mark each tube with the sample location.
   b) If testing will be performed on site, test as soon as possible after taking sample. If testing cannot be done within an hour, place sample in refrigerator or freezer.
   c) If the sample is allowed to reach room temperature, bacteria will multiply, causing an increase in the endotoxin levels, thereby giving an inaccurate report of the endotoxin level in the sample.

C. Proper LAL Sampling Procedure - On Site Gel Clot

The gel clot test, USP bacterial endotoxin test (BET), was the first in vitro toxicity test to replace and animal test for release of a pharmaceutical product. This test is easy to perform and requires little equipment. Gel clot is the reference method. Other LAL methods such as chromogenic and kinetic methods are alternative methods accepted by the FDA.

1. A small quantity (typically 1 ml sample) is mixed with an equal quantity of LAL reagent in a small glass reaction tube.

2. The reaction mixture is incubated for an hour at 37°C in a water bath or dry block heater.

Figure 18.1

Monitoring Schedule

MEASUREMENT	SAMPLE	MINIMUM FREQUENCY
pH*	RO Feed Water Post Acid Injection Dialysate	Weekly Continuous-check Daily Every Patient shift
Free Chlorine • polyamide w/carbon • thin film composite w/carbon • cellulose acetate w/carbon • cellulose acetate w/o carbon	Post-Worker Carbon Post-Worker Carbon Post-Worker Carbon RO Feed & Product Water	Daily Daily Daily Daily
Chloramines	Post Worker Carbon Post Polisher Carbon	Per Shift If Worker Fails
Conductivity/TDS - RO	RO Product Water	Continuously/Daily
Resistivity - DI	DI Product Water	Continuously/Daily
Hardness	Post Water softener	Daily
Radiant Energy Output	UV Effluent	Continuous Check Daily
Pressure	Pre and Post All Components	Daily
Temperature	Post Temperature Blending Valve	Continuous Check Daily
Bacteria	Final Product Water Dialysis Machine Reuse Area Bicarbonate Station	Monthly Monthly Monthly Monthly
Pyrogens (LAL)	Final Product Water Dialysis Machine Reuse Area Bicarbonate	Monthly Monthly Monthly Monthly
AAMI/ANSI Analysis	Final Product Water Tap Water	Yearly Yearly

3. At the end of the incubation period, each tube is removed and read as positive or negative. A positive is indicated by a solid gel that remains intact in the bottom of the reaction tube when the tube is inverted 180 degrees.

4. Assays are performed by titrating the sample to an end point (last positive test in a series of decreasing sample solutions). Assays performed on two-fold serial dilutions have an error of plus or minus two-fold from the endotoxin concentration at the end point.

VII. Monitoring the Water Treatment System

A. Who Is Responsible?

Monitoring of water purity level is considered to be the sole responsibility of the physician in charge of hemodialysis or the medical professional designated by the physician as the person in charge.

B. On-Site Monitoring Schedule

It is difficult to generalize about monitoring schedules. The necessary frequency of monitoring will vary from facility to facility and from component to component. AAMI has made some recommendations concerning certain processes, such as deionization and reverse osmosis.

C. Microbiological Monitoring (LAL)

1. Should be performed at least monthly

2. Total viable microbial counts shall not exceed 200/ml in water used to prepare dialysate.

D. Chemical Contaminants Monitoring (AAMI)

1. Should be performed at least yearly if prepared by DI or RO... more frequently if prepared with lesser level of treatment

2. Must meet AAMI maximum levels of chemical contaminants

E. Chlorine/Chloramine Monitoring

Municipal water contains chemicals such as free chlorine and chloramines. Chloramines are a more stable and potent form of chlorine which is often added by the municipal water system, or can form naturally in the water lines when chlorine comes in contact with organics. These chemicals are added to suppress bacterial growth. They must be removed from the water before it is used for dialysis treatment; otherwise damage to the equipment (especially RO membranes) can occur. More importantly, these chemicals can lead to patient fatalities or injury by severe, hemolytic damage to patient red blood cells from chloramines.

F. Chlorine/Chloramine Removal

1. CDC, FDA and AAMI all recommend the use of two carbon adsorption beds (one worker and one polisher) in series. The exception to this is portable and home dialysis water treatment systems.

2. A sample for testing should be taken after the water has passed through the worker tank (first tank) to insure no chloramine is present. The amount of chloramine in the water can be calculated by measuring the total chlorine present, then subtract the free chlorine. AAMI guidelines recommend chloramine levels of <0.1 mg/L.

3. If analysis of the water sample detects excessive chloramine levels, a second sample should be taken after the water has passed through the polisher tank (second tank).

4. If a second analysis on the water (after passing through the second polisher tank) also shows levels equal to or greater than 0.1 mg/L (0.1 PPM), the product water must not be used for dialysis. If this test shows water has less than 0.1 mg/l (0.1 PPM) of chloramine, the water can be used for dialysis but the worker tank should be replaced within 72 hours.

VIII. Disinfecting the Water Treatment System

Defining disinfection...

Sterilize To make free from all (100%) micro-organisms

Sanitize To clean and reduce bacteria substantially (70%)

Disinfect To destroy most (99%) of the bacteria that cause sickness or disease.

A. Why Disinfection Is Important

1. Hemodialysis water purification and delivery systems, bicarbonate mixing and delivery systems, hemodialysis machines and the dialyzer itself are physically complex systems which potentially provide many hiding places and breeding grounds for harmful bacteria, mycoplasma and fungi. Many harmful organisms can grow in these systems, even though the level of nutrients available may be quite low.

2. Identifying, monitoring and removing these potentially harmful contaminants is a critical element for the nephrology technician's duties. Understanding which contaminants are harmful (and at what levels), where they can come from and why they are harmful are also useful knowledge in the quest to provide a higher quality of care for every patient.

3. A thorough understanding of the monitoring procedures, frequency of testing, acceptable limits and actions to be taken when a problem is identified will ensure the safety of the patients and proper functioning of all systems. Malfunction of a system or human error during the purification process can cause (and has caused) patient fatalities or serious injury.

B. Areas That Should Be Disinfected

1. The water treatment system

2. The distribution system

3. The system for mixing water and dialysate concentrate

4. The dialysis machine to pump the dialysis through the dialyzers

C. Proper Disinfection Schedule

Daily Bicarbonate Mixing Tank Dialysis Machine

Weekly Water Distribution System

Monthly Reverse Osmosis System

These are recommended frequencies, but each individual center should establish their protocol based on their own experience and verification by testing.

D. Disinfecting with Chemical Germicides

1. Chemical agents that are commonly used in dialysis facilities include...

   - Chlorine (household bleach)
   - Hydrogen Peroxide/Peracetic Acid/Acetic Acid (PAA)
   - Formaldehyde
   - Glutaraldehyde

2. The two most common germicides are Chlorine and Peroxyacetic Acid (Minncare & Peracidin are two of the name brands)

E. Formula for Using the Right Amount of Chemical

1. Chlorine (cannot be used on RO membranes)

   Objective 500 PPM for 2 hours
   (min. level to burn out endotoxin)
   Dilutions 1% = 10,000 ppm
   Chlorine Bleach = 5%
   5% x 1,000 ppm = 50,000 ppm
   50,000 ppm ÷ 500 ppm = 100 dilution

   Ratio = 1:100
   (1 part chlorine bleach in 100 parts water)

2. Peroxyacetic Acid (PAA)

   Objective 5000 ppm for 1/2 hour
   (min. level to burn out endotoxin)
   Dilutions 1% = 10,000 ppm
   100% PAA 100 x 10,000 – 1,000,000 ppm
   1,000,000 ppm ÷ 5,000 ppm = 200

   Ratio = 1:200
   (1 part PAA in 200 parts water)

F. Procedure for Disinfecting with Chemical Germicide

1. Take a sample of water for an LAL/Endotoxin test. Determine if there are any components that may be harmed by the effects of chlorine or PAA. Your reverse osmosis membranes, and deionizer (DI) exchange tanks may need to be isolated. (Do not reinstall old DI tanks).

2. Determine how much chlorine or PAA to use (regular household bleach will be fine for chlorine). You need to know how big your holding tank is, and what size piping you have. For every 100 gallons, use 1 gallon of chlorine; for every 200 gallons, use 1 gallon of PAA. Below is an example to use as a guide:

   a) If your holding tank has a "spray ball" on the return loop, the holding tank can be drained to 1/5 volume to save disinfectant.

   b) One gallon of water is contained in the following number of feet foreach of the different pipe sizes:

PIPE SIZE	1 GALLON = # FEET
3/4"	43
1"	24
1-1/2"	10

   Example: 250 gallon holding tank and 300 feet of 1" pipe loop.

   Holding Tank (50 gallons) and piping (12.5 gallons) = 62.5 gallons

   Chlorine (1:100) ~ 62.5 ÷ 100 = .625 gallons of chlorine bleach

   PAA (1:200) ~ 62.5 ÷ 200 = .3125 gallons of PAA

   c) Recirculate in the piping system and let soak for at least 1 hour.

   d) After it has soaked, drain the system, refill and flush the system out with water from your reverse osmosis or deionizer until your test shows no chlorine or PAA in the system.

   e) Take another LAL sample.

G. Chemical Germicide (Disinfectant) Concentration Testing

1. The Purpose for Testing

   To ensure that the prepared solutions are at the proper concentrations. This allows the user to know that...

a) The germicide has been correctly prepared

b) The solution has not degraded during storage

c) The test strips can be used to ensure the presence of the disinfectant in the solution and ensure the absence of the germicide after the rinse cycle.

2. Locations for Testing

   a) Dialysis machines

   b) Reverse osmosis equipment

   c) Reuse dialyzers

3. Proper Rinsing

   a) Important in maintaining minimal concentrations of the chemical

   b) Eliminates patient complications due to chemical toxicities. The most common toxicities of germicides include allergic reactions and hemolysis. In rare causes, the consequences can be fatal.

4. Chemical Germicides (Presence or Absence) in Hemodialysis is Critical

   a) The chemicals which are routinely used to clean and disinfect these dialysis systems are potentially harmful to the patient due to their inherently toxic nature.

   b) Care givers must be properly trained to administer the tests and accurately interpret them.

   c) Tests and procedures must be accepted by the FDA for use tests, positive and negative controls should be included in the procedure and all results should be logged and recorded.

5. Acceptable Dialysis and Water System Disinfectant Tests

   a) Tests for disinfectants used by the dialysis unit or disinfectants added to the local water supply by water treatment plants or the hospital central water supply should ideally be an FDA registered test specifically for hemodialysis use and/or a standard water industry test.

   b) If specific hemodialysis claims or water testing claims are not made by the manufacturer of the test in the accompanying product labeling it is the responsibility of the hemodialysis user to initially verify the performance of the test for the specific hemodialysis application. Such use of a testing product in a manner not recommended or documented in its labeling is sometimes called "OFF-LABEL USE."

   c) The manufacturer does not test the test product for hemodialysis applications. It is the responsibility of the Hemodialysis User to confirm that each new lot of the product received is performing in the same matter as the initially qualified lot. This re-testing is important because manufacturers often make improvements or changes in their products which enhances performance for their product claims; but could cause problems for an Off-Label user.

   d) Never depend on the oral assurance from a colleague that they "have used a product successfully for years" unless it meets Hemodialysis or Water Industry Standards, or is tested by a facility first with appropriate controls and standards.

6. Disinfectant Tests no Longer Appropriate for Use in Hemodialysis Facilities

   The following tests were commonly used "off-label" to test for residual disinfectants and the presence of disinfectants prior to the introduction of test kits specifically designed for hemodialysis use. These "off-label" tests do not meet AAMI Guidelines or current industry standards. Their use could allow potentially hazardous levels of disinfectants to come in direct contact with the patient's blood during the hemodialysis treatment.

7. Appropriate Suppliers

   There are many appropriate sources of hemodialysis and water testing products. Specialty suppliers for test products include Serim Research, Integrated Biomedical Technology, Hach and LaMotte. Disinfectant suppliers such as Minntech, Alden, HDC and Fresenius supply appropriate strips for their disinfectants. Water treatment companies such as AmeriWater, U.S. Filter, Marcor, ZyzaTech supply or recommend appropriate water tests.

H. Disinfecting with Ozone

Ozone is becoming more popular for disinfecting in dialysis. It offers better disinfecting, without residue. This saves a lot of time from rinsing out chemical disinfectants.

1. Ozone is recognized by the US EPA as a viable water treatment alternative to chlorine, and the FDA has added ozone to its list of disinfectants approved "Generally Recognized as Safe."

2. It is the most powerful and rapid acting oxidizer disinfectant produced, and will oxidize all bacteria, endotoxin and biofilms in piping and water systems.

Figure 18.2

Inappropriate Disinfection Tests

Test for:	Inappropriate Test	Actual Sensitivity of Test for Target Disinfectant**	Guideline Sensitivity AAMI or Industry
Residual Bleach - Machines (Chlorine /Amuchina)	HemaStix* (or any Occult Blood urine strip)	3-5 ppm or higher	0.5 ppm
	Starch Iodide Paper (Dip and Read Technique)	8-10 ppm or higher	0.5 ppm
	Blood Glucose Test Strips	There are now many different brands- some which may react in 5-10ppm range and **some which will not react at all**	0.5 ppm
Residual Formal-dehyde	CliniTest* tablets (Urine Glucose Test)	80-160 ppm	5 ppm (3ppm California)
	CliniStix* Strips (Urine Glucose Test)	Does not react with Formaldehyde at all (3 deaths resulted from use of this test in 1 instance)	5 ppm (3ppm California)
Residual Peroxide (Residual Peracetic Acid)	Starch Iodide Paper	25 to 1000ppm depending on the amount of Peracetic Acid remaining in the rinse solution	3 ppm
Peracetic Acid Potency	Starch Iodide Paper	A very crude indicator of the presence of peracetic acid - Turns a dark blue/purple at about 100ppm and turns slightly darker as concentrations reach 500-1500ppm	Solutions below 500ppm should always show negative color

*   *Registered Trademark of Bayer Corporation*

** *As different manufacturer's products may use different formulas and changes are made to products there is no assurance that "off-label" tests will not perform **worse** than these stated values*

3. Ozone is 52% stronger and 3,125 times faster (in water) than chlorine as a disinfectant.

I. *Disinfecting with Heat*

This method of disinfection is most common in Europe. In the US, it is not a commonly practiced method, but is slowly gaining popularity. In order to do heat disinfection, all the pipes and its components must be compatible to withstand steam and its high temperature. Since this is not a chemical disinfection all the components must be heat compatible, with more expensive piping materials,which would result in an increase in capital expense. Maintaining and monitoring a minimum temperature for a specified length of time is critical for successful disinfecting with heat or heat/citric acid.

References

DePalma, John R. "Dialysis-Induced Fever," *Contemporary Dialysis & Nephrology,* December 1988.

AAMI Standards and Recommended Practices, Reference Book *American National Standard for Hemodialysis Systems.*

American National Standard for Water Treatment Equipment for Hemodialysis Applications, RD62:2001.

Diane Dolan, *Contemporary Dialysis & Nephrology,* September 1993

Outline Summary

I. Why Proper Monitoring and Disinfection Is Important

A. Patient Exposure Level

B. Unknown Chemicals in Municipal Water

C. Membrane Technology

D. High Flux & High Efficiency Dialyzers

E. Reuse Blood Leak

F. Reuse Cleaning

G. Bicarbonate Mixing

II. Water Testing Methods

A. AAMI Analysis

   1. Performed Yearly

   2. If Problems, More Often

   3. Tap Water Changes

B. Plate Count Measures Live Bacteria

   1. Membrane Filtration Technique

   2. Dipstick Devices

   3. Pour Plate Technique

   4. Preferred Method Spread Plate

      a. Measured with pipette

      b. Trypticase soy agar

      c. Incubate

      d. Recommended counts

C. LAL (Limulus Amebocyte Lysate) Measures Endotoxin

   1. Measured in EU/ml

   2. Toxic compounds

   3. Dead bacteria = endotoxin

III. Comparing Endotoxin Testing with Plate (Colony) Count

A. Colony Count Measures Live Bacteria

B. LAL Measures Endotoxin Strength

C. Colony & LAL Both Recommended

IV. Why Endotoxin Testing Is So Important

A. Pyrogenic Reactions

B. Ways Endotoxin Enter Blood Stream

   1. High Levels in Dialysate

      a. High flux membrane permeability

      b. High flux membrane absorb

      c. Endotoxin break through

   2. Rinsing of Dialyzers in Reuse

C. Ways Endotoxin are Created

   1. Improper disinfection

   2. Ultra-Violet light

V. What's a Safe Level?

A. AAMI Recommendations

B. Bacterial Endotoxins

C. New AAMI Standards

D. Properly maintained equipment

VI. All About LAL Sampling

A. Locations for taking your LAL sample

   1. Final product water

   2. Re-use area

3. Dialysis machine
4. Bicarbonate mixing station
5. Return water from recirc loop

B. Proper LAL Sampling Procedure - Outside Lab
1. Disinfect sample port
2. Flush port for three minutes
3. Clean catch specimen
4. Prepare for shipment
   a. Cold pack
   b. Test within hour or place in freezer
   c. Room temperature causes inaccurate results

C. Proper LAL Sampling Procedure - On Site Gel Clot
1. Mix in tube
2. Incubate
3. Positive or negative
4. Assay

VII. Monitoring Your Water Treatment System

A. Who is responsible?
B. On site monitoring schedule / chart
C. Microbiological Monitoring
1. Performed at least monthly
2. Acceptable level

D. Chemical Contaminants Monitoring (AAMI)
1. Performed at least yearly
2. Acceptable level

E. Chlorine/Chloramine Monitoring
F. Chlorine/Chloramine Removal
1. CDC, FDA, AAMI recommendations
2. Worker/polisher testing procedure
3. If testing fails
4. Replacing tanks

VIII. Disinfecting Your Water Treatment System

A. Why Disinfection is Important
1. Eliminate toxic substances
2. Health risk to patients

B. Areas That Should be Disinfected
1. Water treatment system
2. Distribution system

3. Dialysate concentrate
4. Dialysis machine

C. Proper Disinfection Schedule
D. Disinfecting with Chemical Germicides
1. Types of germicides
2. Most common germicides

E. Formula for Using the Right Amount of Chemical
1. Chlorine
2. Pereocetic Acid (PAA)

F. Procedure for Disinfecting with Chemical Germicide
1. Review components for compatibility
2. Determine amount of germicide
   a. Spray ball
   b. Pipe size
   c. Recirculation
   d. Soak, drain, flush
   e. LAL Sample

G. Chemical Germicide (Disinfectant) Concentration Testing
1. Purpose for Testing
   a. Germicide correctly prepared
   b. Storage degradation
   c. Presence/absence of disinfectant
2. Locations for Testing
   a. Dialysis machines
   b. Reverse osmosis equipment
   c. Reuse dialyzers
3. Proper Rinsing
   a. Maintain minimal concentrations
   b. Eliminates chemical toxicities
4. Chemical Germicides (Presence or Absence) in Hemodialysis is Critical
   a. Properly trained caregivers
   b. Tests and procedures FDA accepted
5. Acceptable Dialysis and Water System Disinfectant Tests
   a. FDA registered
   b. "Off-Label Use"
   c. Manufacturer not responsible
   d. Appropriate controls and standards
6. Disinfectant Tests No Longer Appropriate for Hemodialysis
7. Appropriate Suppliers

H. Disinfecting With Ozone
   1. FDA, US EPA accepted
   2. Powerful oxidizer
   3. Strength and time
I. Disinfecting with Heat

Chapter 19
Statistics in Dialysis

Contributing Author:
John A. Sweeny, CHT, CBNT

Chapter Outline

I. Introduction

Statistics is defined as the study of observed data in a systematic method to learn the general behavior of a system. The application of statistics or statistical methods to assist in decision-making first began as the term implies in dealing with affairs of state. Today statistical methods are utilized in fields ranging from business and economics to biochemistry and meteorology.

A good example of the power of statistics as a mathematical tool would be the answer to a question such as; "What's the average age of a human being in the United States?" Ideally, the answer could be found by asking everyone his or her age (all 270,000,000 of them!). Practically, the time and manpower needed, let alone the fact that some people would lie, make this basically impossible. Instead, a sample might be taken by asking 100,000 people to answer the question. By applying statistical methods, an answer could be determined from this sample. More importantly, not only could the answer be found, but the degree of error in that answer. It's no wonder the census is done only once every ten years. Thanks to statistics, the census bureau was able to calculate the answer to the question. The median age in the United States for 1997 was 34.9 years, up from 32.9 years in 1990 when everyone was counted.

In the area of dialysis, statistical methods are applied to determine such things as the median age of ESRD patients in different areas of the United States or the expected clearance of urea for a particular model of dialyzer. Virtually every dialysis study published in one of the various dialysis journals contains statistical analysis used to support the conclusions draw by the authors of the study.

The information that follows is intended to introduce the student to some of the statistical terms and concepts used to analyze data. A list of the texts used to prepare this article are listed at the end of this section and can be reference for further study.

II. Basic Terminology

Statistics is applied to a collection of what is referred to as *raw data*. Raw data is data that has been collected, but not arranged, sorted or grouped into any classification or category. An example of this type of data would be the height of the dialysis patients collected as they arrive for their treatment at the dialysis center. This collection of data may be done as a method of determining the average height of ESRD patients in the United States. In this example the data collected at the center would be called a *sample* because it is only part of the total data for all of the patients in the United States called a *population* or *universe*. By applying statistics

to the sample, a conclusion can be drawn about the average height of the entire population. Granted, to know the true average height of all ESRD patients in the United States, all the patients would need to be measured. This would be quite an undertaking involving considerable time, personnel and energy. By applying additional analysis, not only can the sample data give us a good estimate of the average height, but just as important, tell us the magnitude of error in our sample results. As one might expect, the larger the sample used, the more reliable the answer obtained and the lower the magnitude of error.

A collection of raw data arranged in order of magnitude is referred to as an *array*. The *range* of the data is defined as the difference between the largest and smallest number in the array. For the height of the dialysis patients mentioned above, if the shortest was 55" and the tallest was 75," the range would be 20."

Raw data is generally grouped into classes or categories to aid in understanding the distribution of the individual elements. In general, the range of the array will be divided into 5 to 20 classes of equal range size. For the patient height data, ten classes with a range of 2" could be used. For our example, Table 1 shows the data collected at the dialysis center broken into 10 classes.

Height (Inches)	Number of Patients	Height (Inches)	Number of Patients
55-57	2	65-67	23
57-59	4	67-69	16
59-61	9	69-71	10
61-63	13	71-73	5
63-65	17	73-75	1

Table 1 – Patient Height by 2" Classes

The distribution of the data shown in Table 1 can be illustrated using a *histogram*. Histograms are a helpful way to "picture" the data. A histogram consists of a series of vertical rectangles representing each class or category where the height of the individual rectangles are in proportion to the number of elements for that particular class. These diagrams are also referred to as *frequency histograms* because they illustrate the frequency that an element will fall into a particular class.

Figure 19.1

Histogram

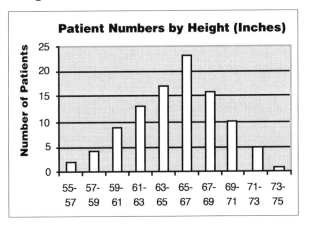

Patient Numbers by Height (Inches)

The *relative frequency* of a class is determined by dividing the number of datum in that class by the total number of datum collected. Because the number of elements in the above example was exactly 100, the frequency percentage for each class will be the same number as the number of elements in each class.

The frequency distribution of data can also provide useful information. When the frequency data is distributed equally on both sides of a center point, a curve representing this distribution would be *bell shaped* or *symmetrical*. In many cases however, the data may not be symmetrical. If more data is to the left or right of the largest class, the data is said to be *asymmetrical* or *skewed*. For the data shown above, the data is skewed to the left and is said to have *negative skewness*. If more data is to the right, the distribution is said to have *positive skewness*. The shape of a frequency curve is not limited to bell shaped curves. The data could be J-shaped (Higher values at one end), U-shaped (lower values in the middle of the range), and multimodal (multiple peaks and valleys across the range).

III. Measuring Degree of Asymmetry

There are several different mathematical methods that can be used to measure the degree of symmetry or asymmetry that a set of data may have. The first and most widely known is the *mean* or *average*. Average is also known as a *measure of central tendency*. Averages of numerical data can be done various ways. The most common average is the *arithmetic mean*. The arithmetic mean is calculated by adding the individual datum together and dividing by the number of datum. For example, the average blood volume for a particular dialyzer model could be calculated from the following data collected for 10 dialyzers.

83mL 87mL 91mL 86mL 84mL 89mL 90mL 86mL 86mL 87mL

Mean = (83+87+91+86+84+89+90+86+86+87)/10 = 86.9 mL

One of the interesting facts about the mean is that if the mean is subtracted from each datum and the results added together the answer would always equal zero. For the dialyzer example above:

(83 – 86.9) + (87 – 86.9) + (91 – 86.9) + (86 – 86.9) + (84 – 86.9) + (89 – 86.9) + (90 – 86.9) + (86 – 86.9) + (86 – 86.9) + (87 – 86.9) = (-3.9) + (0.1) + (4.1) + (-0.9) + (-2.9) + (2.1) + (3.1) + (-0.9) + (-0.9) + (0.1) = 0

Another term that is often confused with the mean is the *median*. The median is not an average, but the middle value in a set of data that has been grouped in order of magnitude. Referring again to the dialyzer volume example, the elements in order of magnitude are:

83, 84, 86, 86, 86, 87, 87, 89, 90, 91

For a collection of an odd number of elements, the middle number would be the median. In other words, if there were 15 elements, the 8th largest would be the median. For the dialyzer data the number of elements is 10. For this or any other situation where the number of elements is even, the median is determined by calculating the mean using only the two middle numbers.

Median = (86 + 87)/2 = 86.5 mL

Mode is defined as the value in a set of numbers that occurs most often. For the dialyzer volumes that number is 86 since it occurs three times. If all the numbers in a set were different, there would be no mode. Further, if several numbers occurred the same number of times, the data set would have multiple modes. When histograms or frequency curves are created for data, the peak of the curve will be the mode for that data.

By calculating the mean, median, and mode for a set of data, the amount and direction of asymmetry can be determined. For data that is symmetrical, the mode, median, and mean will all be equal. For asymmetrical data sets, if the median and mean are to the right of the mode, the data is skewed to the right. For the opposite case where the median and mean are to the left, the data set is skewed to the left. For data sets that are only slightly skewed and have only a single mode, there is a simple approximant relationship between mode, median, and mean:

Mean – mode ≈ 3(mean – median).

For the dialyzer volume data, the mode was 86, the mean 86.9 and the median 86.5. From the above formula we have:

$$86.9 - 86 \approx 3(86.9 - 86.5)$$

$$0.9 \approx 3(0.4)$$

$$0.9 \approx 1.2$$

IV. Measure of Dispersion

Statistically, data can not only be measured for its central tendency, but also for its degree of *dispersion* or *variation*. Both terms are used to describe the amount of deviation of the individual elements from their mean value. One of these measures has been discussed previously, range. Data with a large range certainly would seem to have a high degree of dispersion, but this measure alone can be deceiving. An example of this would be the set of data shown below for the clinical measure of a particular dialyzer's K_{UF} over a series of treatments arranged into an array.

5.7, 9.8, 10.1, 10.4, 10.7, 10.7, 11.0, 11.4, 14.6

The range for this data is $14.6 - 5.7 = 8.9$ mL/hr/mmHg(TMP). Notice that the two values on each end of the array appear to be extremes compared to all the other values. If it were not for them, the range would only be $11.4 - 9.8 = 1.6$ mL/hr/mmHg(TMP). It may well be that these two extremes are the result of incorrect clinical data taken during the treatments, or possibly a calculation error. Fortunately, there are other methods that can be applied to better indicate the actual dispersion.

The simplest way to determine the degree of dispersion other than range is *mean deviation*. Mean deviation is a measure of the average difference between each data point and the mean for the entire sample. The mean is calculated for the sample and then the differences found for each element. All the differences are expressed as absolute values and totaled. The total is divided by the number of elements to obtain the mean deviation. The absolute value of a number is the magnitude of the number expressed as a positive number. Positive numbers are unchanged when expressed as absolute values, but negative numbers are expressed as positives. Placing a vertical line just before and after the number notates the absolute value.

A few examples are:

$$|+7| = +7 \qquad |-6| = +6 \qquad |-4.567| = +4.567$$

For the K_{UF} data, the calculation is:

Find the mean.

Mean $= (5.7 + 9.8 + 10.1 + 10.4 + 10.7 + 10.7 + 11.0 + 11.4 + 14.6)/9 = 10.49$

Take the difference between each element and the average and express each answer as an absolute value.

$$|5.7 - 10.49| = 4.79 \quad |9.8 - 10.49| = 0.69 \quad |10.1 - 10.49| = 0.39$$

$$|10.4 - 10.49| = 0.09 \quad |10.7 - 10.49| = 0.21 \quad |10.7 - 10.49| = 0.21$$

$$|11.0 - 10.49| = 0.51 \quad |11.4 - 10.49| = 0.91 \quad |14.6 - 10.49| = 4.11$$

Find the mean deviation.

Mean deviation $= (4.79+0.69+0.39+0.09+0.21+0.21+0.51+0.91+4.11)/9 = 1.32$

The mean deviation indicates that the variation in the dialyzer's K_{UF} is +/- 1.32 mL/hr/mmHg(TMP) from the average value of 10.49 mL/hr/mmHg(TMP). This result is better than the use of the range as an indicator because all of the elements are part of the calculation as opposed to only two when the range is determined. There's a simple rule in statistics that states that the larger the sample, the better the results.

Another method of determining dispersion is *standard deviation*. Standard deviation is similar to mean deviation in that a mean (average) must be calculated and the difference between each element and the average determined. Once these values are known, the differences are squared and their average determined. The square root of this average is defined as the standard deviation.

For the dialyzer K_{UF} data, the differences were:

$$(5.7 - 10.49) = -4.79 \quad (9.8 - 10.49) = -0.69 \quad (10.1 - 10.49) = -0.39$$

$$(10.4 - 10.49) = -0.09 \quad (10.7 - 10.49) = 0.21 \quad (10.7 - 10.49) = 0.21$$

$$(11.0 - 10.49) = 0.51 \quad (11.4 - 10.49) = 0.91 \quad (14.6 - 10.49) = 4.11$$

Note that absolute values are not needed since each difference will be squared, creating all positive numbers.

Squaring each difference yields:

$$(-4.79)^2 = 22.94 \quad (-0.69)^2 = 0.48 \quad (-0.39)^2 = 0.15$$

$$(-0.09)^2 = 0.01 \quad (0.21)^2 = 0.04 \quad (0.21)^2 = 0.04$$

$$(0.51)^2 = 0.26 \quad (0.91)^2 = 0.83 \quad (4.11)^2 = 16.89$$

Calculating the mean of the squared differences yields:

$$(22.94+0.48+0.15+0.01+0.04+0.04+0.26+0.83+16.89)/9 = 4.62$$

Taking the square root of the mean of the differences gives:

Standard deviation $= (4.62)^{1/2} = 2.15$

The use of standard deviation is the most widely used measure of dispersion.

In nature, the distribution of data will follow a pattern called a *normal distribution*. This distribution is a bell shaped curve resulting from studies of large samples of data. The normal distribution is symmetrical in shape, which means that the mode, mean, and median are all equal in value. Refer to the illustration below. An simple example of data that would fit this type of curve would be a collection of leaves from a tree. Most of them would be collected near the average size, but there would still be some that deviated from the average.

If the size of the leaves were recorded and a standard deviation calculated it would be found that 68% were within one standard deviation of the average. 95% would be within two standard deviations, and 99.7% within 3 standard deviations. By knowing the expected type of distribution, there is no need to strip the tree of all its leaves to determine the true average size. A small sample could be taken and analyzed to see that it matched the normal distribution curve.

An example of the use of statistics in the field of dialysis relates directly to the monitoring of adequacy of dialysis. One of the key factors is the expected dialyzer clearance. How can you be sure the dialyzer you just removed from its sterile package will perform to the standards that came as an information sheet in the box? The manufacturer of the dialyzer has derived the clearance numbers for each of its models through extensive testing to establish an expected distribution of values. Once this is done, testing a sample of dialyzers from each lot and comparing the data against the known distribution curve for that dialyzer type, validation of proper performance can be assured. Statistical methods are even used to determine the sample size necessary to obtain the degree of accuracy desired.

Figure 19.2

Normal Distribution Curve

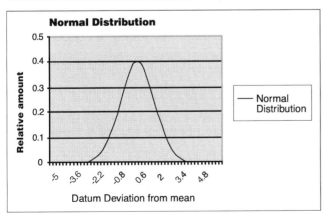

This type of sampling and comparing results to expected values is referred to as statistical decision making. In our example, there is a statistical hypothesis made that all production dialyzers of a particular model or size will yield a prescribed clearance within a certain range or standard deviation. The purpose of sampling is to determine if the latest batch of dialyzers will meet the clearance requirement. Simply put, should they be rejected or passed as acceptable. This type of statistical decision is called a *null hypothesis*. The term comes from the concept that the sampling and testing is being performed to determine if rejection or nullification of the dialyzers is necessary.

When sampling is done, obviously only a fraction of the dialyzers will be tested. This means that there is a possibility that there will be error in the test results. It's possible that the only dialyzers selected randomly for testing were the low clearance ones. There are two possibilities labeled *Type I* and *Type II* errors. A Type I error occurs when we reject the dialyzers when they should have been accepted. In statistical terms, we reject the hypothesis when we should have accepted it. A Type II error occurs when we accept the dialyzers as good when we should have rejected them. In other words, we accept the hypothesis when we should have rejected it.

In order to minimize the chance of error, a range of values or a fixed number of standard deviations may be assigned as the basis for acceptance or rejection. This value is generally picked such that the chance of error is minimized to a value of five or in some cases even one percent. If our hypothesis was that all dialyzers should have a clearance value under test conditions for urea of 235 mL/min, the probability that the sample would yield this number would be very small, and all the dialyzers would be rejected. If instead, a range is selected based on prior experience such as 220 – 250 mL/min, the probability of acceptance will be higher and the hypothesis more realistic. Assigning the accepted range is referred to as a *level of significance*. If the level of significance is 5%, then the chance that a Type I error will occur is only 5 out of 100 times or 1 in 20. This is written as "p < 0.05". For a level of significance of 1%, the condition would be expressed "p < 0.01." Another way of stating this is that the sampling results should not be in error with respect to the hypothesis 99 out of 100 times.

In many cases, the level of significance is expressed in units of standard deviations. For test results that fit a normal distribution, the percentages of data within different multiples of standard deviation are known. These are:

1 Standard Deviation = 68.27%
Significance Level = 31.73% = p < 0.3173

2 Standard Deviations = 95.45%
Significance Level = 4.55% = p < 0.0455

3 Standard Deviations = 99.73%
Significance Level = 0.27% = p < 0.0027

For a 5% level of significance, the error allowed would be +/- 1.96 standard deviations. Returning to the dialyzer hypothesis, if the mean value is 235 mL/min and the standard deviation is determined to be 10 mL/min. The range of acceptable clearance values to yield a level of significance of 5% would be:

10 mL/min X 1.96 = 19.6 mL/min.

Lowest Value = 235 – 19.6 mL/min = 215.4 mL/min.

Highest Value = 235 + 19.6 mL/min = 254.6 mL/min.

The acceptable clearance range would be from 215.4 mL/min to 254.6 mL/min. In nature, there are no perfect answers, but thanks to statistical methods, we have a tool that enables us to estimate error and make decisions that will minimize it.

Bibliography

Theory and Problems of Statistics, Murray R. Spiegel, 2nd Edition. McGraw Hill Publishing, Schaum's Outline Series, Copyright 1988, ISBN 0-07-060234-4

Elementary Statistics for Business, James C. Terrell, W. B. Saunders Company, Copyright 1979, ISBN 0-7216-8797-0

Dictionary of Scientific and Technical Terms, Daniel N. Lapedes, Editor in Chief, McGraw-Hill Book Company, Copyright 1978, ISBN 0-07-045258-X

The World Almanac and Book of Facts – 1998, Robert Famighetti, Editorial Director, K-III Reference Company, Copyright 1997, ISBN 0-88687-820-9

Chapter 20
Anemia Management

Contributing Author:
Patricia Samec, RN, BSN, CNN

Chapter Outline

I. Anemia

I. Anemia

A. Causes In Renal Failure

1. Erythropoietin (EPO) produced in normally functioning kidney to stimulate bone marrow to produce red blood cells (RBC) – This function greatly decreased in renal failure.

2. Blood Loss (1cc blood loss – 1 mg iron loss)
   a) Blood left in dialyzer
   b) Blood sampling
   c) Blood loss from GI tract
   d) Blood loss from access
   e) Blood loss from surgery (declots or other procedures)
   f) Blood loss from other sources

3. Iron Deficiency
   a) EPO requires iron to make RBCs
   b) Blood loss

4. Uremic Toxins
   a) Inhibit EPO
   b) Accelerates destruction of RBCs

5. Infection / Inflammation
   a) Reduced response to EPO
   b) Accelerates destruction of RBCs

6. Renal Bone Disease (Hyperparathyroidism)
   a) Increases bone marrow fibrosis
   b) Inhibits production of RBCs

7. Vitamin Deficiency

8. Aluminum Toxicity

9. Hemolysis
   a) Related to contaminates in the dialysate
   b) Related to mechanical trauma to blood cells
      (1) Poorly functioning blood pump
      (2) Excessive suction at arterial access site
      (3) High blood flow through small needle
      (4) Malfunctioning catheter
   c) Drug induced

10. Co-morbid Conditions
    a) Malignancy
    b) Other Diseases

B. Treatment

1. EPO Therapy
   a) Hemoglobin (Hgb) or Hematacrit (Hct) monitored per unit protocol, usually every two weeks, or oftener if Hgb >10 or Hct >30.
   b) Initial dose of EPO based on weight of patient and target level of Hgb/Hct and patient's current Hgb/Hct. Recommended starting dose is 50 to 100 Units/kg of body weight, three times a week.
   c) Target Hgb level is 11-12. Target Hct is 33-36
   d) Response to EPO is not immediate. It takes a minimum of two weeks to see a change in the patients Hgb/Hct
      (1) Do not adjust the dose of EPO more often than every four weeks unless clinically indicated
      (2) If target Hgb/Hct is not achieved, increase dose by 10-25%
      (3) If Hgb/Hct goal is exceeded, or is trending towards maximum range, decrease dose by 10-25%
      (4) Holding a dose of EPO is not generally recommended because it can cause a dramatic drop in Hgb/Hct

2. Minimize Blood Loss (Important role of PCT)
   a) Loss of residual blood in the dialyzer and tubing
      (1) Give complete washbacks
      (2) Evaluate anticoagulation
      (3) Report poorly functioning access
   b) Blood sampling
      (1) Correct drawing of labs to minimize redraws
      (2) Proper handling of labs to minimize redraws
   c) Blood loss from GI tract
      (1) Monitor occult blood loss
   d) Blood loss from access or blood circuit
      (1) Proper tubing/needle connections to prevent disconnection
      (2) Careful monitoring when clamps are applied post treatment, or when patient is holding sites, to prevent blood loss
      (3) Patient/family teaching so that they are knowledgeable about what to do if bleeding from site

e) Blood loss from surgery

   (1) Monitor Hgb/Hct more frequently after recent surgery

f) Other blood loss

   (1) Report any knowledge of any other blood loss, such as nosebleeds, cuts, etc. to the team leader.

3. Assess Iron Stores and Correct Iron Deficiencies

  a) Ferritin level indicates stored iron

  b) Transferrin Saturation shows available iron for RBC production

  c) EPO is ineffective if patient is iron deficient

  d) Iron is most effectively replace with IV iron given during dialysis

4. Provide Adequate Dialysis to Remove Uremic Toxins

  a) Follow dialysis prescription

    (1) Full treatment time

    (2) Ordered blood flow rate and dialysate flow rate

  b) Monitor adequacy of dialysis

    (1) Correct drawing of pre and post blood samples

    (2) URR > 65

    (3) Kt/V > 1.2

5. Discover and Treat any Source of infection/Inflammation

6. Treat Renal Bone Disease

  a) Control phosphorous

  b) Maintain Serum Calcium between

  c) Vitamin D Therapy

  d) Parathyroidectomy (in sever cases)

7. Correct Vitamin Deficiency

8. Treat Aluminum Toxicity (rare today)

9. Prevent Hemolysis

  a) Monitor water treatment

  b) Proper machine maintenance

  c) Monitor access problems

10. Treat Co-Morbid Conditions

11. Blood Transfusions

  a) Indicated if

    (1) Large blood loss

    (2) Hgb/Hct low and patient symptomatic (chest pain, short of breath, extreme fatigue)

Chapter 21

How to Assess Your Renal Unit's Environment to Pass Inspections

Contributing Author:

Gerald Dievendorf

Chapter Outline

Introduction

Types of Surveys

Introduction

Section 1881(b)(1) of the Social Security Act (the Act) requires facilities to be approved to participate in the end stage renal disease (ESRD) program. The regulations at 42 CFR(Code of Federal Regulations) Part 405.2100, Subpart U, specify the Conditions that facilities must meet to achieve and maintain approval.

The purpose of this document is to provide suggestions and checklists for you to use to perform your own self-assessment, i.e., conduct your own mock internal surveys as a dry run, and otherwise maintain your facility in compliance with applicable environmental codes. When conducting surveys in accordance with the protocols, we look to the substantive requirements in the statute and the regulations to determine whether a citation of noncompliance is appropriate.

The focus of this document is limited to environmental issues that are commonly evaluated during the course of a federal or state survey. Accordingly, **this is not meant to be a comprehensive surveillance tool** for that reason. Other federal "Conditions of Participation" affecting certification in the dialysis program are not covered except as they relate to physical environment. In addition, be aware that some of what follows is interpretive in nature and is meant to be used only as a guideline.

Remember, the only person that wants you to be in compliance more than you, is the surveyor!

Types of Surveys

There are several types for surveys and a different protocol for each type of survey. Federal surveys include Basic, Supplemental, and Initial Surveys. State Agencies, under an agreement with the Centers for Medicare & Medicaid Services (CMS), formerly known as the Health Care Financing Administration, surveys for compliance with the federal code. State Agencies therefore, may cite both federal and state code on any given survey. In addition, State Agencies may come in for state purposes only or federal surveyors may come in to validate their performance.

Basic Surveys are used for re-certification, and therefore assumes that the facility is fully established with a performance history. These surveys involve observing areas and actions, interviewing patients and staff, and reviewing records and documents. All of these are focused most on patient care and outcomes.

Supplemental Surveys are initiated when Condition-level (or suspected Condition-level) problems are noted while conducting the Basic Survey. The Supplemental

Survey protocol is used to identify underlying problems or structural weaknesses in the operation of the dialysis facility that have or could produce Condition-level deficiencies. The Supplemental Survey is organized around Conditions for Coverage for each respective area covered in the outcome-oriented Basic Survey. The Supplemental Survey can be used in whole or in part to augment the Basic Survey.

Initial Surveys are used as the first surveys for new ESRD suppliers. This initial protocol can also be used for facilities that are changing ownership/management or location/services. The focus of the survey will be basic safety and health standards emphasizing review of documents and protocols, observing the site, and interviewing staff.

I. State Agency Pre-survey Preperation Done Off-site

Prior to each survey surveyors review the facility's survey and certification file and facility profiles generated by other organizations. Profiles from other organizations include, but are not limited to, profiles developed by the ESRD Networks and the National Surveillance of Dialysis-Associate Diseases Form (CDC-537) developed by the Centers for Disease Control and Prevention (CDC). This review includes the following:

A. **Facility File:** the facility's history for any prior survey and certification issues. If there have been past environmental indiscretions, you should ensure that any of these issues would not result in repeat deficiencies. Repeat deficiencies may result in enforcement action being taken. Therefore you should review the results of previous Federal and/or State surveys and any complaint investigations for environmental issues. Ensure that these documents are kept on file by your facility.

B. **Profile from the CDC:** information from the National Surveillance of Dialysis-Associated Diseases Form (CDC-53.7). This includes information on the prevalence of HBsAg-positive patients, the prevalence of pyrogenic reactions, reuse techniques, water treatment techniques, and the type(s) of dialyzer(s) used in the facility. Get a copy and review it for environmental issues. It will give you a heads up on the survey team's focus.

II. Surveyor Tour for Observations

After brief introductions, the survey team will begin with observations within the facility, record reviews, and interviews with patients and staff. Surveyors are taught to get a quick overall impression of the facility before proceeding. The observational tour enables the surveyor to make assessments about the physical layout of the facility and determine if the physical layout is designed with consideration of infection control, safety, and emergency preparedness. The purpose of the observational tour of the dialysis unit is to make initial assessments of:

- the cleanliness and infection control practices of the facility;

- the safety and emergency preparedness of the facility and staff;

- the appropriateness of the patient treatment area; and

- the character of patient/staff interactions.

Although these observations are grouped under the initial tour, these areas may be observed in greater depth at any point in the survey. If surveyors see problems in any of these areas, they will proceed to review related policies and procedures. Therefore, ensure that your policies and procedures are up to date.

III. Governing Body and Management – CFR405.2136

The governing body is responsible for the health care and safety of the patients. Included in these responsibilities is the maintenance and implementation of policies and procedures that ensure a safe environment for patients and staff. To ensure compliance, ask yourself the following:

- How does the governing body ensure that the facility is a safe place to dialyze and that the patients, staff, and equipment are prepared for emergencies?

- How do the policies and procedures ensure a sanitary and safe environment?

- How does the facility routinely test for hepatitis and other infectious diseases?

- How does the facility ensure adequate training for staff in infection control and prevention?

- What supervision and oversight is provided for staff to ensure that the policies and procedures for sanitation and infection control are followed?

IV. Physical Environment – CFR405.2140

Observe cleanliness (V145, V380, V387), infection control and prevention practices (V380, V388, V394, V395, V396, V397) of the facility to assess whether the facility is sanitary and that it follows procedures that should lead to the prevention and control of infection.

A. Building and Equipment – CFR405.2140

Basic questions to ask yourself:

- Is the facility equipped and maintained to provide a sanitary and safe environment?

- Is the facility's temperature and ventilation adequately monitored?

- Is waste storage and disposal appropriately handled?

- Is the medical director monitoring the development and implementation of policies and procedures regarding cleanliness and infection control?

- Are storage areas sanitary?

- Are clean supplies and waste separated appropriately? (V394).

- Does the patient reception/waiting area have adequate space for wheel chair storage?

- Are patient restrooms available, clean, and handicapped-accessible?

B. Water – CFR405.2140(a)(5)

Water quality is of vital importance to a dialysis facility and to the patient. The hemodialysis patient's blood can be exposed to toxic contaminants if they are present in the water through water mixed with dialysate, water mixed with reprocessing germicides, and water flushing out dialyzers. Contamination of the water system with organic and inorganic chemicals, bacteria, and endotoxins can result in adverse patient reactions such as hemolysis, bacteremia, pyrogenic reactions (fever, chills, nausea), or death. Some contaminants can cause chronic health defects (e.g., aluminum) and others can be fatal (e.g., fluoride).

An ESRD facility must monitor the quality of the water used in treatments and monitor the equipment used in water treatment. The Association for Advanced Medical Instrumentation (AAMI) has published guidelines for water treatment and for reprocessing dialyzers. The ESRD regulations have incorporated by reference the AAMI recommended guidelines for the reuse of hemodialyzers but not AAMI's guidelines for water treatment. The regulations require water that is biologically and chemically compatible with acceptable dialysis techniques. The reuse regulations require that the quality of water used for reprocessing must have less than 200 colony-forming units of bacteria per milliliter (cfu/mL) and/or less than one nanogram of bacterial endotoxin per milliliter (ng/mL).

Assessment of the water treatment system consists of observations and interviews in the water treatment area at this time (V386, V216). During our review of operational records, we review records of water specimen analysis and equipment maintenance (V217, V218, V252, V253, V254) and also look in patient medical records for patient blood chemistries and symptoms as part of our review of clinical records. (V146, V338, V294).

1. Water Treatment Area and Equipment

   • Ensure that the components of the water treatment and distribution system are compatible and will not leach toxic elements, i.e., that your system does not use copper, zinc, brass, or aluminum components after the first processing element in the dialysis water treatment system.

   • Determine that there are no stagnant flow areas in the fluid distribution system that can not be easily sanitized. Ensure that sampling ports are located after each component of the water treatment system.

   • Review your procedures for how the bicarbonate concentration is prepared and stored. Are the containers used in the preparation or delivery of bicarbonate concentrate rinsed and completely drained at the end of each day? Are they disinfected periodically?

2. Staff questions

   Ensure that the responsible person is prepared to answer the following:

   • Who starts the system?

   • Who tests the water?

   • How often do you test for chlorine/chloramines?

   • What are the accepted limits?

   • What do you do if you exceed those limits?

   • Do you ever put the water treatment system in by-pass?

   • Who determines if the system goes into by-pass?

   • What happens to reuse if this occurs?

   • Who does this when you are not there?

   • Which contaminants are common in your local water?

   • Does your local water department require a back flow preventor?

   • How would your local water department contact you in the event of an emergency or change?

3. Other related questions that may be asked of Management:

   • How does the facility test hemodialysis fluids (i.e., water for dialysate, water for reuse, dialysate) for chemical, bacterial, endotoxin concentrations?

   • How does the medical director document his/her review?

   • What limits are set up by the facility?

   • What action is taken if the chemical, bacterial, and/or endotoxin analyses reveal levels of toxins above specified limits?

   • Where do you document corrective action for results that are not within standards? Examine the results of water analysis. If the water microbial assay results do not seem credible (e.g., consistent reports, "no growth") surveyors will want to consult with the off-site laboratory doing the tests. Ensure that you have this information handy.

   • How does the facility ensure that the water used for dialysis treatments is biologically and chemically acceptable? (V380)

   • What test results and equipment maintenance schedules are maintained?

   • How does the facility meet the water treatment standards that are a part of the Association for the Advancement of Medical Instrumentation guidelines on the Recommended Practice for the Reuse of Hemodialyzers? (V200)

4. Records of analysis of water specimens and equipment maintenance.

   • What documentation does the facility have for maintenance, calibration checks, and testing of the water treatment system?

   • Which tests are done daily or prior to each patient shift?

   • What records does the facility maintain for disinfection and for test results of disinfection? (V386)

C. Favorable Environment for Patients – CFR405.2140(b)

   • How does the facility ensure that fire regulations and fire management procedures are followed properly?

   • Are ventilation and temperature control mechanisms within the facility appropriate and adequate? If you can smell vapors from disinfectants then the surveyors can too. Be prepared to answer how the facility determines the appropriate temperature for both patients and staff. (V392, V224, V226).

- How does the facility ensure the surveillance of patients for safety while they are receiving dialysis treatments?

- Is the patient treatment area set up safely and appropriately? (V145, V381, V387).

- Is the patient's arm and hand free of blood?

- Are clamps available to the patient for emergency takeoff?

D. Contamination Prevention – CFR405.2140(c)

The Survey team will look for evidence of people following the Universal Precautions for infection control and prevention developed by the CDC and regulated by the Occupational Safety and Health Administration (OSHA) requirements. To ensure compliance, ask yourself these questions:

- How are infections and infection rates in the facility monitored and reported?

- How does the facility ensure that universal precautions for infection control are followed?

- How does the medical director ensure adequate training of the staff in sanitation and infection control?

- Does staff wear and change gloves after each exposure to blood and body fluids?

- Does staff wear and change protective clothing (including face/eye protection) appropriately?

- Are the hand-washing procedures appropriate?

- Is there evidence of the prevention of cross contamination? (V388, V394, V395).

- Are appropriate measures taken to prevent cross-contamination between the isolated area and the regular patient care area or among the patients and staff in the isolated area? (V145, V380, V388).

- Are clean supplies kept away from splash areas around sinks? (V394, V395).

- Are paper towel holders, soap dispensers, and trashcans placed appropriately around the sinks?

- If hepatitis B-infected patients will be treated in the facility, observe how cross-contamination will

be prevented. (V110, V380) Note the area of patient treatment.

- Is there adequate space between patient chairs to provide emergency care in the event of an emergency, such as a drop in blood pressure, nausea, and/or vomiting.

- What method does the facility use for disposal of infectious/contaminated materials.

- Are waste containers for trash placed and used appropriately?

- Are the sharps boxes for needles placed and used appropriately? (V394, V395).

- What does the facility do to prevent and control the spread of infections?

- What are the facility's policies and procedures regarding hepatitis testing and control among patients and staff?

- How does the staff collect and dispose of waste?

- How does the staff dispose of needles?

- When and where is protective clothing worn?

- Where is protective clothing stored during breaks? (V110, V380)

- Are medications, laboratory specimens, and food stored in separate refrigerators?

- Are staff food items kept out of the patient care area?

E. Emergency Preparedness – CFR405.2140(d)

To ensure compliance, ask yourself these questions:

- How does the facility ensure that all electrical and other equipment is free of defects?

- How does the facility annually review and test the emergency procedures for fire, natural disasters, and equipment failure?

- How does the facility guarantee that personnel are knowledgeable and trained in their respective roles in emergency situation?

- Observe the safety and emergency preparedness of the facility. Is the facility safe and are staff and patients prepared for emergencies? (V145, V380).

- Are fire extinguisher(s) and a plan for dealing with a fire or other emergencies visible.

- Is there evidence that the staff participates in fire drills?

- Is there evidence that patients understand how to cope with fire or other emergencies? (V382).

- Ask random staff and patients if they know where the fire extinguishers are and if they know what to do in the event of a fire.

- Is emergency equipment in the facility fully equipped and available in the unit? (V403).

- Is the physical layout of the facility designed for safety and emergencies?

- Can all patients be observed? (V391)

- Is there adequate space between patient chairs to provide emergency care in the event of a drop in blood pressure, nausea, and/or vomiting? (V145), V389).

- What emergency equipment is available in the unit?

- Is there a call system or other mechanism in the patient restroom to allow needed help to be summoned? (V110, V380)

F. Dialyzer Reuse – CFR405.2150

It is of paramount importance that the reprocessing of each dialyzer be done in an appropriate and consistent manner. Expect that surveyors will conduct a "flash" survey of the actual reprocessing activity at the beginning of the survey. The purpose of the "flash" survey of the reuse process is to determine the actual state of the reprocessing area and the behavior of the facility personnel before the facility adjusts to your presence. Is your reuse technician prepared to answer surveyor questions regarding the process? After the flash inspection, there will be a more thorough survey of the reuse area. (V226, V227, V229, V230, V293)

G. Reprocessing Area

To ensure compliance, ask yourself these questions:

- Is the area clean and sanitary?

- Is there adequate of ventilation? Vapors from reprocessing materials must be maintained below potentially toxic levels. Formaldehyde vapors should be monitored at least monthly and whenever indicated by the discomfort of the personnel (V230). Testing for air quality for any disinfectants used should be in accordance with OSHA standards (V293). Be prepared to document steps utilized reduce exposure to toxic fumes, i.e., maintaining covers on the containers of germicides and mixing disinfectants carefully. Make sure that the technician is aware of these measures and is implementing them.

- Ensure that there are visible, tangible separations between storage for new dialyzers, reprocessing dialyzers, and used dialyzers awaiting reprocessing (V227).

- Ensure that durable gloves, eye protection (goggles or face shield, eye-wash station), and protective clothing (impervious apron) are available and used during reprocessing (V229).

H. Reprocessed and Stored Dialyzers

1. The survey team will inspect dialyzers that have been reused and are in storage. (V237, V256, V257, V258, V259, V260, V261, V262, V264, V266). To ensure compliance, ask yourself these questions:

- Observe that the external surfaces (jackets) of the reprocessed dialyzers are clean with no visible blood and no leaks or cracks (V256, V258).

- Observe that dialyzer labels (including at least the patient's name, the number of previous uses, and the date of the last reprocessing) are properly applied, legible, and complete (V237, V262).

- Determine that the blood and dialysate ports are capped with no evidence of leakage (V261).

- (NOTE: Caps supplied with the disinfectant peracetic acid and hydrogen peroxide (Renalin) are vented to release under pressure.)

- Observe that the dialyzer headers are free of all but small peripheral blood clots (V243, V260).

- How do you ensure that dialyzers are free of visible, clotted blood, except for a few clotted fibers? (V243).

- How do you ensure that dialyzers contain ample amounts of disinfectant and a minimal air pocket.

2. Technician Interview

Surveyors may question personnel involved in reprocessing regarding adequate training and/or experience to perform the assigned tasks. Sample questions that they may be asked (and you should have them prepared to answer) include the following: (V209, V210, V211) Ensure that the responsible staff can answer the following:

- Can you describe the reprocessing procedures for dialyzers?

- What is the average total volume of disinfectant used for reuse each day?

- How long is the disinfectant stable after it is mixed?

- Once a dialyzer is reprocessed, how long must it remain on the shelf before being used?

- What would you do if you ran out of disinfectant?

- What would you do if the concentration of disinfectant is unacceptable?

- What would you do if you don't have enough time for the disinfectant to sit in the dialyzer?

- What would you do if you don't have enough room in the storage area?

- What would you do if you noticed that the port caps had popped off of the reprocessed dialyzer during storage?

- Where do you record the date of each reprocessing step?

- Where do you record the results of testing device performance and safety?

- What are the risks and actions associated with the toxic substances used in reprocessing?

- What protective clothing do you wear and why?

- What do you do in the event of a large/small spill of toxic substances?

- Ask the technician to show you the location of equipment used to handle a toxic spill.

- Ask the technician to describe the storage and handling of reprocessing chemicals.

- Where do you store the reuse chemicals?

- Is the temperature correct in the storage area?

- Where are the written procedures for the handling and safe storage of reprocessing chemicals?

- How do you ensure that toxic vapors from disinfectants are monitored as necessary?

- What steps are taken if the staff complaints of discomfort from vapors?

- What happens when a patient has an adverse reaction to a dialyzer?

- How is the reused dialyzer investigated and where is this documented?

- Describe your training and certification for working with reprocessing.

- What procedures do you follow to ensure that the disinfectant solution is mixed thoroughly?

- Describe your training and/or experience to perform the assigned tasks. (V200, V430).

- How long is the disinfectant stable after it is mixed?

- How long can a reprocessed dialyzer remain on the shelf before being used?

- What would you do if you ran out of disinfectant?

- What would you do if the concentration of disinfectant in dialyzers after storage is too low?

- Ask the technician to describe the risks and actions associated with the toxic substances used in reprocessing.

- What toxic substances do you work with?

- Which personnel are aware of the risks and actions necessary in the handling of toxic substances?

- Are there certain temperatures that must be maintained in the storage area?

- How does the facility verify the membrane integrity of the dialyzers?

- Is pressure testing and/or leak testing done on every dialyzer to verify its membrane integrity? (V248, V249)

- How many times do you refill the dialyzer with germicide in order to ensure that the effluent (final) germicide concentration in the dialyzer is within 90 percent of the intended use concentration.

- How do you determine the adequate volume for filling the dialyzer?

- Since the dialyzer fibers are wet with other liquids when you begin to fill it with disinfectant, how do you know when the concentration of germicide in the dialyzer is adequate to disinfect the dialyzer? (V253)

3. The Process

Surveyors will observe the reprocessing of dialyzers if the timing is appropriate including cleaning, performance testing, and disinfection. Reprocessing must be observed before the survey is completed.

- Ensure that proper disinfectant solution concentrations are achieved.

- Ensure that dialyzer port caps are in contact with a disinfectant for a specified time period (V295).

- Ensure that dialyzers and headers are rinsed with treated water (not tap water) until the effluent is clear and the dialyzer is free of visible clotted blood (V240, V241, V242, V243).

- Ensure that the dialyzer ports are disinfected and capped with new or disinfected caps (V295).

- Is the outside of the dialyzer being cleaned with a low-level disinfectant? (V255).

- Is your storage area designed to minimize deterioration, contamination, and breakage? (V227)

- Does your facility have a system in place to flag dialyzers of patients with similar last names to alert care givers? (V234, V235, V236, V237, V262, V266, V267)

- Does the facility have operating manuals for automated reprocessing equipment, or complete process protocols developed by the facility for manual reprocessing equipment?

- Do you maintain records that can determine how each dialyzer was reprocessed?

- Who performed the procedure?

- When was the dialyzer reprocessed?

- Are dialyzers tested for performance?

- What test results are achieved?

- What do logs of discarded dialyzers reveal as the reasons for discard?

- Are these records accurately and completely maintained? (V222, V223, V224, V225)

4. The Procedures

A dialyzer failure is the unexpected failure of a dialyzer to perform safely and effectively. Such failures include inadequate clearance or inadequate ultrafiltration performance and blood or dialysate leaks. Failures include a TCV less than 80 percent of the reference TCV and more than a few clotted blood fibers in a dialyzer. These are outcome measures that should be monitored by the facility (V245, V246, V247, V249, V276, V280, V282). Questions for the Medical Director may include the following:

- What parameters has the facility established for dialyzer failures?

- How are these parameters measured?

- How do you validate that TCV measures efficacy?

- How do you assess the adequacy of your dialysis treatments?

- How is reuse considered as part of reviewing adequacy of dialysis?

- How many pyrogenic episodes were there in your facility during the last year?

- How were they investigated?

- What is the mean, median, and range of reuses?

- How do you know that a dialyzer has failed?

- How do you record dialyzer failures? To whom do you report dialyzer failures?

- What do you do with a dialyzer that has failed?

- How do you introduce a new dialyzer if one fails?

- What do you do if the patient comes in the next day and reprocessed dialyzer isn't ready?

- Who starts the system?

- Who tests the water?

- When do you test for chlorine/chloramines?

- What are the accepted limits? What do you do if you exceed those limits?

- Do you ever put the water treatment system in by-pass?

- Who determines if the system goes into by-pass?

- What happens to reuse if this occurs?

- What contaminants are common in your local water?

- How does the facility test hemodialysis fluids (water, dialysate) for chemical, bacterial, and endotoxin concentrations?

- How often is each test done?

- How does the medical director document his/her review?

- What action will be taken if the chemical analysis reveals levels of toxins above AAMI specified limits?

The Survey Exit Conference

The general objective of the exit conference is to communicate informally with the facility representative about preliminary observations and findings at the end of the survey. Surveyors may either describe the requirements within which you are not in compliance and the findings that substantiate the deficiencies, or inform you that requirements appear to be met based upon a preliminary analysis of the findings of the Basic Survey protocol.

A formal statement of deficiencies (if any) will be mailed. If surveyors identified an immediate and serious threat to patient health and safety, you will be so advised as well as the significance of finding(s) that could affect your continued certification in the program and the need for immediate corrective action.

Ensure that you understand each of the issues noted at the conference, especially if you are told that one of the conditions of participation in the federal program is not substantially in compliance. Failure to demonstrate substantial compliance with all conditions of compliance will eventually result in decertification from the program and loss of Medicare reimbursement. If any of the items was corrected "on-the-spot" it may still be cited, but the prompt correction will be noted.

References

Interpretive Guidelines for ESRD Facilities, January 1998.

Chapter 22
Professional Boundaries

Contributing Author:
Karen Crampton, ACSW

Chapter Outline

I. Professional Boundaries

I. Professional Boundaries

The concept of boundaries is defined differently from person to person and culture to culture. In order to provide optimal patient care, the concept of professional boundaries requires a universal understanding in the dialysis setting. Professional boundaries address relationship limits between patients and care providers. The challenge is understanding and abiding by the limitations of this relationship for the greater good.

Providing chronic medical care to patients is an intensely interpersonal dynamic. Dialysis patients are unique since they may receive care from the same medical personnel for 5, 10, 20, or more years, 3 or more times per week. Due to the frequency and duration of dialysis treatments the setting potentially contributes to strong personal relationship development. This relationship, if appropriate, can have a positive impact on patients or if inappropriate, can contribute to disruptive situations in the dialysis unit. The challenge is to develop relationships that are therapeutic. In order to develop therapeutic relationships with patients multiple variables must be considered.

A. Evaluate the Atmosphere

Some patients enjoy the reciprocal relationships and joking with staff that helps them cope with their treatment. The joking and camaraderie contribute to a pleasant atmosphere that helps make the time on dialysis go faster. Both patients and staff admit they prefer this jovial atmosphere; however, there is potential risk in this type of environment. Despite good intentions, this jovial atmosphere can easily turn hostile if appropriate professional boundaries are not maintained. This is where confusion enters.

Boundaries and professionalism may be defined differently by members of the same staff. It has become clear that asking someone to be professional is too subjective. In a professional relationship standards of ethics and conduct are upheld. Professionals accord appropriate respect to the fundamental rights, dignity, and worth of all people. In a professional relationship the rights of individuals to privacy, confidentiality, self-determination, and autonomy are respected. Further expectations are outlined in policy and procedure manuals such as policies on attire, gift acceptance, the exchange of goods and services etc. Once staff understand expectations they can begin to work on an atmosphere that is professional *and* comfortable for them and for patients.

B. Evaluate Relationships/ Boundaries

As soon as a staff member spends personal time with a patient, exchanges goods and services, shows favoritism, or establishes a friendship, they exchange their professional relationship for an emotional one. There are consequences to the blurring of boundaries and unprofessional relationships. The same patient that enjoyed a joke on Monday may become agitated and act out on Wednesday over the same joke. Such acting out behaviors may include obscenities and threats. The reverse side for staff is that they lose their ability to respond objectively due to the friendship they chose to develop versus a professional relationship. *In a friendship the focus goes back and forth, from one person to the other. With a patient and caregiver, the focus should always remain on the patient.* When objectivity is lost, staff respond out of emotion, exacerbating the situation. Responding to a problematic situation as a professional means that a staff person might try to de-escalate a patient's anger or request assistance from others. Responding as a friend may incite feelings in the employee of anger, betrayal, or hurt.

A violation of boundaries that occurs frequently is when staff assist patients with personal matters outside of the dialysis setting.

C. Recognize the Imbalance of Power

The imbalance of power is signified by the fact that staff provide life-sustaining treatment to patients with the use of complex equipment. With this, the health care provider has tremendous influence over their patients, whether they believe it or not. When a relationship is strictly professional, it has checks and balances that help prevent patients from getting upset with staff interactions. As soon as the relationship becomes emotional and personal, the professional relationship is lost and the checks and balances which protect the patient are no longer viable. Staff now respond as though the patient were their "friend" instead of their patient for whose care they are responsible. It is possible to maintain a warm and caring professional relationship with patients that make them feel cared for while respecting professional boundaries.

D. Recognize the Risk

Patients are at risk due to violated boundaries whether or not we acknowledge it. For every good deed performed outside of the professional realm the negative ramifications can far out weigh the benefits. Professional codes of ethics subscribe to this concept. Patients aren't the only ones at risk as a result of boundary violations. If a staff member committed a boundary violation consequences could include disciplinary action, sanctions against professional licensure, or ultimately termination. Professionals should avoid developing personal relationships with patients as it is a conflict of interest. Also, they should be alert to and avoid conflicts of interest that interfere with the exercise of professional judgement.

Furthermore, staff put themselves at risk for liability as a result of after hours contact. If a patient was to pursue litigation, the staff may not have legal support from their employer because they were not acting in the capacity of an employee.

E. Be Respectful – Be Respected

What is the goal of the clinical staff? It is to provide optimal dialysis in order for patients to have quality of life. Relationships are an important element; it makes people feel cared for. A positive professional relationship with patients can be managed and should be a goal for every staff member. Mutual respect is another goal. Many disruptive situations in dialysis units are a result of someone feeling disrespected. Unintentional disrespect is often the outcome of and response to the personal relationship instead of the professional one. The familiarity that grows between staff and patients contributes to a relationship that may be so comfortable at times that responses are personal instead of professional. For instance, the staff person who is over involved with the patients is more likely to argue with a patient and feel angry or hurt. Conversely, the patient may feel free to cross the boundary with the staff because it has been part of the norm for treatment and they view themselves as a peer. In situations where patients cross the line, it is incumbent upon the staff to set limits respectfully by reminding them what is and what is not acceptable.

F. Identify Your Role in Unprofessional Boundaries

Barnsteiner, RN and Gillis-Donovan, RN state, "Professional nursing in any setting is emotionally complicated. It requires an ability to be meaningfully related to a patient and family yet separate enough to distinguish one's own feelings and needs. Nurses, willing caretakers by professional choice and emotional style, are suited for most of what the job requires. Their care taking style, however, includes varying degrees of a need to be needed, which increases their susceptibility to getting caught in intense relationships." Some might say, "Not me" or "It's not a big deal" however, we owe it to our patients to be introspective about ourselves and our own needs so we do not blur relationships and send mixed messages. Dialysis staff should have a heightened awareness, due to chronicity, of the potential for personal relationships instead of professional ones even though they seem harmless.

G. Misconduct

In a professional relationship the patients' rights are respected. Staff should not engage in inappropriate personal relationships with patients or their families. Misconduct includes but is not limited to:

- Gift giving, including material items or services
- Sharing detailed information about one's personal life
- Promoting one's personal beliefs such as religion or politics
- Attending social events with patients
- Developing personal relationships such as friendships or intimacy
- Exchanging goods or services

H. Teamwork

In order to provide an optimal atmosphere for patients, staff should function as a team. The ability to work together is *strengthened* by the following:

- Consistency in enforcing policies
- Educational opportunities to strengthen professionalism
- Learning how to graciously refuse gifts
- Agree as a group not to buy or sell from patients, even the smallest items
- Be aware that eyes and ears see and hear everything, so make good use of breaks

The ability to work together is *weakened* by the following:

- Speaking in a foreign language (unless used for translation)
- Sexual innuendo or harassment
- Discussion of personal matters on the treatment floor
- Discussion of staff conflicts
- Swearing or offensive language
- Criticism

I. Conclusion

Some staff justify that their friendship is just what a patient needs; it isn't, patients come to dialysis for dialysis treatment. Inappropriate relationship development is a shift away from patient needs to one of staff needs, introducing risks to patients that they should not be subjected to. Patients have the right to professional care.

It may also be beneficial to discuss the "fishbowl" setting of dialysis and acknowledge the challenges of working under the constant eye of patients and others.

The Master's prepared social worker in each unit has been trained in the area of interpersonal relationships/dynamics. They can be a resource to help identify relationships that are more than therapeutic as well as assist in the development of unit standards. Staff need to feel empowered to alter their style and supported over the loss of personal relationships with patients.

Bibliography

1. Doner-Kagle J., Northrup-Giebelhausen P.: *Dual Relationships and Professional Boundaries.* NASW CCC, Code: 0037-8046/94: 213-219.

2. Gillis-Donovan J., Barnsteiner J.: *Being Related and Separate: A Standard for Therapeutic Relationships. The American Journal of Maternal Child Nursing.* 223-228, July, 1990.

3. Thorne S.E., Robinson C.A., *Health Care Relationships: The Chronic Illness Perspective. Research in Nursing & Health* 11, 293-300, 1988.

4. 1995 Delegate Assembly: Revision of The Code of Ethics. NASW News, Jan. 1996.

5. Greenfield Health Systems' Relationships Policy, 2001

Chapter 23
History of Dialysis

Contributing Authors:

John Sweeny BS, CHT, CBNT
Narayan Venkataraman, MSc, BE

The earliest known scientific theories and attempts to create an artificial kidney device arose in the 1850s. Thomas Graham, Professor of Chemistry at Anderson's University in Glasgow, coined the term "dialysis" in 1854 in a paper entitled "The Bakerian Lecture – On Osmotic Force". He noticed that crystalloids were able to diffuse through vegetable parchment coated with albumin (which acted as a semi-permeable membrane). He called this process "dialysis". Using this method he was able to extract urea from urine[15]. Dialysis is a Greek word meaning "loosening from something else".

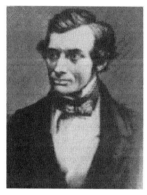

Fig 23.1 Dr. Thomas Graham

Prior to his work in understanding the dialysis process, Graham is credited in 1833 with one of the fundamental diffusion principle that bares his name. Graham's Law states, "*The rate of diffusion of a substance is inversely proportional to the square root of the masses of the molecules or the molecular weights.*" It is this principle which explains why the diffusion of urea (molecular weight of 60 daltons) across a semi-permeable membrane will be greater than that of creatinine (molecular weight of 113 daltons) even if the concentration of each substance are equal.

Also in the middle 1850s, an improved membrane material, collodion, began to be used in diffusion studies. Collodion was made by mixing cellulose with nitric acid to form cellulose nitrate. When cellulose nitrate was deposited onto a surface from a solution of 60% ether and 40 % alcohol, and then allowed to dry, collodion membrane was produced. It is interesting to note that collodion because of its high nitrate content had explosive properties and was also referred to as guncotton. It was this material that Jules Verne used to fuel his rocket in his famous novel "From the Earth to the Moon" written in 1865. In 1855, a German physiologist, Adolph Fick used this membrane in his studies of diffusion and is credited with the discovery of another basic principle referred to as Fick's Law: "*The rate of diffusion of a solute is directly proportional to the concentration difference from one area to another.*" During a dialysis treatment, the rate of toxin loss is always greatest at the beginning of the treatment and decreases as the blood concentrations are lowered.

In 1913, Jacob J. Abel, Leonard G. Rowntree, B. B. Turner and colleagues constructed the first artificial kidney. Their studies were performed at the pharmacological laboratories of the John Hopkins University in Baltimore, Maryland. They

used hirudin, produced from leeches obtained from Parisian barbers, as an anti-coagulant and actually had to interrupt their research during World War I when their supply of leeches from Europe became limited. They passed animal blood from an arterial cannula through celloidin tubes that were contained in a glass "jacket". The glass jacket was filled with saline or artificial serum. They coined the term

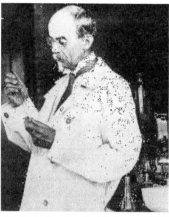

Fig 23.2 Dr. Jacob Abel circa 1913
An early Pioneer in Haemodialysis

"artificial kidney" and referred to the process known today as hemodialysis as "Vividiffusion". Blood was returned into the vein of the animal via another cannula[15]. The inventors wrote: "this apparatus might be applied to human beings suffering from certain toxic states, especially if due to kidney damage, in the hope of tiding a patient over a dangerous chemical emergency." The apparatus was never used to treat a patient[25].

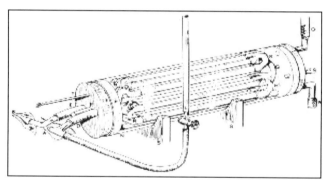

Fig 23.3 Vividiffusion Apparatus of Abel, Rowntree and Turner. *Consisted of a glass outer jacket with 16 celloidin hollow tubes. A forerunner of the modern hollow fiber dialyzer.*

George Haas (1886-1971) working at the University of Giessen in Germany performed the first successful human dialysis in the autumn of 1924[23]. The dialysis was performed on a patient with terminal uremia "because this was a condition against which the doctor stands otherwise powerless" [15]. The dialysis lasted for 15 minutes, and no complications occurred. Dr. Haas is also credited with being the first person to use heparin as an anticoagulant in 1928 although it would be several years before it became the preferred anticoagulant for clinical use.

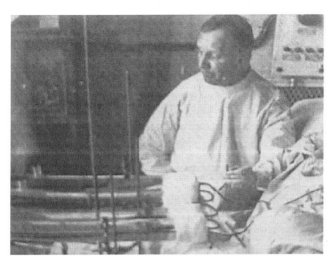

Fig 23.4 George Haas oversees dialysis of a girl in 1926
The semi-permeable membranes were celloidin tubes.

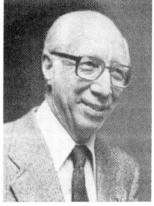

Fig 23.5
Dr. Willem Johan Kolff,
MD, PhD

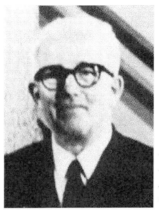

Fig 23.6
Hendrik Berk –
Dr. Kolff's Associate and
Collaborator

Mr. Berk provided Dr. Kolff with the practical mechanical
knowledge and talent that was required to bring Dr. Kolff's
inventions to life.

During the 1930's, Heinrich Necheles was performing dialysis studies at Peking University in China. He was using sheep peritoneum as his membrane. This membrane,however would expand when blood pressure was applied increasing the amount of blood required to perform his experiments. To correct this problem, he took sheets of screening and wired them together to create flat sections of membrane. It was this design that led to the development of the flat plate dialyzer several years later. Necheles was also the first experimenter to add a "clot catcher" to his venous return line, a priming solution chamber to his arterial line, and to use a gas heater to control the temperature of the dialysis bath.

Dr. Willem Kolff, who was living in German occupied Holland, developed the first workable artificial kidney during World War II over the period 1943-1945[11]. His rotating drum artificial kidney consisted of 30-40 metres of cellophane tubing in a stationary 100-litre tank. The effective size of this membrane was 2.4 square meters and clearances were measured in the 140 to 170 mL/min range comparable to standard dialyzers of the 1980's. This device resembled a drum barrel made of slats with open spaces between the slats. Cellophane "sausage" casing was wound around the drum. The lower portion of the drum, which was suspended length-wise in a half-barrel reservoir, was lowered into a dialysis bath. This procedure required 2.5 liters of blood circulation outside the body during dialysis and required priming with blood transfusions. Either metal tubes or glass tubing was used to create a blood access in an artery and a vein, and could be used only once per pair of blood vessels. Neither blood pumps nor plastic tubing was used to connect the blood accesses to the cellulose sausage casing. It was Kolff who made clinicians and experimentalists interested in the treatment of uremia, and this machine that delivered effective haemodialysis treatments [15].

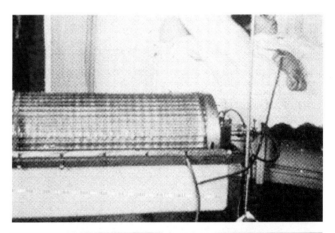

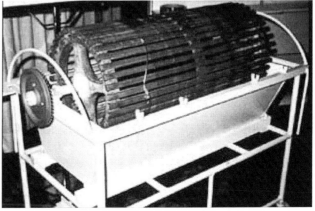

Fig 23.7 Dr. Kolff's Rotating Drum Kidney

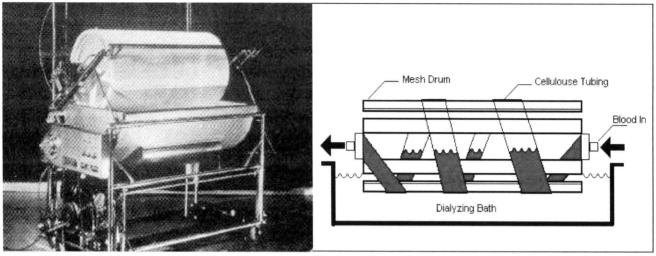

Fig 23.8 Dr. Kolff's Rotating Drum Kidney

Rotating Ford water pumps permitted the drums to rotate at either end, enabling the blood to flow through. Blood was "pumped" using the patient's heart and blood pressure into the cellulose casing, and was propelled from one end of the drum to the other, by the rotation of the drum. Blood was then collected in a glass cylinder with an open nipple at the lower end. Rubber tubing connected the patient's venous access to the glass cylinder. By alternatively lowering and raising the cylinder, blood was collected and drained back into the patient's vein.

Over the 17-month period from March 1943 until July 1945, Dr. Kolff dialyzed 16 patients without success. His 17th patient, Sophia Schafstadt, a 68 year old housewife began treatment with a urea level of 300 mg/dL, about three to four times higher than that of a typical dialysis patient today. Dr. Kolff lowered her toxins, and she became the first human being ever to be successfully dialyzed until kidney function returned. The date in 1945 of this success is of particular interest in light of recent events. It was September 11th.

Following WW II, Dr. Kolff migrated to the United States, bringing three of these machines with him. The machines were used in this country as models for more advanced "rotating drums." Kolff came to Mt. Sinai Hospital in New York City to train two doctors, Alfred P. Fishman and Irving Kroop. They successfully dialyzed the first patient in the United States on January 26th, 1948. The patient diuresed eight hours after the treatment. An interesting footnote to this history is the fact that the first patient dialysis in the United States should have been back in May of 1947, but the patient diuresed at the sight of the equipment!

Once in the United States, Kolff began searching for someone to assist him in developing an improved rotating drum. During a visit to Boston, he met Carl Walter, a surgeon at Peter Bent Brigham Hospital. Carl Walter was the founder of Fenwal Laboratories, later to become a division of Baxter Travenol in 1959. Mr. Walter enlisted the help of an engineer named Edward Olson to work with Dr. Kolff to create the Kolff Brigham kidney. Approximately 40 units were produced between 1949 and 1962, and shipped around the world. The price of one of these units was $5,600 in 1950. Olsen was still receiving requests for parts as late as 1974.

In 1946 Nils Alwall produced the first dialyzer with controllable ultra-filtration in Lund, Sweden at the University Hospital. It consisted of 10-11 meters of cell-ophane tubing wrapped around a stationary, vertical drum made of a metal screen [15] – resembling a rotating drum device stood on its end. Unlike the Kolff rotating drum, the blood membrane remained

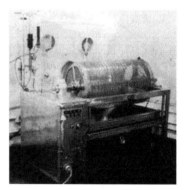

Fig 23.9 The Kolff-Brigham dialyzer, 1950. A modified version of the original rotating drum kidney

stationary while the dialysate moved pass the tubing. Dr. Alwall later enclosed his coil dialyzer so that a negative pressure could be applied to the dialysate. In doing so, Alwall became the first person credited with creating a negative pressure dialyzer. He also opened the first dialysis treatment facility in 1950.[1]

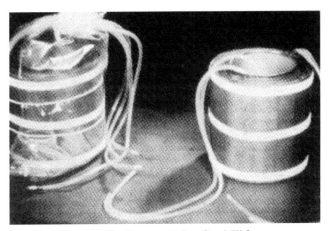

Fig 23.10. An Alwall dialyzer in the 1950s. The dialysis tubing was wound around the vertically mounted screen. Dialysate circulated around this at variable pressure. (Courtesy: Dr N. Hoenich)

The late 1940's was definitely an exciting time in the development of dialyzers. Depending on the particular article, a variety of different individuals could be given credit for the creation of the first practical dialyzer. The literature in general is not very helpful for two reasons. The first is (as Alwall pointed out in one of his articles), most researchers did not publish immediate results of their work until they had sufficient data to prove their experiments were valid. This delay in publication could be as long as 5 years. Secondly, World War II dramatically limited the ability of individual researches to communicate with each other and hence, most developers were operating independently from each other. Probably the fairest thing that can be said is that the artificial kidney was a simultaneous invention. The credit can be shared by Nils Alwall in Sweden, Willem Kolff in Holland, Gordon Murray in Canada, and Leonard Skeggs and Jack Leonards in the United States.[24]

The Skeggs/Leonards dialyzer incorporated flat sheets of membrane sandwiched between rubber gaskets. Each set of gaskets and membrane were separated by metal plates to keep the blood compartment from expanding during use. It was this parallel plate design that was improved upon by others and culminated in the mass production of flat plate dialyzers by Gambro and other companies.

Gordon Murray's dialyzer was similar to Alwall's design except that it used smaller diameter tubing, and as a result, had a lower total surface area. Murray used his dialyzer in conjunction with a pulsing blood pump that created turbulence in the blood flow and thereby increased the dialyzer's performance. Dr. Murray is credited with having performed the first dialysis treatment in North America.

In spite of Dr. Kolff's success with his rotating drum, he realized that dramatic reductions in size would be necessary if dialysis was ever to be made available as a general therapy. He was familiar with the design of Alwall's coil and decided to pursue this format for his next generation kidney. He convinced the Singer Sewing Machine Co. to create a sewing machine that would stitch two coils of membrane between fiberglass screening that was wrapped around a tin can. The tin can was an orange juice can from the Dole Fruit Company and Kolff referred to his final product as his "Orange Juice Kidney".

Once Kolff had his twin coil dialyzer completed, he was faced with the challenge of finding a company willing to manufacture the device as well as a create the necessary ancillary hardware so it could be utilized. After approaching several companies without success, he met with William Graham, Senior Chairman of Baxter Healthcare Corporation. William Graham was a chemist and understood the concepts of diffusion, osmosis, and ultrafiltration. He realized the potential Kolff's coil had and agreed to develop the system that Kolff required. The first commercially produced dialyzer, the U200A, complete with tank system was introduced into the marketplace on October 30, 1956. The dialyzer including its bloodlines was $59.00. Thanks to inflation, today's price would be $366.47. The stainless steel batch tank held 100 liters of dialysate that was pumped through the dialyzer. Because the blood flow resistance in the coil was high, a Sigmamotor blood pump with "rolling fingers" was used to push the blood through the tubing.

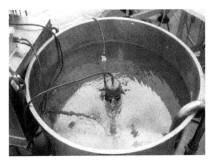

Fig 23.11 Dr. Kolff's 'Orange Juice Can' Kidneys

Fig 23.12 Modified Kolff tank with hollow fiber kidney

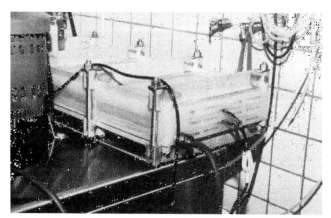

Fig 23.13 Two layer Kiil Board Dialyzer, 1964. This dialyzer built in layers with sheets of cellulose separating the blood compartments and the dialysate compartments, was the forerunner of the flat plate dialyzer.

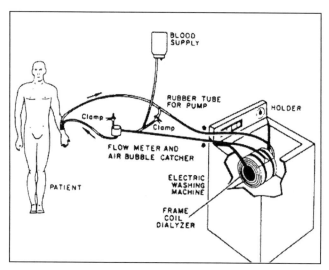

Fig 23.14 Maytag Dialysis. During the Korean Conflict two ingenius Army Physicians rigged up a crude dialysis machine made from a common washing machine. This photo, however, is a circa 1961 drawing of a Japanese home dialysis machine created from a Maytag washing machine.

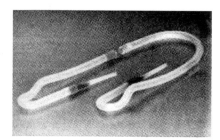

Fig 23.15 The Scribner/Quinton Shunt

In the late1950's, on the west coast of the United States, dialysis was being accomplished using the Kiil dialyzer developed by Fredrick Kiil of Norway. His design allowed for a small priming volume and little internal blood flow restriction. Blood flow rate could be maintained using arterial pressure and hence, a blood pump was not required to deliver a treatment.

The first patients treated by dialysis were all believed to have acute renal failure. The methods in use for getting adequate flows of blood into the machine exhausted veins and arteries very quickly, and only a few dialysis treatments could be undertaken. The major problem that prevented consideration of using dialysis for treatment of patients with End Stage Renal Disease (ESRD) was that there was no means to establish a "permanent" blood access. The development of methods to use blood vessels repeatedly while preserving them made it possible to contemplate keeping a few patients alive for longer periods even though they had permanent renal failure.

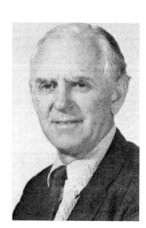

Fig 23. 16 Belding H. Scribner, MD circa 1974

In the mid-50s, teflon and silastic were invented. These proved to be relatively safe plastics, and they enabled Dr. Belding Scribner and engineer Wayne Quinton to create the first tubing that served as a "permanent", at least long lasting, blood access. The arteriovenous shunt, as described by Quinton and Scribner (1960) was the key development.

The first all Teflon shunt was implanted in Clyde Shields, a machinist, by surgeon Dr. David Dillard on March 9th, 1960. This first shunt lasted only three months before it required replacement, but considering the fact that an acute patient lasted only about three weeks, the improvement was dramatic. A second patient received a shunt just 13 days later, and a third patient was cannulated in May.[28] The real testimony to the brilliance of Dr. Scribner and the stamina of Clyde Shields is the fact that this first patient lasted 11 years on dialysis. Clyde Shields survived a series of complications including malignant hypertension (controlled by proper ultrafiltration), gout (dialyzed twice a week instead of once), peripheral neuropathy (increased dialysis time to three times per week), metastatic calcification (patients put on antacids), and iron overload (regular transfusions eliminated).

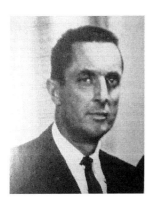

Fig 23.17 Mr. Clyde Shields – 1st Successful Chronic Dialysis Patient. This photo was taken in 1966 after five years of dialysis therapy. At the age of 39, in March of 1960, Mr. Shields had a Teflon AV shunt surgically implanted in his right arm. He lived for over 11 years, passing away in 1971 at the age of 50 due to an MI.

In 1961, Wayne Quinton discovered a way to extrude silicone so that the inner surface would not cause clotting. By using the silicone to support the Teflon tips inserted into the blood vessels, so the tips would remain still and not gouge the interior wall of the vessel. This silicone/Teflon combination improved the life of a cannula by a factor of ten.

In the 1960s, many advances were made in hemodialysis. The first outpatient hemodialysis center was established in Seattle, in 1962. Home hemodialysis also began.[29]

Home hemodialysis was introduced to overcome the difficulties in providing adequate facilities in hospitals for the increasing number of patients being put forward for treatment. If a relative provided help for the patient, it could be carried out without the use of doctors, nurses or hospital premises, extending the number of patients that could be treated, as well as being better for the patient. The first patients dialyzed at home were treated in Japan, using domestic washing machines to stir the dialysate. This went unnoticed in the West at the time. However in 1965 at the American Society of Artificial Internal Organs meeting, reports of home hemodialysis of four patients in Boston (Hampers et al) and two in Seattle (Curtis et al) were supplemented by a report from Nose (supported by Kolff) of his earlier experience, and by a report of two patients treated at home in London (Shaldon). All reported success and plans to expand their programs.

The Redy machine was semi-portable and was suitable for younger patients (under 45) who were waiting for transplantation. No home adaptation was needed. Older patients awaiting transplantation would be placed on standard home dialysis. The Redy machine was also used on those who were going on holiday. It used 5.5 liter of water and re-regenerated the dialysis fluid in a charcoal column. (Hospital HD used 180 liter of water for each dialysis). The charcoal column would convert urea to ammonia. The toxins went into a cartridge and clean water was re-cycled [websites]. It was not very efficient. In the UK, outbreaks of hepatitis accelerated

home hemodialysis programs, as it became a priority to reduce the risk of cross-infection.

Despite the growth of dialysis in the 1960s, dialysis programs were limited in number and size, and every patient who needed dialysis was not accepted. It was necessary for hospitals to form patient selection committees to choose which patients would go on dialysis and which ones would not. Patients had to meet very rigid requirements to be chosen.

By 1963, Dr. Scribner recognized the need to reduce the labor of performing treatments through the automation of the process. He enlisted the help of engineer Dr. Albert L. Babb. Dr. Babb developed a proportioning system using chemical feed pumps produced by the Milton Roy Co. It was Dr. Babb that gave us the ratio of 34:1 (water : acetate concentrate) that is still used today to proportion acid concentrate and water.

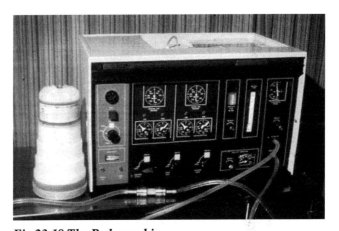

Fig 23.18 The Redy machine

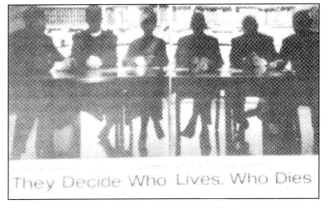

Fig 23.19 Dialysis Treatment Selection Teams. Prior to January of 1973, dialysis was available on a very limited basis. There were few machines and for most patients, no way to pay for the treatments. The Medicare ESRD Act passed in November of 1972 remedied that situation.

Milton Roy Company was founded by Milton Roy Sheen and his son Robert T. Sheen. The elder Sheen had passed away by the early 60's, but Robert Sheen being a chemical engineer, was very interested in the concept of using his company's pumps to create a dialysis machine. Working with Dr. Babb's prototype "Mini – I" which was a single patient system for home use, the company introduced the Model A to the market in 1964. It sold for $7,200 and featured automated hot water disinfection (called sterilization back then), automatic alarm testing, variable Sodium, remote patient control, and a wooden veneer so it would look good in the home. Milton Roy Co sold its medical division to Extracorporeal in the 1970's, and Johnson and Johnson then acquired the company in 1978. In 1984, the division was sold to Baxter Healthcare. The location of the production facility was not a business decision, but came about because Robert T. Sheen liked to go fishing. Milton Roy Co was located outside of Philadelphia, Pennsylvania, but Mr. Sheen kept his fishing boat in St. Petersburg, Florida. When it came time to start a medical division, Sheen decided to move all the company executives to Florida so he could better pursue the hobby he loved. Today, Baxter is producing its 9th generation of single patient systems, the Baxter Meridian, in the Tampa Bay area of Florida about 10 miles from where Mr. Sheen kept his boat.

The Model A system was designed to work with a Kiil dialyzer to perform nocturnal home hemodialysis. The Kiil Dialyzer was developed in 1959 by Fredrik Kiil of Norway. His dialyzer was an improvement on the parallel plate design of the Skeggs-Leonards dialyzer that had four layers that needed to be assembled. The Kiil required only two layers to be sandwiched together, however, each layer had a larger surface area and a large metal frame to clamp the polypropylene "boards" together. The total weigh of the unit was about 100 pounds.

While Scribner was growing his ESRD patient population in Seattle, Washington, Dr. Richard Drake was beginning to develop his program just to the south in Portland Oregon. Drake recognized that a single patient machine was necessary to automate the dialysis process. Although the Milton Roy Model A was being utilized by Scribner's group, it was expensive and in the 60's, funding was very limited. Dr. Drake desired a simpler machine and turned to his neighbor an inventor by the name of Charles Willock.[7] Mr. Willock, working in his basement, designed a dialysis machine with fixed proportioning to meet Dr. Drake's requirements. With the addition of Bob Smith, the DWS Company was formed. The first Drake-Willock machine, the Model 4002 came to market in 1964. DWS Inc. was sold to Becton Dickinson and Company in 1977 and became B-D Drake Willock.

Meanwhile, Cordis Dow introduced the first hollow fiber dialyzer on the market in 1968. The hollow fiber design quickly became the preferred dialyzer replacing both coils and flat plate designs. In July of 1983, Dow Chemical purchased Cordis's interesting the company and created CD Medical Inc. CD Medical then proceeded to acquire B-D Drake Willock from Becton Dickinson in 1984. The evolution of companies continued in 1990 when Althin Medical purchased CD Medical to form Althin CD Medical, Inc. The name was simplified in 1993 to Althin Medical Inc. Finally, in 2000, Baxter Healthcare acquired Althin Medical. The end result of this long chain of company acquisitions is that the Milton Roy Model A and Drake Willock Model 4002 final were brought together under one roof.

The table of machines below lists the various dialysis machines sold in the United States beginning with the Milton Roy Model A.

COMPANY	MODEL	YEAR
Milton Roy	Model A	1964
Drake Willock	DWS-4002	1964
Drake Willock	DWS-4011/4015	1966
Milton Roy	Model B	1967
Travenol	RSP	1967
Drake Willock	DWS-4215	1969
Milton Roy	Model BR	1970
Drake Willock	DWS-4216	1972
B. Braun	HD 103	1972
Cobe	Centry	1972
Cobe	Centry 2	1975
Gambro	AK-10	1977
Extracorporeal	SPS-350	1978
Cobe	Centry 2 – Rx	1980
Cobe	Centry 2000	1981
Cobe	Centry 2000 – Rx	1983
B. Braun	HD-secura	1984
Travenol	SPS-450	1984
Fresenius	A1008	1984
Drake Willock	DWS-480	1984
Fresenius	2008C	1984
Fresenius	2008D	1986
Cobe	Centrysystem 3	1987
Travenol	SPS-550	1988
Fresenius	2008E	1988
Baxter	1550	1991
Althin	System 1000	1991
Fresenius	2008H	1992
Althin	Ultratouch 1000	1995
B. Braun	Dialog	1995
Althin	Tina	1997
Baxter	Meridian	2000

The Brescia Cimino forearm fistula (1966), which did not require exteriorized pieces of plastic, was a major advance in blood access. The idea of performing. side-to-side anastomosis using an artery and vein came to Dr. Cimino from his experiences as a medical student at the Bellevue Blood Bank in New York City. Surgeon Kenneth Appell working closely with Dr. Cimino created the first fistula. The expansion of the vein enabled Dr. Cimino to use 14 gauge needles to obtain blood flows of 200 – 350 mL/min. Patients preferred this form of access in spite of the need for needle insertion at each treatment. Reasons given included ability to swim and bathe without the need to protect the access site, no anxiety regarding possible thrombosis, and reduced chance of infection. Today, fistulas and grafts are the vast majority of all blood access types used for hemodialysis.

The Landmark legislation in 1972 made it possible for Medicare to pay for 80% of treatment costs for both dialysis and transplant patients. This new law removed financial barriers to treatment and helped dialysis facilities expand with more equipment for patients. Patient selection committees became a thing of the past.

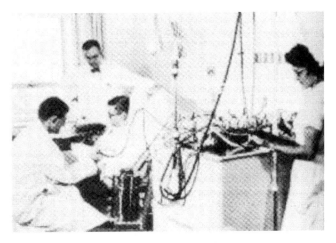

In the 1980s-1990s, computerized hemodialysis machines, better dialyzers, and improved monitoring and safety devices reduced treatment times, gave doctors better ways to monitor treatment, and made possible a more normal life for patients. Due to the many advancements made in dialysis therapy, ESRD patients can now lead healthier and more normal lives. Research and development continues to improve the quality of care for ESRD patients.

References

1. Alwall, Nils, *On the Organization f Treatment with the Artificial Kidney and Clinical Nephrology in the 1940's and Following Decades – A Contribution to the History of Medicine*, Three parts:

   I.   The Nineteen-Forties, Dialysis & Transplant, Volume 9, Number 4, April 1980, pp 307-311.

   II. Turn of the Decade 1949/1950, Dialysis & Transplant, Volume 9, Number 5, May 1980, pp 475,476,508.

   III. The Nineteen Fifties, Dialysis & Transplant, Volume 9, Number 6, June 1980, pp 559-563,565,566,569.

2. Bone JM, Tonkin RW, Davison AM, Marmion BP, Robson JS. *Outbreak of dialysis-associated Hepatitis in Edinburgh, 1969-1970*, Proceedings of the European Dialysis and Transplant Association. 1971; 8: 189-97.

3. Lucien Craps, *The Birth of Immunology*, Sandoz, 1993.

4. Curtis FK, Cole JJ, Fellows BJ, Tyler LL, Scribner BH, *Hemodialysis in the home*, Transactions of the American Society of Artificial Internal Organs 1965; 11:7-10 (see accompanying articles and discussion pages 3-17).

5. Colin Douglas, *The Houseman's Tale*. Canongate, 1975.

6. Daugirdas, John T., Todd S Ing. *Handbook of Dialysis*. 2nd edition. Little, Brown and Co. Boston/ New York/ Toronto, 1994.

7. Drake, Richard F., *Dialysis: Early Years in Oregon*, Dialysis & Transplantation, Volume 11, Number 4, April 1982, pp 220-222.

8. Eady R. *The dawn of dialysis: reminiscences of a patient*. British Journal of Renal Medicine. Summer 2001, pages 21-24.

9. Haeger Knut, *The Illustrated History of Surgery*. Harold Starke, London, 1989.

10. Hampers CL, Merril JP, Cameron E. *Hemodialysis in the home – a family affair*. Transactions of the American Society of Artificial Internal Organs 1965; 11:3-6 (see accompanying articles and discussion pages 3-17)

11. Keck PS, Meserko JJ, *Willem J. Kolff: Pioneer in Artificial Organ Research*, Proceedings of the American Academy of cardiovascular Perfusion, Volume 6, January 1985

12. Kuss, Rene, Pierre Bourget, *An illustrated history of organ transplantation. The great adventure of the century*. Sandoz, 1992.

13. Lambie AT. *A nephrologist's tale*. Proceedings of the Royal College of Physicians of Edinburgh. 1990; 9: 362-372.

14. Marmion BP, Tonkin RW. *Control of hepatitis in dialysis units*. British Medical Bulletin. 1972; 28 (2): 169-79.

15. Maher, John F., *Replacement of renal function by dialysis*. 3rd edition. Kluwer Academic Publishers, 1989.

16. McBride, Patrick T., Genesis of the Artificial Kidney BAXTER Healthcare Corp, 1987.

17. McGeown, Mary G., *A brief history of transplantation*. British Transplantation Society. 26 February, 2001

18. Merrill JP. *Should your hospital have a haemodialysis unit?* Hospital practice. February 1968, pages 23-29.

19. Murray JE. *Human organ transplantation: background and consequences. Science* 1992 256:1411-6

20. Nose Y. *Home dialysis*. Transactions of the American Society of Artificial Internal Organs 1965; 11:15 (see accompanying articles and discussion pages 3-17)

21. Nose Y. *Home hemodialysis: a crazy idea in 1963*: a memoir. ASAIO Journal 2000; 46:13-17

22. Parsons FM. *Origins of haemodialysis in the United Kingdom*. British Medical Journal. 1989: 1557-60.

23. Paskalev, Dobrin N., *Georg Haas (1886-1971): The Forgotten Hemodialysis Pioneer,* Dialysis & Transplantation, Volume 30, Number 12, December 2001, pp 828-832.

24. Peitzman, Steven J., *Science, Inventors, and the Introduction of the Artificial Kidney in the United States,* Seminars in Dialysis, Volume 9, No 3, (May-June) 1996, pp 276-281

25. Robson JS, Dudley HAF. *Report on the United Kingdom artificial kidney units*. The Royal Infirmary of Edinburgh. August, 1958.

26. Robson JS. *Advances in the treatment of renal disease*. The Practitioner. Symposium on advances in treatment, 1969; 203: 483-93.

27. Robson JS. *Medicine yesterday and today*. Inaugural Lecture No 63. 24 January, 1978.

28. Scribner, Belding H., Babb, Albert L., *Chronic Hemodialysis in Seattle: 1960-1966, Part I,* Dialysis & Transplantation, Volume 11, Number 3, March 1982, pp 223,228,229.

29. Scribner, Belding H., Babb, Albert L., *Chronic Hemodialysis in Seattle: 1960-1966 Part II,* Dialysis & Transplantation, Volume 11, Number 4, April 1982 pp 324-329.

30. Sinclair ISR, Henderson MA, Simpson DC. *Fluon arterio-venous shunt for repeated haemodialysis*. Lancet. 19 August, 1961: 410.

31. Starzl TE. *The development of clinical renal transplantation*. American Journal of Kidney Diseases. 1990; 16 (6): 548-56.

32. Tenckhoff H, Shilipetar G, Boen ST. *One year's experience with home peritoneal dialysis*. Transactions of the American Society of Artificial Internal Organs 1965; 11:11-14 (see accompanying articles and discussion pages 3-17)

Websites

www.hdcn.com, www.shodor.org, www.kidneyetn.org, www.shodor.org, www.renux.dmed.ed.ac.uk, www.baxter.com, www.fresenius.de, www.edren.org, www.communities.msn.com, www.renalweb.com, www.sin-italia.org, www.gambro.com

and, some related websites with contents not explicitly stated to be copyrighted.

The National Association of Nephrology Technicians/Technologists was founded as a profession-al, non-profit organization in 1983 to serve the needs of tech-nicians and technologists as their own group, versus relying on the support or services of other organi-zations. As we head toward the millennium, the roles of the technician and technologist continue to grow and expand. In keeping with this trend, NANT has grown as a presence in the nephrology community and in its educational offerings.

Goals of NANT

In order to provide quality service to its members, NANT has established the following goals: To set forth high quality standards in the dialysis in-dustry; promote the recognition, job security and employment opportunities of nephrology technologists and tech-nicians; educate dialysis practitioners; stimulate research; disseminate new ideas; and address technician and tech-nologist practice issues. NANT contin-ues to strive to accomplish these goals and expand its role into the nephrology community.

NANT Chapters

To meet the local needs of its members, NANT has five regions: the Northeast, Southeast, North Central, Northwest and Southwest. Each region is directed by a Regional Vice President. Through the cooperation of the Regional Vice Presidents, NANT's Director of Chap-ter Activities and the National Office, local area chapters are provided with the information and assistance to de-velop and grow. Chapter involvement provides the best forum for involving practitioners in the regular exchange of ideas and opinions.

NANT Educational Events

Education and accreditation have become more important issues in in-dividual career development and the structure of the technician's and tech-nologist's role in a unit. In recognition of this trend, NANT has expanded the content of its National Symposium to offer concurrent sessions. This new and expanded format enables NANT to offer a variety of sessions for all skill levels.

In addition, NANT offers regional educational programs. These presenta-tions include lectures by industry experts and hands-on workshops with vendors presenting state-of-the-art equipment. The success of this pro-gram has prompted an expansion of the topics covered and the regions in which these meetings are offered.

NANT as a Resource in the Industry

NANT provides the following resourc-es to the nephrology community.

Continuing Education Units (CEUs)
NANT provides CEU certificates for local meetings, corporate programs and nephrology-related professional volunteer organization and health care facility programs. To find out more about the CEU approval process and fees, please contact our National Office.

Educational program listings
NANT's National Office has a list of programs in the United States that pro-vide academic training for a career in nephrology.

Job descriptions
Considering the wide spectrum of technological expertise required within the dialysis facility, NANT has adopted two separate and distinct prac-titioner job descriptions: the Renal Di-alysis Technician and the Nephrology Technologist.

The job profiles that NANT has created for these distinctions include: occupational description, job descrip-tion, employment characteristics and educational programs.

www.dialysistech.org
The NANT web site is a valuable re-source for the nephrology community, providing the latest information on in-dustry and legislative issues. Members can access information on upcoming events and participate in NANT-spon-sored educational discussion forums.

Additional resources and technical expertise
Many of NANT's board members play an active role in other industry orga-nizations. This involvement enables NANT to keep abreast of industry trends, legislative issues and develop beneficial, cooperative relationships with other organizations and associ-ations; allowing NANT to combine strengths for the benefit of the field of nephrology. NANT members have

access to the technical expertise of other members. The National Office can direct member inquiries to appro-priate parties.

Membership Benefits

▪ Discounted registration fees for NANT-sponsored symposiums, NANT-sponsored regional meetings and workshops

▪ *NANT News*, our bimonthly newsletter

▪ Complimentary one-year subscrip-tions to industry publications including:
   *Contemporary Dialysis &
      Nephrology
   Dialysis and Transplantation
   Nephrology News and Issues*

▪ Discounts on NANT publications

▪ Access to educational opportunities to expand your skills

▪ The opportunity to participate in a national forum that can communicate positions and statements to industry and government leaders

▪ The opportunity to participate on a local level through NANT chapters

▪ Access to information that can shape your career and role in the field of ne-phrology

▪ Access to forums for networking with peers

How to Join

NANT's individual membership is $50.00 per year. To join, complete the application on the reverse side and for-ward it with your payment to NANT's National Office.

For additional information, or details on corporate memberships, please contact our National Office at 937.586.3705, toll-free at 877.607. NANT or fax 937.586.3699.

Membership Year

Your membership payment is for the 12-month period following the receipt of payment. Please allow four to six weeks for the processing and mailing of new member materials.

Members of NANT include:		**...and people involved in these areas:**	
▪ Technicians	▪ Nurses	▪ Patient care	▪ Equipment maintenance
▪ Technologists	▪ Administrators	▪ Reuse	▪ Administrative areas
▪ Supervisors	▪ Physicians	▪ Transplantation	

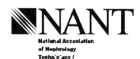

NANT MEMBERSHIP APPLICATION

National Association of Nephrology Technicians / Technologists

The Future in Renal Technology

Please return this form with your payment to:

PO Box 2307
Dayton, OH
45401-2307

Phone:
937-586-3705

Toll-free:
877-607-6268

Fax: 937-586-3699

nant@nant.meinet.com

www.dialysistech.org

General Information

Please type or print

_____
Date

_____
Name

Home address:

_____
Street address

_____
City / State / Zip

_____
Country

_____
Area code / Phone

Work address:

_____
Position / Title

_____
Employer

_____
Department / Division / Facility

_____
Street address

_____
City / State / Zip

_____
Country

_____
Area code / Phone

_____
Area code / Fax

Preferred mailing address: ☐ Home ☐ Work

Type of membership you are applying for:

☐ **Full ($50.00)**
You must be a staff technician, equipment technician, chief technician or LPN/LVN to be eligible for this voting category of membership.

☐ **Associate ($50.00)**
All others, except students, are eligible for this non-voting category of membership.

☐ **Student ($35.00)**
Limited to full-time students only; copy of current student ID must accompany application. This is a non-voting membership.

Personal Data

What is your gender?
F ☐ Female   M ☐ Male

What year were you born?

_____

Are you certified?
1 ☐ BONENT   3 ☐ NNCC
2 ☐ NNCO   4 ☐ Other_____

How long have you been involved in dialysis? Check only one.
1 ☐ 1 – 5 years   3 ☐ 11 – 15 years
2 ☐ 6 – 10 years   4 ☐ Over 15 years

What best describes your position? Check only one.
A ☐ Staff technician   F ☐ RN
B ☐ Equipment technician   G ☐ Administrator
C ☐ Chief technician   H ☐ Supervisor
D ☐ LPN/LVN   I ☐ Student
E ☐ Physician   X ☐ Other_____

What type of organization is your primary employer? Check only one.
A ☐ Hospital/University   D ☐ Manufacturer/Supplier
B ☐ Chain affiliation   X ☐ Other_____
C ☐ Free standing unit

In what areas of dialysis are you involved? Check all that apply.
A ☐ Patient care   D ☐ Equipment maintenance
B ☐ Reuse   E ☐ Transplant
C ☐ Administrative   X ☐ Other_____

In what areas of dialysis are you employed? Check all that apply.
A ☐ Chronic   C ☐ Acute
B ☐ Home training   X ☐ Other_____

Method of Payment

(Federal ID # for voucher use only: 14-1722307)

☐ Payment enclosed
(Make checks payable in US funds to: NANT)

☐ Please invoice against Purchase Order #:

_____

☐ To pay for membership by credit card, please visit www.nant.biz. Credit card transactions will only be accepted via www.nant.biz